Developments in Animal and Veterinary Sciences, 6

Trends in veterinary pharmacology and toxicology

OTHER TITLES IN THIS SERIES

Developments in Animal and Veterinary Sciences, 6

Trends in veterinary pharmacology and toxicology

Proceedings of the first European Congress on
Veterinary Pharmacology and Toxicology

held from 25 to 28 September 1979
in Zeist, The Netherlands
Organized by the European Association for
Veterinary Pharmacology and Toxicology

Edited by

A.S.J.P.A.M. van Miert
*Instituut voor Veterinaire Farmakologie en Toxikologie, Veterinaire Faculteit,
Rijks Universiteit, Biltstraat 172, Utrecht, The Netherlands*

J. Frens
*Instituut voor Veterinaire Farmakologie en Toxikologie, Veterinaire Faculteit,
Rijks Universiteit, Biltstraat 172, Utrecht, The Netherlands*

F.W. van der Kreek
*Ministerie van Volksgezondheid en Milieuhygiene, Dokter Reyersstraat 10,
Leidschendam, The Netherlands*

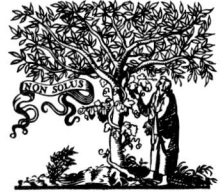

ELSEVIER SCIENTIFIC PUBLISHING COMPANY
Amsterdam — Oxford — New York 1980

ELSEVIER SCIENTIFIC PUBLISHING COMPANY
335 Jan van Galenstraat
P.O. Box 211, 1000 AE Amsterdam, The Netherlands

Distributors for the United States and Canada:

ELSEVIER/NORTH-HOLLAND INC.
52, Vanderbilt Avenue
New York, N.Y. 10017

Library of Congress Cataloging in Publication Data

European Congress on Veterinary Pharmacology and
    Toxicology, 1st, Zeist, Netherlands, 1979.
    Trends in veterinary pharmacology and toxicology.

    (Developments in animal and veterinary sciences ; 6)
    Bibliography: p.
    Includes index.
    1. Veterinary pharmacology--Congresses. 2. Veter-
inary toxicology--Congresses. I. van Miert, A. S. J. P.
A. M. II. Frens, J. III. van der Kreek, F. W.
IV. European Association for Veterinary Pharmacology
and Toxicology. V. Title. VI. Series.
SF915.E95 1979   636.089'51   80-16069
ISBN 0-444-41878-4

ISBN 0-444-41878-4 (Vol. 6)
ISBN 0-444-41703-6 (Series)

Printed in The Netherlands

CONTENTS

Poster Session. Chairman: F.W. van der Kreek

INTRODUCTION

The first European Congress on Veterinary Pharmacology and Toxicology was held in the Netherlands in September 1979. It was organized under the auspices of the European Association for Veterinary Pharmacology and Toxicology (EAVPT).

As such this doesn't mean anything more than that another congress has convened with all the ingredients that are accompanying such a happening.

However, there is more to it than just that. The congress was a sign that the EAVPT - that was started in 1978 - has reached maturity. For a long time the present members of this association had the feeling of being in between Scylla and Charybdis, not making their voice heard enough in the veterinary sciences in general, nor in the pharmacological/toxicological field.

It is hard to define a veterinary pharmacologist or toxicologist. Since it is a wide ranging discipline, every veterinarian will have to deal with it at one time or other. It not only encompasses the fundamental aspects of these sciences, but also the clinical field is closely interwoven with pharmacology and toxicology. In legislation of veterinary drugs a background in this field cannot be missed, while residues of drugs play an important role in health aspects of the human population and the environment.

One of the main objectives of the congress was to bring together the workers of the several subdisciplines of the complex field of veterinary pharmacology and toxicology, so that they were able to get acquainted and share their views. More than 150 people from 24 different countries did come. This made it possible that the problems that were felt could be discussed in a wide forum, and it was found that these problems were not unique to the individual.

The background of the participants was as diverse as the subjects that vigated in the congress. People from universities, government and industries were present as well as clinicians, pathologists and non-veterinary scientists. Apart from the formal sessions, there was enough time available for informal contacts, especially since the participants were housed at the conference centre Woudschoten, where the congress took place. With enough time on their hands and no place else to go, many happy discussions resulted from this set up.

The programme of the congress started out with the official opening by his Excellency van der Stee, minister of Agriculture and Fisheries. This by itself signifies the importance that was attached to this meeting. In his speech he stressed one of the main themes of the congress in asking to contribute to the broadening and harmonization of skills in the countries of Europe by exchange of data on scientific research projects and ideas.

In an introduction to the programme by the Minister of Health and Environmental Protection, Dr. Ginjaar, it was asked of the EAVPT to give attention to the implementation of EEC directives and the problems connected to it, like the danger that good pharmaceutical products with only a limited demand may disappear from the market and of the effects drugs and their metabolites may have on the environment.

All these aspects were indeed incorporated in the congress, not only via speakers that were experts in their field, but also in workshops and a poster session.

The subjects that were dealt with in this congress were of a very diverse nature. Sessions ranged from clinical toxicology to the relevance and future trends of research and from legislation to teaching. In all a total of 44 invited papers was given, divided into 11 sessions. Both fundamental and clinical pharmacology/ toxicology was brought into the picture, all with a veterinary relevance. It was a pleasure indeed to see eminent toxicologists attending a session on rumen pharmacology, and legislators taking part in the discussion on the relation of pharmacology to immunology.

The workshops that were organized served their purpose in that everybody had a chance to give his views on the subject under discussion. Most of the time some general agreement could be reached. The poster session gave individuals a chance to talk on their own projects and many people took this opportunity. The discussions that ensued sometimes went on into the small hours of the night.

Although it are the participants who make the congress, the organizing committee, consisting of J. Frens, W.F. Böhne, H. Heinrich, F.W. van der Kreek and A.S.J.P.A.M. van Miert, owes a great deal to those who helped to make it run as smoothly as it did. Without trying to the complete, special thanks is due to Marlou Berkhout, Cock van Duin, Carl Eustatia, Co Eyndhoven, Ineke van Holsteijn, Chris Maas, Hetty van Peet, Felice and Ruud Woutersen.

The organization of the congress would have been impossible without the support of our sponsors and the wise counsel of one of them.

The organizers are grateful for the tolerance that was shown in respect to the absences and preoccupations which naturally resulted from the organization of this congress.

Special thanks are due to Miss C.Z. Troost, Miss P.J.van der Laan and Miss C.W.P. van Vliet for technical assistance in preparing the proceedings of this congress.

J. Frens.

X

SPONSORS

The congress was made possible with support of
ACF Chemiefarma NV
Aesculaap BV
Bayer Nederland BV
Beecham Veterinaire Producten
Eli Lilly Benelux
Faculty of Veterinary Medicine, Utrecht University
FIDIN
Intervet Nederland BV
Merck Sharp and Dohme BV
Ministry of Agriculture and Fisheries
Ministry of Education and Science
Ministry of Health and Environmental Protection
Pfizer BV
Royal Netherlands Veterinary Association
Upjohn Nederland
Wellcome Nederland BV

TOXICOLOGICAL RESEARCH AT THE UNIVERSITY OF UTRECHT ON CHEMICAL POLLUTION AND
WILD LIFE

H. VAN GENDEREN

Institute of Veterinary Pharmacology and Toxicology, University of Utrecht.
172 Biltstraat, 3572 BP Utrecht (The Netherlands)

ABSTRACT

In three examples of mass poisoning of birds with pesticides in the Netherlands
in the years of 1965-1970 it is shown that extreme environmental factors and
particulars of behaviour have acted together with the poisons to produce a
calamity. Very often, mixtures of chemicals were involved.

This experience led to the study of the toxicological relevance of adaptive
mechanisms which are insufficiently challenged in the usual toxicity tests. Three
examples are given; conditioned behaviour in rats, rotary flow experiments with
fish and functioning tests of the immune system in rats.

In other experiments, the joint action of mixtures of large numbers of
aquatic pollutants has been studied at the level of the LC50.

INTRODUCTION

In the years of 1963 and after, the ornithologists in the Netherlands became
aware of a spectacular decline in the abundance of birds of prey and fish-
eating birds. Similar observations had already been made elsewhere and following
the appearance in 1962 of Rachel Carson's "Silent Spring" the idea was generally
held that the use of pesticides was responsible.

Clearly an investigation of the local situation was indicated. After a first
survey with chemical residue analysis of birds found dead in the field it was
confirmed that we had indeed a problem with chlorinated hydrocarbon pesticides,
methylmercury and also with polychlorinated·biphenyls (Koeman et al., 1966).

One of our objects for study was the buzzard (Buteo buteo). Field observations
were made with the help of many amateur ornithologists, residues were determined
and we learned the importance of the relationship between body burden and response.
In 16 buzzards found dead an average residue of 17.9 ppm (range: 7.8-31.2)
dieldrin was found in the liver. In some animals, in addition heptachlorepoxide
was present. It was necessary to find the relationship of residue (body burden)

and response. A level of 15-20 ppm in the liver in different experimental animals appeared to be a lethal concentration.

It could be established beyond doubt that this was a case of mass-poisoning by the seed dressing agents dieldrin and heptachlor, through a short food chain with voles, woodmice and seed eating birds between the dressed seed and the buzzards. This information was used with success to terminate the permission to apply these agents for seed dressing (Koeman et al., 1967).

In the next bird, I want to discuss, the fish eating sandwich tern (Sterna sandvicensis), the situation proved to be more complicated (Koeman, 1971, Koeman et al., 1972). The size of the breeding colonies, particularly at the island of Griend, had declined considerably in the past few years. In the birds found dead the body burden for any of the pesticides dieldrin, telodrin, endrin, DDE and PCB's was much higher than in live animals of the same age and colony, but not high enough to explain beyond doubt that one of these insecticides was the cause of poisoning. Emaciation by any other cause would also give rise to a higher residue in the liver as a result of its release from the depot fat. If, however, we considered the action of dieldrin, telodrin and endrin to be additive on the basis of its LD50, we could calculate for the dead birds a body burden for the "dieldrin toxicity equivalent" that was enough to be lethal. As an example, in a series of dead chicks an average of 29.1 ppm for the dieldrin toxicity equivalent (range 8.9-51) was found in the livers.

Still the difference in body burden between alive and dead birds was rather high. Further observations in the field gave the answer. Most killing, particularly in chicks, occurred after periods of stormy weather, when the parents were not able to get food for the chicks. The chicks used the yolk residue much quicker than normal and were killed by the redistribution of the insecticide mixture. No killing occurred when the catch of fish was abundant.

It is of interest to note that in this case the poisoning was by a mixture of environmental contaminants through the food chain and we had the additional factor of bad weather.

In the study of a third species of birds, the eiderduck (Somateria mollissima), other complications arose (Koeman et al., 1972). Many female birds died in the period shortly after hatching their young. During breeding the female does not take food. In trying to explain the loss of birds two interesting observations were made, first a high infestation with enteric parasites when the animals began to eat after the long period of starvation and second a much higher level in blood of chlorinated hydrocarbon insecticides and pcb's after the same period of starvation. In this case it seems that emaciation from breeding, blood loss and epithelial damage from enteric worms and high burden of insecticides act together to kill the animals. From observations of dying and dead animals and the similarity with the poisoned terns we concluded that in at least part of animals the insecticides gave the finishing stroke.

So far, our field studies had been limited to the level of animal populations. At this level e.g. parasites are dealt with as biotic factors of the environment. We know very little of effects of poisons as the higher level of ecosystems, with parameters such as diversity, primary production etc. Since observations on the diversity of bird species in relation to the use of insecticides for tsetse control in Nigeria were made by Koeman et al. (1971). There is still a long way to go before we may speak of toxicology at the ecosystem level.

In the meantime many things have changed. The chlorinated hydrocarbon insecticides are not a manace to wild life in our country any more. Governmental institutes are now active in this field, particularly the toxicological department of the Central Veterinary Institute (CDI) and the Research Institute for Nature Management.

THE ENVIRONMENT IN THE FIELD AND IN THE LABORATORY

From our experience with these and other cases of mass-poisoning we have learned that poisoning in the field is very different from experimental poisoning in the laboratory.

Toxicity testing programs for new chemicals very often are poorly adapted to the toxicological situation of wild life, even if the environmental fate of the compound has been properly attended to

1e. the experimental animals in a toxicity test are protected against: changes in temperature and humidity, parasites, predators, infectious diseases, etc. In nature animals should be able to survive the extremes in the environmental factors which are characteristic for the ecosystem they live in;

2e. toxicity studies are mainly concerned with the relation of dose and response; either acute or chronic. The no toxic effect level refers to the concentration in the feed, or the daily intake. For the observations in the field, however, the only useful parameter is the body burden (residue, concentration in blood) and the "no toxic effect body burden". For the aquatic environment the concentration in water may be the most relevant parameter.

In addition, the problems of joint action of chemicals in mixed exposures (as usual under natural conditions) are hardly dealt with.

For survival under natural conditions a number of adaptive mechanisms have been identified which are (for vertebrates) summarized in table 1.

We would like to know if chemical pollutants of the environment may interfere with the functioning of these adaptive mechanisms at dose- or body burden-levels which are considered to be no effect levels in the usual toxicity test. The results will briefly be reported of three different series of experiments made in the approach to this problem.

Finally, some results of experiments with mixtures will follow.

Table 1   Adaptive mechanisms to the environmental challenge

1. homeostatic mechanisms
   to compensate for variable envir. factors,
   such as temperature, humidity, availability
   of food, etc.

2. responses to extreme environmental conditions,
   involving "stress", through:
   a. nervous system, adaptive behaviour;
      fight and flight
   b. adaptive hormone system; gluco-corticoid
      release, etc.
   c. immune system

3. induction of biotransformation enzymes

4. additional mechanisms critical for survival:
   a. hemopoietic
   b. blood clotting
   c. wound healing
   d. foreign body reactions
      etc.

Part of this work refers to fish as the experimental animal, because the aquatic environment is most exposed to chemical pollution.

BEHAVIOURAL TESTS

These studies were made by Musch (1974) with rats and dieldrin as the main drug. Dieldrin acts on the nervous system and the characteristic effect after both acute or chronic exposure is convulsion. Below the dose level of convulsions the animals look normal.

The results of a number of well-known behavioural tests with rats at a dose level which did not produce convulsions or other visible abnormalities are presented in table 2.

Table 2   Adaptive behaviour and dieldrin

Rat (dieldrin: acute 6-12 mg/kg;
   semichronic 20 ppm in feed)

Criteria:

1. Open field (acute): more "immobility"
   and less "rearing"

2. Conditioned avoidance
   a. acquisition (acute) retarded
      some "freezing responses"
         (semichron.): decreased
   b. performance (acute) less responses
         (semichron.): normal
   c. extinction (acute): some retardation
         (semichron.) normal

3. Reinforcement schedules (acute): decreased
   response rates in most animals

It may be summarized from these observations that dieldrin at that dose level produced a decreased frequency of responses and gave occasionally omissions of response. Both these effects and changes in the electro-encephalograms, observed elsewhere, are suggestive for a condition similar to that of epilepsy with occasional episodes of petit mal.

Still, effects are irregular and there is a large variability between individuals. Some improvement was obtained in later experiments with fish, when a program of reversal of conditioned avoidance was used.

It is of interest to note that the dose levels of dieldrin were higher than the no effect level for enzyme induction in the liver and other effects in the liver.

To sum up our experience of this and other tests: behavioural tests in the context of toxicology are very time consuming, the results, if any, are difficult to quantify and also to qualify in terms with a broader meaning than the performance in a specified test. The usual conditioned avoidance test is not a severe enough challenge to adaptive behaviour to detect small defects; perhaps the reversal of conditioned avoidance is a more critical test.

ROTARY FLOW

The second method of testing I would like to mention is that of the rotary flow in fish as developed by Lindall and Schwanbom in 1971. In this test a fish is placed in streaming water in a glass tube. The tube is turning round on its axis and as a result of the friction of water against glass the water will move in a spiral flow. The fish will keep its normal position as a results of its righting reflexes. Now the speed of rotation of the cylinder is gradually increased until a speed is arrived at which the fish will turn round and lose control of its position. This is the critical number of rotation per minute for that fish. Lindahl and Schwanbom could demonstrate that sublethal poisoning with methyl mercury in fish resulted in a lower critical number of r.p.m. They obtained a residue-response relationship on that basis.

We have used this method with dieldrin with irregular effects at sub-lethal dose levels. This was unexpected because we knew from earlier work with dieldrin that the muscular force in rats was affected at sublethal dose levels. On the other hand, with parathion, after a two month exposure period, in goldfish a nice concentration response curve was obtained (Leeuwangh et al., 1974). The response began to be significantly different from controls when the acetyl-cholinesterase activity of the brain was at 41 per cent of its normal activity. This is a confirmation of a more general experience that a deterioration of the functioning of the brain does not appear before at least half of the acetyl-cholinesterase activity is inhibited.

To conclude, we consider this a most valuable extension to standard toxicity tests in fish; it is quantitative and it covers several functions of the nervous system and striated muscle at the same time.

IMMUNOTOXICITY

The results to be presented are mainly from studies by Seinen (1978). Initially, our interest in immunosuppression as a toxic effect was raised in the work on the toxicity and mode of action of polychlorinated biphenyl preparations by Vos (1972). Later on, it appeared that the property of immunosuppression was also present in some of the widely used organotin compounds. Some of the results of Seinen's experiments are presented in table 3.

Table 3. Immunotoxicity

Rat. Dialkyl tin compounds (semichronic)

Criteria: affected:

    thymus weight and histopathology
    spleen weight and histopathology
    delayed type hypersensitivity to
    tuberculin
    humoral antibody formation (less)

     not affected:

    carbon clearance

In vitro:
    cytotoxicity to lymphocytes and
    thymocytes,much less to cells from
    bone marrow

Particularly, dibutyl- and dioctyl tin dichloride were active immunosuppressing agents. It appeared to be the result of a relatively specific cytotoxic action on the thymocytes of rats. The action is less specific in mice and guineapig, but human lymphocytes are equally sensitive as those of the rat.

It is concluded that in dibutyl- and dioctyl tinchloride immunosuppression is the most sensitive criterium of effect. At an immunosuppressing dose level probably nothing would happen in the usual toxicity test, particularly when S.P.F. animals are used. Of course, in nature a defective immunosystem would be disastrous. I would like to support the recommendation of Seinen that in the usual three-months toxicity test in rats at least thymus weights should always be determined.

Work on immunosuppression in fish is in progress.

MIXTURES

The problem of mixed exposure to chemicals is most apparent in polluted surface waters and the experiments to be reported deal with fish as the experimental animal. The study is from Könemann (1979).

For a large percentage of chemical pollutants in surface waters, the toxicity is of the "unspecific" type and nearly wholly determined by the partition coefficient between n. octanol and water. They have a similar action. For 50 of such chemicals, belonging to the chlorobenzenes, chlorotoluenes, aliphatic chloro-hydrocarbons, alcohols, glycolderivatives and others the acute LC50 for guppies was determined. Equitoxic mixtures were prepared and for these also the joint LC50 was determined. It appeared that the LC50 for the mixture of the 50 compounds corresponded to nearly 1/50th of the LC50 for each of the compounds present. This is a clear example of joint action with "concentration addition", and it is important to note that each compound contributes to the total toxicity of the mixture at a concentration (2% of the LC50) which is usually not considered to be of interest.

When compounds with each a very different specific action were mixed at equitoxic concentrations the joint effect was much less than calculated on the basis of concentration addition. Further work is in progress.

REFERENCES

Koeman, J.H. and Van Genderen, H.: Some preliminary notes on residues of chlorinated hydrocarbon insecticides in birds and mammals in the Netherlands. J.appl.Ecology 3, (suppl. 99-106), 1966.
Koeman, J.H., et al.: Vogelsterfte door landbouwvergiften. Landbouwvoorlichting 24, 399-404, 1967.
Koeman, J.H.: Thesis Utrecht, 1971.
Koeman, J.H., et al.: Faunal changes in a swamp habitat in Nigeria sprayed with insecticide to exterminate Glossina. Neth.J.of Zoology 21, 443-463, 1971.
Koeman, J.H. and Van Genderen, H.: Tissue levels in animals and effects caused by chlorinated hydrocarbon insecticides, chlorinated biphenyls and mercury in the marine environment along the Netherlands coast. In: "Marine Pollution and Sea Life" (FAO conference), pg. 428-435. Fishing News (Books) Ltd, Rosemount Avenue, West Byfleet, Surrey, England, 1972.
Könemann, H.: Toxicity tests in fish with mixtures of more than two chemicals. To be published in 1979.
Leeuwangh, P. and Siligardi, M.: Internal report, 1974.
Lindahl, P.E. and Schwanbom, E.: A method for detection and quantitative estimation of sublethal poisoning in living fish. Oikos 22, 210-214 and 354-357, 1971.
Musch, A.: Gedragsveranderingen als toksikologies kriterium voor de werking van dieldrin bij de rat. Thesis Utrecht, 1974.
Seinen, W.: Immunotoxicity of alkyltin compounds. Thesis Utrecht, 1978 and Tox.appl.Pharmacol. 42, 213-224, 1977.
Vos, J.G.: Thesis Utrecht, 1972 and Tox.appl.Pharmacol. 21, 549-555, 1972.

TRENDS IN RESEARCH ON VETERINARY PREVENTIVE MEDICINE OF RELEVANCE
TO PHARMACOLOGY

J.M. PAYNE
Agricultural Research Council, Institute for Research on Animal
Diseases, Compton, Nr. Newbury, Berkshire, RG16 ONN, (U.K.)

ABSTRACT

   National research institutes are entering a difficult time because
of restricted funding. Thus increased planning and collaboration is
vital. High priorities for veterinary research include complex
infection of young animals, premature culling due to mastitis, lameness and production disease, and zoonosis. Much that has been
achieved requires application. In particular improvements in
veterinary preventive medicine involve a combination of guidelines
for eradication, vaccination, husbandry improvement and possibly
also the breeding of superior stock. In the long term future progress
depends on new breakthroughs in fundamental science.

INTRODUCTION

   I welcome the opportunity of presenting this subject from the point
of view of national research institutes. Other aspects relating to
university and commercial institutes are being considered by my
colleagues, Drs. Van Genderen and Marsboom. The time is appropriate
because we are at a point where existing ideas need reconsideration.
Various factors impose this need for fresh thought. Firstly, there
is restriction in the supply of funds for research. Thus research
institutes may seek to increase their collaboration both with
commercial firms and also with other national research institutes in
the European Community. Some already have done so and have planned
conjoint projects on a European basis. Secondly, there have been
spectacular advances in both fundamental and applied science which
need development for practical use. The technology already exists
to prevent many diseases but it awaits application. We must realise
that it is not enough to discover a promising antigen; we must go

further and at an early stage assess the feasibility for meeting
legislative requirements, and with profit for the manufacturer.
Thirdly, we need to foster a background of good fundamental science.
Our preoccupation with planning and applied science may obscure the
scientific breakthroughs which lead to future progress. In this
respect, public relations are important because many people fear
scientific progress and need re-awakening to the exciting possibilities
of new fundamental discoveries.

This paper discusses research in national institutes under three
main headings:
1. Which diseases merit priority?
2. How can new methods of preventive medicine be successfully applied?
3. What predictions can be made for new developments?

1. MAIN AREAS MERITING HIGH PRIORITY IN VETERINARY RESEARCH
Priorities have changed because several diseases can now be prevented
using existing knowledge. However a residue of very important
problems remains. These fall into three main groups.
a. Complex infections of mucosal surfaces such as the alimentary
   canal, respiratory tract, the udder and the eye.
b. Diseases limiting productive life - including infertility and
   premature ageing of key organs and tissues.
c. Zoonoses including hazards from toxic residues in human food.

a. Complex infections of mucosal surfaces
No-one needs reminding of the severe losses associated with diarrhoea
and pneumonia in young animals. Modern research shows that the
causes are more complex than realised because so many pathogens have
been identified in outbreaks. Unfortunately the problem is intractable
because many of the pathogens defy isolation and culture, so that new
techniques had to be developed to show their presence. Electron
microscopy became a vital tool to reveal rotaviruses, coronaviruses
and the calici-like virus (Newbury agent) in the faeces of scouring
calves.

Respiratory disease in calves is another complex infection in which
we have now identified at least four primary pathogens, notably,
Mycoplasma bovis, M. dispar, parainfluenza-3 virus and respiratory
syncytial virus.

The question arises - how can such complex infections be prevented?
We are achieving modest success with vaccines prepared against some
key patnogens, especially those involved in respiratory disease.

Less headway has been made with the viruses associated with enteritis
though some interesting developments have been made in the prevention
of diarrhoea caused by Escherichia coli. The so-called K88 antigen,
which is a virulence determinant causing adhesion to the mucosal
surface and enteritis in piglets, can be used to give protection
via antibodies in the colostrum. Also it is possible to breed
piglets with a high degree of heritable resistance.

Another complex disease of a mucosal surface is mastitis of dairy
cows. Antibiotics and improved hygiene aimed at limiting the transfer
of infection from cow to cow give benefit, but the disease persists
and an especially severe and dangerous form associated with coliform
bacteria is becoming common. Unfortunately only very few coliform
bacteria are needed to initiate the infection - and as this pathogen
heavily contaminates the environment of cubicles and yards it is
not surprising that the disease is prevelant. No effective specific
immunity has yet been initiated within the udder. But a promising
way ahead may be to investigate the role of non-specific immunity
because some cows have naturally high resistance to the disease, and
this seems to be hereditable in part. The feasibility of inducing
an effective degree of non-specific immunity needs urgent investigation

b. Diseases limiting productive life

Infertility is probably the major cause of culling in dairy herds.
New endocrinological knowledge will no doubt help to alleviate some
of this. Methods for pre-determining and synchronising oestrus will
ease problems of detecting cows for service. However, recent work
reveals that infertility in high yielding dairy herds may be
associated with fatty change in the liver. This so-called "fatty
liver syndrome" disrupts glucose and protein metabolism leading to
hypoglycaemia and hypoalbuminaemia - all of which correlate
statistically with failure to conceive. Thus active research into
the pathogenesis and prevention of fatty liver is of very high
priority.

Another factor limiting productive life is premature senility of
key organs and tissues. Bones may lose 16% of their mineral during
one lactation and if this is not replaced in the dry period then
osteoporosis follows. Muscles too are involved. If skeletal muscle
is lost to provide for the energy and protein needs of lactation,
regeneration tends to be incomplete. Loss of bone and muscle will,
in the long term, lead to lameness and the need for premature
culling. Thus ageing is a most important subject for new research.

c. Zoonoses including hazards from toxic residues

There has been considerable public concern about the potential dangers of microbiological and toxicological agents in human food. Some of this may be exaggerated but nevertheless the development of better ways of monitoring food products for pathogens and toxic residues is of high priority. Surprisingly, improved methods of detection can have unfortunate repercussions because some modern techniques are so sensitive that they can reveal very low levels of contamination indeed. As few as 4 salmonellae/100g. of slurry or sludge can be detected and in the case of chemical residues immuno-assay techniques reveal anabolic steroids in meat down into the picogram range. Such accuracy misleads the public into the belief that there are actual and imminent dangers. Unfortunately we do not know the minimum levels needed to cause a real hazard and it is as important to investigate this aspect as to improve our methods for detecting the mere presence of potentially harmful agents.

Many zoonoses are well-known but still merit high priority for research. Salmonellosis is one of the most studied which still merits high priority to devise ways of preventing spread through the food chains leading to man. Proper processing of animal feed, farm-yard slurry or human sewage sludge may help but potentially important ways of limiting spread might be to improve the detection of sub-clinical carriers of infection and to boost immunological resistance by vaccination.

2. NEW METHODS OF PREVENTIVE MEDICINE

Basically there are only four ways to prevent disease. We may aim for complete eradication either on a national or a local level, we may use vaccination or other specific prophylaxis, we may lay down guidelines for improved husbandry and feeding, or finally we may attempt to breed stock which have a high resistance to disease.

Some may feel that eradication is not relevant to a conference on pharmacology, but this is not so. Rarely can eradication start without initial reduction in the weight of infection in the population - either by vaccination or chemotherapy. We could eradicate many diseases using only existing knowledge but there are limiting factors - for instance persistance of infection in the environment or in wild animals - but even if complete eradication of the aetiological agent is impossible it may still be feasible to eradicate a disease as a clinical entity using specific prophylactic agents. Examples include the distemper complex in dogs and clostridia.

diseases.

Modern immunology opens up new possibilities for specific prevention of disease, even for those complex infections of mucosal surfaces mentioned earlier in this paper. Antigens against the primary pathogens involved in respiratory disease show promise in small-scale field trials. Also new possibilities emerge for protecting young animals by vaccinating the mothers who transfer passive immunity via the colostrum. In this respect the virulence determinants or the K88, K99 antigens on coliform bacteria seem particularly promising for the prevention of neonatal scours in piglets and calves.

Vaccination is not the only specific method of preventing disease. Production disease demands a different approach. An example is parturient hypocalcaemia in the dairy cow for which analogues of vitamin D_3 offer improvements on older methods. Another example is the specific prevention of trace element deficiencies by the use of soluble glass depots given subcutaneously.

Rarely, if ever, is there a simple way of preventing a disease using one single agent. Almost always there has to be a complex plan of action involving a strategy of attack. A very good example of this is the 10-point plan devised for the prevention of ketosis in dairy herds. This involves the regular use of a diagnostic procedure to detect preclinical cases, a sequence of steps to improve management and feeding combined with specific methods for treatment. Multicomponent guidelines of this kind are used increasingly in modern preventive medicine. They usually involve a combination of diagnostic test, improved husbandry together with specific prophylaxis and treatment when needful.

Breeding for resistance to disease is usually too cumbersome for application in large domestic animals. However, three recent developments indicate that we need to revise this view. Firstly pigs can be bred which are resistant to coliform scours caused by E. coli carrying the K88 virulence determinant. This virulence determinant is a protein which adheres the coliform bacteria to the mucosal surface of the intestine, but some pigs are superior in that they resist the adhesion. A specifically devised test using a preparation of "brush borders" from mucosal cells has revealed that adhesion/non-adhesion to the K88 virulence determinant is inherited along simple Mendelian lines, adhesion being dominant and non-adhesion being recessive. It is now possible to genotype boars to be used for breeding. The second example is scrapie. This disease, which involves slow degeneration of neurones in the brain of sheep, is caused by a transmissible agent. However, some sheep are resistant in the sense that they do not succumb to experimental challenge within their normal life span - or show a very prolonged incubation period. Again straightforward Mendelian principles are involved with susceptibility being dominant and resistance being recessive. The third example is mastitis in cows where the daughters of certain bulls have been shown to have an unduly high incidence of mastitis compared with others. Although mastitis could not be eradicated by a breeding programme, it might be possible to avoid breeding from bulls conferring undue susceptibility. The tentative conclusion about the potential value of breeding for preventing disease is that it adds another tool in the overall strategy of prophylaxis alongside eradication, specific therapy and guidelines for improved husbandry.

3. PREDICTIONS FOR FUTURE DEVELOPMENTS

   The need to increase collaboration between national research institutes and pharmaceutical companies has been mentioned already. In very general terms research institutes study the aetiology of disease, then develop diagnostic tests and attempt to find antigens of potential promise as vaccines. On the other hand pharmaceutical companies concentrate on new products such as vaccines, chemo-therapeutic agents and the like. Their major concern is to prove the efficacy of their products and to ensure safety in use. Obvious common ground for collaboration is in the development of antigens towards the formulation of effective vaccines. There might be collaboration in working out the strategy for practical application. However, these are not new ideas. Potentially fresh ground for collaboration involves work in new and hitherto neglected areas.

   One exciting new area is that of non specific resistance to infectious disease. We know that several factors suppress macro-phage function but little is known of how to improve phagocytic activity in key organs such as the udder. This could have value in the prevention of mastitis.

   Another new and relatively unexplored field is that of recovery from disease. Enteritis can have devastating effects on growth but factors affecting recovery are little known - treatments aimed at improving recovery would be most valuable. In fact ill thrift in growing stock though common is so ill defined that it has escaped investigation. The work will inevitably be long term and fundamental so that quick empirical results are unlikely. It may involve detailed study of factors initiating cell division in response to tissue damage and also of the control of tissue and organ size.

The two examples of non specific resistance and of growth in recovery from disease emphasise the importance of fostering good and well directed fundamental science. Fundamental science is the origin of our future technology on which we all depend.

RESEARCH IN VETERINARY CLINICAL AND FUNDAMENTAL PHARMACOLOGY AND TOXICOLOGY
RELEVANCE AND FUTURE TRENDS : LEGISLATIVE ASPECTS

Pr. G. MILHAUD - Service de Pharmacie et Toxicologie
Ecole Nationale Vétérinaire d'Alfort - 94704, Maisons-Alfort-France

ABSTRACT

Although all the laws on veterinary medicinal products have the same aim, the practical requirements of the national authorities can be very different, and are bound to influence the trend of research and its practical carrying out.

Thence, an approximation of the laws of the different countries is highly desirable.

In the veterinary field, the aim of research is not only to discover new medicines (active ingredients or pharmaceutical forms) but also to be able to market them. For research to be able to develop and for laboratories to expand, new products must be, periodically, launched on the market.

Prior to world war II, veterinary therapeutics was essentially an individual business, frequently based on medicines not prepared in advance. The latter have been, little by little, superseded by propietary medicinal products, prepared in advance, which, in many countries have failed to be submitted to any legislative constraint as to their preparation and sale.

In recent years, treatments provided to a large number of animals has considerably developed, resulting in new therapeutic practices and new pharmaceutical forms such as medicated feedstuffs. The different countries have set up more or less exhaustive and binding regulations.

In the US, FDA has progressively set up a more and more sophisticated system. The state laboratories in the East countries have to carry out tests on most of the medicines they use. In Europe, several Council Directives are being drawn up in order to harmonise the regulations in the different countries of the EEC. We will essentially refer to these proposals to try and find out the influence of regulations on research.

All regulations have the same objectives :

1°/ to ensure the quality of medicines by setting up analytical control tests.

2°/ to guarantee their activity thanks to pharmacological and clinical informations.

3°/ to ascertain innocuity or, at least, a satisfactory tolerance in the animal treated.

4°/ to protect man, either as a user of medicines or as a consumer of animal-
based foodstuffs.

The means used to reach such objectives are more or less efficient. The turnover of veterinary medicines is modest and consequently, the amount of money to
spend on research is necessarily limited. Moreover, regulations can favour certain
types of products at the expenses of others, for instance medicated feedstuffs
products not prepared in advance instead of propietary medicinal products. As a
result, the definitions to be found as a preamble to any regulations and the sco-
pe of a text must be studied with the greatest care.

The definition of the very word medicine is of importance : the EEC directive
n° 65/65 of january 26th, 1965 simultaneously defines the human medicine and the
veterinary medicine as any product or composition meant for the prevention or
treatment or diagnosis of human or animal diseases. Any medicine meant for animals
will be called veterinary medicinal product.

The proposed directive for veterinary medicines defines various types of products :

- the propietary medicinal product,
- the ready-made veterinary medicinal product,
- the premix for medicated feedingstuff,
- the medicated feedingstuff,

and stipulates that the provisions of the directive apply to premix for medicated
feedstuff and not to medicated feedstuff. Consequently there remains to know exactly where the line must be drawn between premix for medicated feedstuff and medicated feedstuff. Now, the present definition of premix for medicated feedingstuff
is "any veterinary medicinal product prepared in advance with a view to the subsequent manufacture of medicated feedingstuffs".

Some people think that the definition primarily concerns active ingredients on
special excipient, manufactured by the pharmaceutical industry for the preparation
of medicated feedstuff. Others, on the contrary, putting the 2 definitions side by
side, consider that a premix for medicated feedstuff must be understood as the
last premix, the one that will be used as the very last mixture with the feedstuff
to obtain the medicated feedstuff.

The second interpretation provides a correct balance between the propietary medicinal product and the premix, whereas the first notably reduces the requirements
and the guarantees demanded from medicated feedstuffs and thus favours the

medicated feedstuff, which is bound to have consequential effects on research in veterinary pharmacology and toxicology.

It is also very important to know where the line must be drawn between medicated feedstuffs and feed additives. The EEC Directive n° 70/524 of nov. 20 [th] 1970 clearly defines the nature of additives ; yet substances which have a medicinal activity at the doses used, such as coccidiostats or dimetridazole are still ruled by this directive.

Finally, if derogations are allowed to pharmacists and veterinarians for the medicines not prepared in advance, active ingredients especially in the form of medicated feedstuff which would never have been authorized, either for lack of information as to their activity or toxicity, or on account of adverse side-effects, run the risk of being used.

On the other hand, it is obvious that the requirements of national authorities as to the control of the quality, activity and toxicity of the veterinary medicines will directly affect research.

In the field of analytical controls, it may be decided to characterize and check the purity of a medicine by simple analytical methods, easy to reproduce and requiring no sophisticated apparatus. In such a case, numerous reactions must be devised, for they are rarely specific and conclusions can be reached only through comparing results. Conversely, more reliable and generally more specific methods can be preferred, such as atomic absorption spectrophotometry, liquid-liquid chromatography or infra-red spectrometry which require very costly equipment but are very time-saving. It is easy to realize the part that pharmacopoeia commissions and national authorities can play in the evolution of analytical techniques and in research.

The definition of 'production batch' has equally big consequences, for it determines the setting up of controls of manufacture which must be carried out on every batch.

As regards activity, authorizations can be with-held if the veterinary medicine has no therapeutic effect or if the applicant has not provided sufficient proof of such effect, based on pharmacodynamic and clinical evaluations. Again, the trend of research will depend on whether the authorities will systematically demand quantitative pharmacological assays and comparative clinical trials or whether they will be satisfied with less precise observations. Also, national authorities requirements as to the data to be provided on the emergence of resistant organisms cannot but have important repercussions on this category of medicines.

Even more than on activity, it is on the assessment of toxicity that the complexity of the dossier to provide will depend. In fact, veterinary medicines hold an unprivileged position, compared to human medicines for it is not only necessary to have guarantees for the treated animal and for the user but also for the consumer of animal-based foodstuffs. Therefore one could envisage requirements exactly similar to those of human medicines and phytosanitary products. Yet this appears unrealistic, since, on the one hand, pharmaceutical companies could not bear the costs entailed, and, on the other hand, it would lead to a thoroughly useless over-protection of the treated animal and of the consumer. Indeed, many medicines are dispensed very unfrequently and are administered long before slaughtering, which means they are very unlikely to be found in the consumer's plate. As regards those which are more frequently administered such as antiparasitory or antibiotic medicines, the fact that several medicines are available for the treatment or prevention of one disease and the fact that man's food is varied, will account for the low rate of risks as to their daily presence in man's diet, reversely to what happens in laboratory animals.

Besides, other factors of protection are to be taken into account, such as the preservation, ripening and cooking of foodstuffs.

After a long debate, a compromise was reached by the working party on Economic Questions for the Directive on analytical, pharmaco-toxicological and clinical standards and protocols of veterinary medicinal products.

A paragraph deals with the studies for toxicity, single-dose toxicity and tolerance in target animals ; another paragraph deals with the study of residues, reviewing the various techniques used to measure the residue levels and the informations necessary to assess their toxicity.

In the course of the discussion, further requirements were introduced in the original text proposed by the Committee. Studies for teratogenicity have been extended to "new molecules with a chemical structure not analogous to known products"; studies for carcinogenicity, initially limited to substances having a close chemical analogy with a known carcinogen or to substances which had given rise to abnormal signs and symptoms during the repeated dose toxicity study were extended to all substances which had given positive or suspicious result in the tests for mutagenic effects. Thence, the tests for mutagenic effects which were optional have become necessary.

Finally, the possibility offered to refer to published data to replace, in some cases, as provided in the Directive, the pharmacological tests and clinical trials, can completely alter the nature of the documents, thence of the tests required by the national authorities.

These few examples show that research in veterinary medicinal products is greatly dependent upon the laws.

The latter determine :

1°/ which type of products or of pharmaceutical forms will be marketed,

2°/ the analytical pharmacological and clinical data necessary for application,

3°/ consequently, the possibility for a firm to market new medicines, thence to survive.

For a new molecule to be profit-earning, it must be marketed in many countries and therefore obtain the necessary authorizations in those different countries. So, it is indispensable, owing to the cost entailed by applications and to the limits of the market, that an approximation of the laws should be achieved. Such harmonization must concern not only the number of tests to carry out but also the protocols for the results to be reliable and accepted in every country. Yet, in this field, as in many others, too great perfectionism would be disastrous, for, in order to avoid a danger which often does not exist, it would freeze research and would deprive veterinary medicine of valuable therapeutical means. Therefore, as recommended in one of the preambles of the proposals for Council Directives, "one must safeguard public health without checking industrial development".

RESEARCH IN VETERINARY CLINICAL AND FUNDAMENTAL PHARMACOLO-
GY AND TOXICOLOGY
THE INDUSTRY POINT OF VIEW

R. MARSBOOM
Janssen Pharmaceutica N.V., 2340 Beerse, Belgium

ABSTRACT

The pharmaceutical industry envisages the future as one of great opportunity
with more difficult challenges and with a greater responsibility toward mankind.
If society really wants its essential health needs to be met quickly and fully, it
should try to create a proper motivating climate in which creative drug research
and development is likely to prosper. These challenges can only be met with the
full cooperation of academia and the government under which we must operate.

Addressing the future research directions from the industry point of view,
is addressing the future of the pharmaceutical industry itself. One of the most
intriguing management phenomena of the late 60s and 70s has been the rapid
spread of the strategic (long range) planning concept. The major reason why
companies have adopted this concept so rapidly is that the idea apparently pro-
mised management that they could now control the destiny of their organisations.
It is clear from all strategic plans, that the pharmaceutical industry will not
have an easy ride in the years to come. In this however we are not alone. Other
industries have their problems as well: some companies will do well and survive.
The saying about the survival of the fittest needs only to be changed to the survival of the smartest.

In spite of the enormous progress made in the last 30 years, there is still no
entirely satisfactory solution for many serious problems in human, veterinary
and plant medicine. Mankind is in need of better therapeutic, prophylactic and
diagnostic drugs and is looking toward the scientific community as a whole and
toward the profession and the industry in particular to provide these better
drugs. Only innovative products are the driving force of the industry.

The lesson we have learned over the past two decades is that biological research cannot be segregated into discrete components. Such a philosophy strengthens the basic concept that there is only one research and also only one medicine, which has human, veterinary and even agricultural components. These components are influenced by the sociological and economical climate of the various geographic areas of the globe. We cannot ignore the trends in research in the various health sectors, because the interaction between these three sectors will necessarily interfere with any cohesive and responsible research program. This means that research workers cannot any longer limit themselves to their own small area of interest or to the screening process they are performing. Also, that most important products will not result any more from "haphazard" findings. This is not an attempt to downgrade the excellent pioneering of the generations before us, but there are no longer simple answers to what appear to be simple problems. It seems apparent that great advances in future drug-research will only be made by using the concept of specific problem oriented research techniques.

The pharmaceutical industry is not a monolithic bloc i.e. all industries are not the same and each industry tries to be personal. But the common basic research organisation within the industry is invariably the same: from the literature over synthesis and analysis to pharmacology and toxicology before ending up into the development and marketing in one or more of the three health care sectors. Drug research is essentially an interdisciplinary endeavour. It is like an orchestra with medicinal chemists, pharmacologists, toxicologists, biochemists, pathologists, clinicians, statisticians, engineers and many other experimental scientists playing their instruments. Conducting such an orchestra is not an easy task. It requires perspective, deep understanding of the problems to be solved together, enthusiasm and above all motivation, the capacity to dream about the ideal wonder-drugs of the future: effective, safe and inexpensive.

The point I would like to make in this connection is that if society really wants its essential health needs to be met quickly and fully, it should try to create a proper motivating climate in which creative drug research and development is likely to prosper. This is why new and superior drugs will only be found by inquisitive and dedicated researchers living in a free world, where ideals and dreams can still come true. They will not be found nor even recognized by complacent and unimaginative bureaucrats, soaked in habits of mind and in excessive regulations cutting down on innovation.

How can we achieve the balance in research we seem to want and need? First, we must ensure that some of our ressources are made available for fundamental projects. This is true for all countries, even the developing countries. At a recent conference held in Belgium concerning health policy for developing nations, the eminent Nobel Price winner Dr. De Duve pointed out that these countries as well as the developed nations would achieve far more if some time and money was set aside to solve problems at the fundamental level. We must stop believing that we are to poor to do fundamental research in any sector or in any country. Rather than hiring someone to develop a vaccine against a given disease, it is better to hire someone to study the organism to learn its inner-most secrets. Once we know the secrets, the vaccine will be a natural by-pro-duct of the research program. The research worker cannot ignore his responsa-bilities when the time comes that his expertise is required in applying his fin-dings. Secondly, industry, government and academia must be drawn together. I have alluded to the fact that research becomes more and more difficult because the disease processes we are trying to solve become more and more sophisti-cated. We must therefore form a compatible research structure that mutually attacks problems, shares knowledge and supports bright scientists and their ideas while being responsive to the needs of the society. Academia has the responsability to train people, government and industry have the responsability to provide opportunities for these people to use their training to be creative. If the pharmaceutical industry had to bear all of the efforts and all of the costs, the research component of new drugs would place an unfair burden on the final users of the drugs. Ultimately then the cost would fall on the governments and therefore on the people through taxation as usual. The point I would like to make in this connection is that it would seem far wiser if industry, academia and government would share in the training and development of people and methods.

What does this all mean in terms of the specific task the pharmaceutical industry has with regard to increasing the worlds supply of food and improving human and animal health? We are there to help and not to exploit misery: in a proper motivating climate the pharmaceutical industry can provide mankind with new and superior drugs. The duty and the right we have to improve the quality of life are only restricted by the steadily increasing R and D costs, resulting merely from unscientific and meaningless regulations: 250 x 10.6 US dollars R and D costs per new product indeed explain why the birth rate of new superior and often badly needed drugs is, in my view at least, incredibly low and still declining.

The veterinary profession in particular can make its most valuable contribu-tions in the area of research. Some of the factors that influence our thinking are:
1. The fact that the world market for AHC products, which is estimated to amount to 3.2 billion US dollars in 1976 and to 5.5 billion in the 90s, is comprised of three major segments: feed additives   46%
                                                 pharmaceuticals   43%
                                                 biologicals-vaccines 11%

2. The fact that we have a highly concentrated business in a fairly narrow geographic area. The North American and the Western European zones account
for some 56% of the world AHC business. In country terms we estimate that
some 15 key markets comprise 2/3 of the available world business

> United States - Canada
>
> Germany, France, United Kingdom, Italy, Spain,
> Benelux
>
> Japan
>
> Mexico, Argentina, Brasil
>
> South Africa
>
> Australia, New Zealand

In practical terms we are particularly interested in the AHC problems of the
North American and the West European zones. The following subjects are fundamental:

a. improvement of husbandry and management

b. improvement of productivity

c. enhancement of immunity.

Husbandry and management cannot be forced on populations directly. Specific
diseases that continue to exist are due to a large part to poor management i.e.
mastitis, MMA, the calf pneumonia-diarrhea complex, baby-pig diarrhea,
mycotic infections particularly in poultry, some parasitic diseases, foot rot,
some forms of infertility. The pharmaceutical industry can provide drugs to
partially substitute for poor management, although this is certainly not the best
or not the final answer. Improving productivity and enhancing resistance or
immunity are also not easy challenges. The pharmaceutical industry can play a
vital role in these developments by learning about biology and by understanding
the mechanism of action. If we know the exact mode of action of compounds like
levamisole in the area of immunomodulation, new compounds that are even more
effective will be easy to formulate. Here again the argument for knowing the
secrets of biology are substantiated and we believe once these secrets solved,
synthetic agents can and will provide protection. Fine technology will substitute
for clever hands.

3. The fact that there is a marked difference in the market structure of the different markets. The basic determinant of the northern hemisphere livestock
systems with intensive stock husbandry is the use of confinement feeding as a
major production technique. So the northern hemisphere market structure is
characterized by a high feed additive segment (55%) and by only 35% pharmaceuticals and 10% biologicals. Companion animal products (pets, equine) will

continue to occupy a small but interesting segment of the AHC business particularly in the western world. Companion animals are a factor in the quality of
life we have or want to have in the future. In an aging population companion animals play an important role in the psychological welfare of these people. Public
health considerations are important here as zoonoses will become increasingly
important. Although several human products can be adapted for animal use, the
industry must show awareness and recognize that some problems of these companion animals are unique. The southern hemisphere is based on extensive stock
husbandry and the market structure is characterized by a low feed additive segment (10-15%) and either a high consumption of pharmaceutical type products
rising to over 80% in Australia and South Africa and based on anthelmintics and
acaricides or a high consumption of biological type products in Latin America
and based on foot and mouth disease vaccine. There is of course a steady evolution in the animal production industry and thus a steady change in the needs for
various product types.

4. The fact that our AHC opportunities lay in two main areas:
- the area of animal disease, or area of therapy, the so-called ethical line
  approached through the veterinary profession
- the area of animal health, or area of prevention, the so-called non-ethical
  line approached through the allied disciplines involved with live-stock production.
For the developing market of the 90s there will be more intensive livestock
production as food demands and food needs are seen to continue to expand. This
feature will shape the market place demand for OTC products i.e. growth pro-
motors in various species: cattle, pig and poultry. This means that we will have
to penetrate this market segment through the non-ethical line. Disease control
will continue to be essential to optimize such production and so we also will
have to penetrate this market segment through the veterinary profession.

.   Besides the already mentioned factors such as: product lines, business concentration, differences in market structure and the reality of prophylactic and
therapeutic medicine, many other factors interfere with the research programs
of the industry i.e. insufficient patent protection, difficulty in hiring qualified
personnel and especially the wave of regulations in the area of control:
one fool can ask more questions than a hundred wise man can answer.
The political commitment to public health care has isolated the pharmaceutical
industry in many countries by increasing requirements on safety, toxicity, efficacy, stability coupled with more guidelines regarding presentation of data and
therefore resulting in more time-consuming and more costly processes to obtain

new drug applications. In an unified Europe old-fashioned import and export barriers are disappearing but replaced by more bureaucracy in a chauvinistic nationalism.

The social goal and scientific innovation of our therapeutics as well as their economic benefits to mankind should be communicated to our customers who have a real desire to better understand. If we do not act, or if we fail to create an environment where the authorities have to follow up with what the society wants and needs, then politicians will act in a very fertile area and legislation people will have to follow into forced directions. We are indeed living in a strange world with its tremendous scientific and technological potential on the one hand, and an even more impressive rapidly growing but suffocating dictatorial bureaucracy on the other. The air is filled with criticism, scepticism, suspicion and empty slogans. Capitalism, free enterprise, the multinationals, imperialism and colonialism are the sources of all evil. The pharmaceutical industry as well as the medical profession are seen as the professional exploiters of human misery. Drugs are dangerous and far too expensive. We need the welfare state, more security, more leisure, less problems, more money. In short: panem et circenses, the old Roman utopia.

I strongly believe that creative thinking and action cannot but suffocate in a world of bureaucratic materialism, where force, power, conspiracy against work and selfishness are the main driving forces and where charity is dead. A society interested in better health care should not allow its mood to be set by the overly suspicious.

Do we really need another World War II to make us understand that all we need to create several other penicillins is to allow crash programs to be carried out. Let us remember what Sir Alexander Fleming once said at a banquet in his honour in New York City: "I appreciate your kind remarks, gentlemen, but I can only think tonight of the thousands of lives that would have been saved had the profession paid attention to my early accounts that appeared in the press and elsewhere before World War II came along to cause them to take it down from the shelf and work with it as a new salvation".

How many penicillins are on our laboratory shelves waiting to be taken down? How much is lost as a consequence of our demotivating, suffocating, delay-producing, dictatorial regulatory systems?

To be specific, let us consider for a moment the amount of problems caused by the various nematodes, cestodes, trematodes, fungi, protozoa, bacteria, viruses, rickettsias and ectoparasites. A number of these infectious diseases can be eradicated with available means. Why are these attainable goals not being pursued more vigorously? Because of ignorance and indifference, not because of unsurmountable technological or socioeconomical reasons. Sometimes we seem to be conspiring against progress. Roundworm, hookworm and whipworm infections still occur, mostly in the third world. Old problems like brucellosis and tuberculosis, that we thought we had solved have reappeared in new and more threatening ways. This, I feel, is a scandal. Filariasis, schistosomiasis, hydatidosis, trichinellosis and so many other parasitoses continue to undermine the productivity throughout Asia, Africa and South America; we are still nowhere in our struggle against trypanosomiasis and East Coast Fever. Drug resistant bacteria and protozoa are spreading. We are in great need of effective drugs against most systemic mycoses caused by Candida, Aspergillus, Histoplasma, Blastomyces, Coccidioidomyces, etc., etc.. Why does it take us so long to find and develop such drugs? Because we fail to create a proper motivating climate in which creative drug R & D is likely to prosper. Let us not only allow but encourage people of good will everywhere - in the pharmaceutical industry, in academia, in medicine, in the government - to take the new penicillins down from the shelf. Let us all stop worrying and quarreling too much about irrelevant details. Let us concentrate on how to increase R & D efficiency rather than on how to create more bureaucracy and spend our energy on a more positive approach towards R & D. If we succeed in creating this new climate, the great beneficiary will be the society.

Let me, in closing, summarize in a few words the classical history of most modern drugs.

Shortly after the announcement of its discovery the new drug often tends to be ignored or met with sterile scepticism: somebody is trying to sell something. The world has been fooled so often in the past, so let us be extremely careful this time and wait for independent confirmation, for more data, more facts, more double and triple blind experiments, absolute proof of safety, etc..

In a second phase, when the obvious facts can no longer be denied, the general feeling changes: there must be something to it, but the whole story is much less important than we were once led to believe. At this stage the usual rumours start spreading about all kinds of mysterious dangers. Smoke is being produced and people start looking for a fire. "This new drug, my friend, is much too toxic to treat your cat with". At this stage too, opinions and convictions tend to vary considerably from country to country.

In a third and final phase then when, many years later, the drug is described in most textbooks as quite effective in the treatment, prevention or diagnosis of a certain disease or symptom and reasonably safe, widely used in practice and promoted on a large scale, published slogans tend to determine general opinion: of course, as we all know, this is the drug of choice for the treatment of this or that condition, but why get excited about it? It is, after all, such an old story.

TISSUE DAMAGE AT THE INJECTION SITE AFTER INTRAMUSCULAR INJECTION OF DRUGS IN FOOD-PRODUCING ANIMALS

FOLKE RASMUSSEN

Department of Pharmacology and Toxicology, Royal Veterinary and Agricultural University, Copenhagen (Denmark)

ABSTRACT

Tissue damage at the injection site has been described after intramuscular injection of antibiotics, chemotherapeutics, vitamins, lidocaine, diazepam, digoxin etc. in food-producing animals.

After intramuscular injection of saline or sterile water little or no tissue reaction has been observed, while vehicles containing glycerol formal or propylene glycol caused damage at the injection site.

Therefore, in order to develop drug preparations for intramuscular administration, which cause minimal tissue damage, it is important to consider all components of the preparation.

INTRODUCTION

It is well known that intramuscular injection of a number of drugs and of vehicles containing glycerol formal or propylene glycol may cause tissue damage at the injection site in both man and animal. In some cases there has been pain, and abscesses, fibrosis and contractures have been observed at the injection site (ref. 1, 2, 3, 4, 5, 6, 7, 8, 9, 10, 11, 12, 13).

RESULTS AND DISCUSSION

Antibiotics and chemotherapeutics

Intramuscular injection of preparations containing streptomycin and/or sodium, potassium or procaine salts of benzylpenicillin has been shown to leave very slight local damage 6 days after injection into cows and swine (Table 1) (ref. 5). However, species variations have been observed and in hens streptomycins caused necrosis at the injection site (Table 1) (ref. 14). Suspensions of benethamine or benzathine salts of benzylpenicillin or penethamate hydriodide in water produced small necrotic areas at the injection site. Histologically there were vascular and fibroblastic proliferation and regeneration of degenerated bordering muscle fibres (ref. 5, 15).

Table 1. Irritative effect at the injection site six days after intramuscular injection of preparations containing penicillins and/
or streptomycin (ref. 5, 14, 15).

Antibiotics	Animal species	Degree of tissue damage	
		macroscopic[1]	microscopic[2]
Penicillins	Cows	o+	o+
sodium, potassium	Hens	o+	o+
and/or procaine	Swine	o+	o+
in water			
benethamine, benza- thine or penethamate hydriodide in water	Swine	++	+++
Streptomycin in water	Hens	++	++
	Swine	o+	o+
Streptomycin and peni-	Cows	o+	o+
cillin-procaine in	Hens	o+	++
water	Swine	o+	o+

[1] Macroscopic changes:
o   no reaction
+   haemorrhage
++ small necrotic areas
+++ pronounced necrotic areas

[2] Microscopic changes:
o   no reactions
+   vascular and fibroblastic proliferation, regeneration in hyalin
degenerated muscle fibres
++ a necrotic area surrounded by a
demarcating zone with pronounced
vascular and fibroblastic proliferation
+++ as ++ but with numerous fagocytic
giant cells and necrotic muscle
fibres with calcifications

In all cases after intramuscular injection of tetracyclines a.o. oxyte-tracycline, rolitetracycline and tetracycline severe reactions with necro-ses and a peripheral zone of haemorrhage, oedema and fibrosis were seen six days after the injection to cows, swine and hens. Fagocytic giant cells and necrotic muscle fibres with calcifications were more pronounced in swine (Table 2) (ref. 5, 14, 15, 16, 17). Similar reactions are seen in swine in-jected with preparations containing erythromycin, spiramycin and tylosin (ref. 5, 15) and in hens injected with spiramycin and tylosin (Table 2) (ref. 14).

Table 2. Irritative effect at the injection site six days after intramuscular injection of preparations containing antibiotics
(ref. 5, 14, 15)

Antibiotics	Animal species	Degree of tissue damage	
		macroscopic[1]	microscopic[2]
Erythromycin in propylene glycol	Swine	+++	+++
Neomycin in water	Swine	+++	+++
Tetracyclines oxytetracycline in water	Cows	+++	++
	Hens	+++	++
	Swine	+++	+++
rolitetracycline in oil	Swine	+++	+++
tetracycline in water	Cows	+++	++
	Hens	+++	++
	Swine	+++	+++
Tylosin in propylene glycol	Hens	+++	++
	Swine	+++	+++

1) and 2) see Table 1.

Histological examination showed changes characteristic of a foreign body
reaction. Phagocytic giant cells and necrotic muscle fibres with calcifications were found especially in the swine.

Chemotherapeutics such as sulphonamides and trimethoprim gave rise to
tissue damage at the injection sites in both swine (ref. 6, 18), hens (ref. 14)
cows and horses (Table 3). Six days after injection of preparations containing sulphadiazine, sulphadimidine, sulphadoxine, sulphamethizole, sulpha-
pyrazole and/or trimethoprim, macroscopic changes-mainly areas of necrotic
muscle surrounded by a haemorrhagic zone, were seen at all injection sites.
Histological examination of tissues six days after injection revealed that
all injections caused necrosis of the muscle fibres. The necroses were surrounded by a fibroblastic and histiocytic demarcating zone with foreign body
giant cells and were slightly calcified. In the periphery of the demarcating
zone there were regenerating muscle fibres.

Thirty days after the injections of antibiotics and chemotherapeutics
causing severe local damage, the injured muscle tissue had been replaced by
scar tissue with small remnants of necrotic tissue. The histological findings
were mainly areas of scar tissue containing islands of necrotic muscle fibres
with foreign body giant cells and marked calcifications (ref. 5, 6, 18).

Table 3. Irritative effect at the injection site six days after intramuscular injection of preparations containing chemotherapeutics
(ref. 6, 14, 18)

Chemotherapeutics	Animal species	Degree of tissue damage	
		macroscopic[1]	microscopic[2]
Sulphadiazine	Cows	+++	
Sulphadimidine	Hens	+++	++
Sulphadoxine	Horses	+++	
Sulphamethizole	Swine	+++	+++
Sulphapyrazole in water			
Sulphadiazine and trimethoprim in water	Swine	+++	+++
Sulphadimidine and trimethoprim	Swine	+++	
Sulphadoxine and trimethoprim in glycerol formal	Cows	+++	
	Horses	+++	
	Swine	+++	+++

1) and 2) see Table 1.

Vitamins

Both water and fat soluble vitamins are known to damage the tissue at injection sites. In 1975 Behrens et al. demonstrated tissue damage in sheep(ref.19
after intramuscular injections of 3 ml fat soluble vitamins A, D_3 and E in
peanut oil or soybean oil. Necrosis was observed at the injection sites and
regional lymphadenitis also occurred. Similar reactions were seen in swine
six days after intramuscular injection of vitamin A (100,000 i.u./ml, 10 ml)
and vitamin D_3 (100,000 i.u./ml, 6 ml), (ref. Rasmussen, unpublished results).
Calcification and necrosis at the injection site have been described after
intramuscular injections of vitamin A and D_3 (150,000 i.u.) in a hydrophilic
vehicle into piglets (ref. 20).

Various drugs

A number of other drugs are known to cause tissue damage at the injection
sites (ref. 9).

After intramuscular injection into steers and swine sodium selenite in
distilled water has resulted in muscular necrosis at the injection sites,
accompanied by haemorrhage, oedema and infiltration of neutrophils (ref. 21).

When preparations of drugs containing lidocaine, diazepam or digoxin were
injected intramuscularly into swine post mortem examination of the injection
sites six days later revealed large-scale muscle tissue necrosis (ref. 12,

22, 23). The volume of the digoxin preparation injected into swine was 1.5, 2.0 or 4.0 ml per site, while the amount of necrotic tissue varied from 36 to 330 cm^3 and were proportional to the volume injected (ref. 22).

Vehicles

Five to seven days after intramuscular injection of saline or sterile water little or no tissue reaction could be observed in swine and rabbits (ref. 18, 23). However, intramuscular injection of vehicles containing 40% propylene glycol, 10% ethanol, 0.3% sodium phosphate and 0.08% anhydrous citric acid in distilled water to swine damaged the tissue. Necrosis was seen in all cases after injection of 1.5, 2.0 or 4.0 ml of vehicle alone, but the amount of tissue damaged was much smaller (2 to 24 cm^3), than after injection of the vehicle containing digoxin (ref. 22).

Table 4. Irritative effect at the injection site three to six days after intramuscular injection of various vehicles (ref. 13, 14, 18)

Vehicles	Animal species	Degree of tissue damage	
		macroscopic[1]	microscopic[2]
Glycerol formal 33 and 50% in saline	Hens	++	++
	Rabbits	+++	
	Swine	+++	+++
Propylene glycol 40% in water	Hens	+++	++
	Rabbits	+++	
	Swine	+++	+++
Physiological saline	Rabbits	o	
	Swine	o	o
Sterile water	Rabbits	+	
	Swine	o	o

1) and 2) see Table 1.

Vehicles containing glycerol formal or propylene glycol caused severe muscle damage at the injection site in swine, hens and rabbits (Table 4) (ref. 12, 13, 14, 18, 22, 23). In experiments on rabbits injected propylene glycol it was observed that the damaged tissue at the injection sites was in most cases well defined by a greyish demarcating zone and consisted solely of necrotic muscle tissue. The damaged tissue after injection of glycerol formal was less firm and contained small amounts of normal fibres localized among necrotic muscle fibres (ref. 13).

Using oil as a vehicle cystic formations were observed in the periphery

of the demarcating zone after injection into swine (ref. 15). Further, parts
of oil may be absorbed to the lymphatics as liquid oil and small oil cycts
may appear in the regional lymph nodes. After very large dosis or repeated
applications oil droplets may be released from the lymph nodes and via the
main lymphatics cause pulmonary oil microembolism (ref. 24).

CONCLUDING REMARKS

The results referred to and discussed above show that both the drug itself and the vehicle used can cause tissue injuries. Furthermore, tissue
damages may vary from one animal species to another and may depend on the
drug concentration and the volume injected. It is therefore important to
consider all these factors when developing new drug preparations for intramuscular administration.

REFERENCES

1. Hanson, D.J., 1961. Local toxic effects of broad-spectrum antibiotics
   following injection. Antibiot. Chemotherapy, 11: 390-404.
2. Hanson, D.J., 1963. Intramuscular injection injuries and complications.
   GP (General Practitioner), XXVII, 109-115.
3. Shintani, S., Yamazaki, M., Nakamura, M. and Nakayama, I., 1967. A new
   method to determine the irritation of drugs after intramuscular injection in rabbits. Toxicol. Appl. Pharmacol., 11: 293-301.
4. Hagen, R., 1968. Contracture of the quadriceps muscle in children.
   Acta Orthop. Scandinav., 39: 565-578.
5. Rasmussen, F. and Høgh, P., 1971. Lokalirritation og koncentrationer på
   injektionsstedet efter intramuskulær injektion af antibiotikaholdige
   præparater på køer og grise. Irritating effect and concentrations at
   the injection site after intramuscular injection of antibiotic preparations in cows and pigs. Nord. Vet.-Med., 23: 593-605.
6. Rasmussen, F., Nielsen, P. and Svendsen, O., 1973. Vævsbeskadigelser
   og koncentrationer på injektionsstedet samt restkoncentrationer i mu-
   skulatur, lever og nyrer efter intramuskulær injektion af injectabile
   sulfadimidini 0,2 g/ml på grise. Tissue injuries, concentrations at
   the injection site and the concentrations in muscles, liver and kidney
   after intramuscular injection of injectable sulphadimidine 0.2 g/ml in
   pigs. Nord. Vet.-Med., 25: 256-261.
7. Kienel, G., 1973. Eine rationelle Methode zur tierexperimentellen
   Prüfung der Lokalen Verträglichkeit von intramuskulären Injektionen.
   Arzneim.-Forsch., 23: 263-266.
8. McCloskey, J.R. and Chung, S.M.K., 1977. Quadriceps contracture as a
   result of multiple intramuscular injection. Am. J. Dis. Child.,
   131: 416-417.
9. Greenblatt, D.J. and Allen, M.D., 1978. Intramuscular injection-site
   complications. J. Amer. Med. Ass., 240: 542-544.
10. Immelman, A., Botha, W.S. and Grib, D., 1978. Muscle irritation caused
    by different products containing oxytetracycline. J. South Afr. Vet.
    Ass., 49: 103-105.
11. Rasmussen, F., 1978. Tissue damage at the injection site after intra-
    muscular injection of drugs. Vet. Sci. Commun., 2: 173-182.

12. Steiness, E., Rasmussen, F., Svendsen, O. and Nielsen, P., 1978. A comparative study of serum creatine phosphokinase (CPK) activity in rabbits, pigs and humans after intramuscular injection of local damaging drugs. Acta pharmacol. et toxicol., 42: 357-364.
13. Svendsen, O., Rasmussen, F., Nielsen, P. and Steiness, E., 1979. The loss of creatine phosphokinase (CK) from intramuscular injection sites in rabbits. A predictive tool for local toxicity. Acta pharmacol. et toxicol., 44: 324-328.
14. Blom, L. and Rasmussen, F., 1976. Tissue damage at the injection site after intramuscular injection of drugs in hens. Br. Poult. Sci., 17: 1-4.
15. Svendsen, O., 1972. Histologiske forandringer efter intramuskulære injektioner med antibiotikaholdige præparater. Histologic changes after intramuscular injection with antibiotic preparations. Nord. Vet.-Med., 24: 181-185.
16. Weber, H.A. and Molenaar, A.P., 1971. Stable solutions of oxytetracycline suitable for parenteral and peroral administration and process of preparation. United States Patent Office, 3: 557,280.
17. Rasmussen, F. and Ladefoged, O., 1974. Tissue damage at the injection site after intramuscular injection of drug preparations formulated by addition of polyvinylpyrrolidone. Acta vet. scand., 15: 636-638.
18. Rasmussen, F. and Svendsen, O., 1976. Tissue damage and concentrations at the injection site after intramuscular injection of chemotherapeutics and vehicles in swine. Res. Vet. Sci., 20: 55-60.
19. Behrens, H., Matschullat, G. and Tuch, K., 1975. Uber die Verträglichkeit öliger Vitaminløsungen beim Schaf nach intramuskulärer Applikation. Dtsch. Tierärztl. Wschr., 82: 27-31.
20. Bille, N., 1970. Hypervitaminosis D og calciphylaxis hos husdyr. Hypervitaminosis D and calciphylaxis in domestic animals. Nord. Vet.-Med., 22: 218-233.
21. Herigstad, R.R. and Whitehair, C.K., 1974. Local and systemic effects of parenteral injections of sodium selenite in cattle and swine. Vet. Med. Small Animal Clinician, 69: 1035-1038.
22. Steiness, E., Svendsen, O. and Rasmussen, F., 1974. Plasma digoxin after parenteral administration. Local reaction after intramuscular injection. Clin. Pharmacol. Ther., 16: 430-434.
23. Steiness, E., Svendsen, O., Rasmussen, F. and Nielsen, P., 1977. Prediction of local damage after intramuscular injection. In: Hans Bundgaard, Per Juul and Helmer Kofod (Editors), Drug design and adverse reactions. Munksgaard, Copenhagen; Academic Press, New York; Nancodo, Tokyo.
24. Svendsen, O. and Aaes-Jørgensen, T., 1979. Studies on the fate of vegetable oil after intramuscular injection into experimental animals. Acta pharmacol. et toxicol., in press.

COMPARATIVE MACROSCOPIC EVALUATION OF MUSCLE DAMAGE IN RATS AND IN CATTLE[+] AFTER INTRAMUSCULAR ADMINISTRATION OF SOME COMMERCIALLY AVAILABLE INJECTABLE MEDICINES

C.A. LADAGE, Th.A. van WALSTIJN and H.A. van RIESSEN
ACF Chemiefarma NV, Straatweg 2, 3600 AA MAARSSEN (The Netherlands)

ABSTRACT

In rats injection of several commercially available medicines frequently used for animals or humans caused damage to the muscle. The reactions were most pronounced for the injectable formulations of levamisole, nitroclofene, pentazocine and thiazinamium.

Injection in cattle of chloramphenicol resulted in muscle necrosis, while the reactions caused by nitroclofene and oxytetracycline were milder.

It is discussed that the quadriceps femoris muscle of rats can be used as a primary screen for muscle damage caused by injectable formulations in cattle.

INTRODUCTION

The predictive value is determined of the use of the muscles of rats for the determination of the muscle damage caused by some injectable formulations in cattle.

The determination of muscle damage in rats (body weight of about 250 g) was performed according to a slightly modified method as used by Kienel (1973, ref. 1).

The muscle damage in cattle was investigated 7 days after intramuscular treatment of 2 cows in the cossum of in the neck (body weight of about 500 kg) with the therapeutic doses of the selected formulations or with the maximum acceptable volume per injection site.

In rats the damaged area was actually measured and expressed as a percentage of the total area, while in cattle the damaged volume was estimated. The nature of this damage was determined only macroscopically.

[+]Experiments in cattle were carried out in co-operation with Dr. J.F.M. Nouws, Meat Inspection Service, Havenweg 2, Nijmegen (NL)

RESULTS AND DISCUSSION

In rats injection of several medicines mentioned in Table 1, with the exception of atropine (No 1) and ergometrine (No 5), caused damage to the muscle (Tables 1 and 2).

The reactions were most pronounced for the formulations of levamisole (No 10), nitroclofene (No 11), pentazocine (No 14) and thiazinamium (No 15). So in rats injection of medicines frequently used for treatment of patients might cause severe reactions. It is known that if necrosis of the rat muscle is observed after injection of e.g. antibiotics, steroids of alkaloids, such compounds precipitate adverse reactions in man (ref. 2).

Not only the muscles of rats are suitable for a reliable prediction of clinical reaction in humans, but also the muscles of other animal species, like rabbits and pigs, as is apparent from experiments with, for example the compounds diazepam, digoxin and lidocain (ref. 3).

Although our results showed that chloramphenicol and diazepam caused somewhat milder reactions in rat muscles than levamisole, nitroclofene, pentazocine and thiazinamium, injection in rabbits or dogs caused muscle necrosis (ref. 4, 5).

In rats, injection of two different formulations of oxytetracycline produced different degrees of muscle damage, because - as also shown in rabbits (ref. 6) -, after addition of polyvinylpyrolydon (PVP), the injectable formulation was less irritant for the muscle.

This influence of PVP in rats has already been reported with regard to the proxyphylline/lithium-hydroxyde formulation of a nitroclofene-related compound (ref. 7). However, injection of relatively large volumes of an analogous formulation in cattle did not confirm the results obtained in rats (ref. 7), although the observation in cattle was restricted to those reactions that were visible on the exterior of the animal.

Also pigs hardly any reduction in muscle damage was found after injection of 10 millilitres of a PVP-containing formulation of oxytetracycline and sulphadimidine (ref. 8), possibly because small injection volumes used in small animals are less toxic for the muscle than large volumes often applied in patients (ref. 3).

For these reasons some injectable formulations of the commercially available antibiotics chloramphenicol (form. No 2) and oxytetracycline (form Nos 12 and 13) as well as of the anthelmintic levamisole (form. No 10) and the anti-liver-fluke compound nitroclofene (form.No 11) were injected in the muscles of the neck or the cossum of cattle (Table 3).

Although damage to the muscle is always reflected by an increased plasma-activity

Table 1 Comparative evaluation in rats of the damage caused to both quadriceps femoris muscles after injection of several commercially available formulations of medicines (DETAILED RESULTS)

chloramphenicol,25%(No2) *1

days pi	damaged mm²	area %
1	20±4	46±8
2	17±2	33±3
4	14±2	28±8
7	11±2	25±7
10	7±1	14±3
14	5±1	10±4
18	3±1	6±3

diazepam,0.5%(No3)

days pi	damaged mm²	area %
1	15±4	28±10
4	9±4	18±5
8	7±2	16±5
11	3±1	7±3
14	2	5
17	1	2

emitine-HCl,3%(No4)

days pi	damaged mm²	area %
1	8±3	18±4
2	11±2	18±5
3	9±2	19±3
8	3±1	8±2
10	1	2

iron-complex,5%(No8)

days pi	damaged mm²	area %
1	3±1	8±2
2	4±1	10±1
3	3±1	7±3
4	3±2	8±5
7	2	6
10	1	2
14	1	2

iron-complex,10%(No9)

days pi	damaged mm²	area %
1	4±1	9±3
2	3±1	7±2
3	3±2	7±1
4	1	2±1

levamisole-HCl,10%(No10)

days pi	damaged mm²	area %
1	18±3	32±9
2	20±7	54±21
3	23±5	53±16
4	16±7	44±24
7	18±4	43±11
10	16±4	33±8
14	12±1	35±5
17	8±1	27±3
21	4±1	11±5

nitrociofene,12.5%(No11) *1

days pi	damaged mm²	area %
1	21±12	43±14
7	21±6	55±21
10	12±3	34±9
14	7±2	19±6
17	12±3	31±9
21	5±4	15±12
24	0	0
25	0	0

oxytetracycline-HCl,5%(No12) *1

days pi	damaged mm²	area %
1	21±4	39±7
2	21±2	40±4
4	12±5	28±12
7	7±2	15±4
8	9±3	16±5
11	8±5	15±10
14	6±3	14±7
16	4±2	8±4
18	2	5

oxytetracycline-HCl,10%(No13) *1

days pi	damaged mm²	area %
1	13±2	26±4
2	12±3	25±8
4	9±3	22±5
7	2±1	5±2
9	3	7

pentazocine,3%(No14)

days pi	damaged mm²	area %
1	17±2	39±10
4	8±1	21
8	9±1	22±2
11	9±1	22±2
14	7±2	16±7
17	4±3	11±10

thiazinamium,2.5%(No15)

days pi	damaged mm²	area %
1	34±1	75±10
4	37±3	100
8	31±9	90±20
11	32±9	95±10
14	18±4	66±22
17	11±1	39±11
21	7±6	21±5
24	7±6	40±39
28	3±1	5±2
30	1±1	6±3

vitamine-B-complex,6.7%(No16)

days pi	damaged mm²	area %
1	12±3	23±5
2	9±3	21±8
3	7±2	16±5
4	6±1	18±5
7	3±1	8±2
9	2	5

Table 2   Comparative macroscopic evaluation in rats of the muscle damage caused to both
quadriceps femoris muscles after injection of several commercially available
injectable formulations of medicines and vehicles.

No	Compound	Tmin days	Sreg days	No	Compound	Tmin days	Sreg days
1	atropine,1%	★1	★1	9	iron-complex,10%	2	★2
2	chloramphenicol,25%	16	12	10	levamisole-HCl,10%	20	6
3	diazepam,0.5%	10½	9½	11	nitroclofene,12.5%	22	12
4	emitine-HCl,3%	7½	5½	12	oxytetracycline-HCl,5%	15	13
5	ergometrine maleate,0.015%	★1	★1	13★3	oxytetracycline-HCl,10%	6½	3½
6	physiological saline,0.9%	★1	★1	14	pentazocine,3%	18	17
7	glucose,10%	★1	★1	15	thiazinamium,2.5%	27	10
3	iron-complex,5%	7	★2	16	vitamine-B-complex,6.7%	6½	5½

★1   · no reactions were observed   Tmin: Number of days after injection in which the degree of
★2   muscle damage was never maximal   muscle damage is minimal
★3   formulation contained PVP   Sreg: Number of days between the degree of muscle damage
                                         being still maximal and becoming minimal

of Creatine-phosphokinase (CPK) (ref. 4, 9, 10, 11), the muscle damage in cattle
was only investigated macroscopically seven days after injection.

The results presented in Table 3 showed that chloramphenicol (form. No 2)
caused, after injection in cattle, severe muscle necrosis and oedema, as already
reported by Nouws & Ziv (1977, ref. 12) and by Ziv (1979, ref. 13). The necrosis
was more pronounced than could be expected from the results obtained in rats.

The opposite applied to levamisole as in one animal muscle degeneration was
observed.

Nitroclofene caused muscle necrosis after injection in the neck. However, the
reactions were much milder if the formulation was injected in the muscles of the
cossum.

The marked demarcation zone indicated that a regeneration proces had developed.
As described by Ladage (1979, ref. 7), these reactions were almost completely
reversible within a couple of weeks of treatment.

The reaction due to nitroclofene might be compared with the reactions caused
by oxytetracycline observed in animal No 56.

The influence of PVP in the formulation of oxytetracycline in reducing the
muscle necrosis in cattle was quite remarkable, so the absence of this influence
in the muscles of pigs (ref. 8) might be a result of species differences.

Table 3   Comparative macroscopic evaluation in cattle of the muscle damage caused after injection in the muscles of the neck or cossum of commercially available formulations of some antibiotics and an anthelmintic in relation to the nitroclofene- containing formulation Distoject R.

Active principle non-proprietary name (code number formulation)	An. No	Injection vol. ml	dose mg/kg	Local reactions 2 days	5 days	7 days	Macroscopic observation of the injection site oedema	muscle degeneration	muscle necrosis	dem. zone	lymphnode	Pes.
chloramphenicol; 25' (1.713-77.11.10)	57	24	10	-	-	-	++ >30 cm; spread over whole neck; haemorrhagic.	-	+++ ~20x7x4 cm. strongly haemorrhagic	-	na	d
No 2	70	24	10	-	-	-	++ ~30 cm; haemorrhagic.	-	+++; ~20x20x3;also between fasci ; strongly haemorrhagic	+?	na	d
levamisole (hydrochloride); 10ᶜ (2.1810-77.12.07958)	49	30	5	-	-	+_	+ ~15 cm.	++;~4x8 cm haemorrhagic - reaction in fat.	+_	-	slightly haemorrhagic	nd
No 10	54	30	5	-	-	+_	+ ~15 cm.	-	-	-	strongly haemorrhagic	nd
nitroclofene; 12% (3.36-28.6.164)	52	14	3	-	-	-	+ ~20 cm between membranes.	- somewhat wet.	++ ~6x8x1 cm; yellow and bordered.	++	somewhat red and enlarged.	nd
No 11	53	14	3	-	-	-	+ ~20 cm between membranes and fasci.; slightly haemorrhagic	- somewhat wet.	++ ~5x12x1 cm; yellow and bordered.	++	na	nd
nitroclofene; 12% (3.36-28.6.164)	47	14*1	3	+_	+oe	-	+ ~5 cm in muscle and fat.	-	+ ø5 cm; yellow and strongly restricted.	+	na	nd
No 11	50	14*1	3	-	+oe	+oe	+ ~10-15 cm.	-	+ ø9 cm; yellow, strongly restricted and cavernous.	++	na	nd
oxytetracycline (hydro-chloride); 5 (4.22-6006)	48	36	3	+_	-	-	+_ ~5 cm; haemorrhagic; green dis-colouration(4x12cm)between fasci	-	? injected intermuscularly	?	na	d
No 12	56	36	3	-	-	-	+ ~10-15 cm; localized.	+(+);~3x5 cm. somewhat wet.	++ ~8x12x1 cm haemorrhagic.	++	na	d
oxytetracycline (hydro-chloride); 10ᶜ (5.2016-80151356)	51	15	2½	-	-	-	+ ~10-15 cm between membranes; haemorrhagic.	-	-	-	little enlarged.	d
No 13	55	15	2½	-	-	-	++ >15 cm between membranes and fasci.; haemorrhagic.	++;~30x0.2 cm; haemorrhagic.	-	-	na	d

*1 : injected in the muscles of the cossum.

Abbreviations and symbols used in Table 3 :

Formulations No	Compound	Composition of vehicle
1.713 - 77.11.10	chloramphenicol;25%	?
2.1810 - 77.12.07958	levamisole(HCl);10%	?
3.36 - 28.6.164	nitroclofene;12½%	DMSO;Cetiol B
4.22 - 6006	oxytetracycline(HCl);5%	propyleneglycol;water
5.2016 - 80151356	oxytetracycline(HCl);10%	polyvinylpyrolydone;water

Local reactions:

±   : some hardening of the muscle
oe   : oedema

Macroscopic observation of the injection site:

Oedema, muscle degeneration and muscle necrosis:
-      : no alterations
±   : minor alterations
+   : alterations clearly noticable
++   : strong alterations
+++   : severe alterations
!   : alterations stronger than +++

Demarcation zone (Dem.zone):
-      : absent
+   : visible
++   : marked

Lymphnodes:
na   : no alterations

Residues (Res.):
nd   : not determined
d   : determined

★1   : formulation injected in the muscles of the cossum

CONCLUSIONS

The use of the rat muscle (quadriceps femoris muscle) for a primary screen of muscle damage in cattle produces reliable results, but it should always be kept in mind that injection of large volumes in cattle may cause more severe reactions, as injection of chloramphenicol in cattle caused more severe reactions than determined in rats. However, the opposite was seen after injection of levamisole.

LITERATURE

1: Kienel, G. (1973), Arzneim.-Forsch (Drug Res.), 23, 263-266.
2: Paget, G.E. and Scott, H. (1957), Brit. J. Pharmacol., 12, 427-433.
3: Steiness, E., Rasmussen, F., Svendsen, O. and Nielsen, P. (1978),
   Acta Pharmacol. et Toxicol., 42, 357-364.
4: Gloor, H.O., Vorburger, C. and Schädeling, J. (1977),
   Schweiz Med. Wschr., 107, 948-952.

5: Hanson, D.J. (1961), Antibiotics and Chemotherapy, 11, 390-404.

6: Immelman, A., Botha, W.S. and Grib, D. (1978),
   J. South African Vet. Ass., 49, 103-105.

7: Ladage, C.A. (1979), Thesis Vet. Fac. Utrecht.

8: Rasmussen, F. and Ladofoged, O. (1974), Acta Vet. Scand., 15, 636-638.

9: Greenblatt, D.J. and Koch Weser, J. (1976),
   New England Journal of Medicine, 295, 542-546.

10: Meltzer, H.Y., Boyer, M. and Mrozak, S. (1970),
    Am. J. Med. Sci., 259, 42-48.

11: Warnock, G. and Ellmann, G.L. (1969), Science, 164, 726-727.

12: Nouws, J.F.M. and Ziv, G. (1977), Refuah Vet., 34, 131-135.

13: Ziv, G. (1979), Künzen Veterinary Institute, Bet Dagan Vet Symp. Rekovat.

LOCAL REACTION STUDIES IN RABBITS AND DOGS

V. Tittes-Rittershaus, H. de Vries and H. de Jong
Research Laboratories, Intervet International B.V., P.O. Box 31, 5830 AA Boxmeer
The Netherlands.

SUMMARY

From a comparative local reaction study in rabbits and dogs, the somewhat contradictory results of two oily preparations were presented. The damaging properties of preparation C were equal in both species while the foreign body reaction found after the injection of preparation A was more severe in a few individual dogs than in rabbits.

This difference may raise doubts whether the rabbits can safely be used to predict reactions in dogs. As a consequence it is suggested that in all cases where foamy macrophages are seen in local reactions of rabbits a particularly low borderline should be drawn for acceptance.

As every evaluation should rely on quantitative data all lesions were scored. The score system used was developed and already useful during preliminary studies.

INTRODUCTION

In the course of safety testing of pharmaceutical products intended for parenteral injection two different preparations were submitted to local reaction tests in two different species. The target animal for these two preparations was the dog but for ethical as well as economical reasons we prefer to use the dog as little as possible. Rabbits are recommended for this type of test by the FDA (ref. 1) as long as 1965 and more recently many references have appeared (ref. 3-7, 9)in which rabbits were the chosen species. However, we have been unable to find any studies comparing the local effects of preparations in dogs and rabbits.

Rasmussen (ref. 8) observed variations between species with respect to the local damage caused by a streptomycin preparation. Behrens (ref. 2) also suggests that the severe local reactions following intramuscular injections of two oily vitamin A preparations in sheep may be due to a special sensitivity in this species. From a comparative study in rabbits and dogs we selected the results of two oily preparations for today's presentation as their effects were to some extent contradictory with respect to the species correlation.

MATERIAL AND METHODS

Preparations

The 2 preparations used were oily compositions with a longacting steroid ester as active compound. They were coded A and C.

Animals

The test animals were 6 white New Zealand rabbits of about 2½ kg kept individually in galvanized iron cages. Six of the 12 dogs were 5 years old beagles while the other six were 6 months old mongrels. All dogs were kept in indoor kennels. The animals were fed species specific pellets and both species were allowed fresh tap water ad libitum.

Test design

Each animal received 4 injections, i.e. controlaterally 2 into each M. sacrospinalis. The preparations were distributed randomly but each animal received both preparations. The injection sites were shaved and injections given under aseptic conditions. The drugs were deposited 8-10 mm deep and a volume of 0,75 ml per injection was given. After 4 weeks the animals were sacrificed by an intravenous overdose of pentobarbitone sodium.

Terminal studies

After the examination of the subcutis the Mm.sacrospinales were removed and sliced transversally into strips 3-5 mm thick. Muscle specimens from the centre of the lesions were fixed in 5 % neutral buffered formalin, processed and 5 μ thick paraplast sections from two different levels of each specimen were stained with haematoxylin and eosin. Slides were read twice, once per drug group and once per animal. The pathologic findings were judged and noted by a score system developed during preliminary studies.

For explanation see graph 1.

Macroscopic lesions were scored + to +++ depending on their extension, i.e. being small and multifocal, reticular or diffuse. One additional score was given for macroscopically recognizable necrosis.

The microscopic scoring was performed under 40 x magnification and the number of scores (+ to +++) depended on the percentage of the field occupied by the lesions.

Where there were indications of severe and possibly progressive pathological changes, for instance, haemorrhage, necrosis, large pseudocysts, marked lymphoid or granulocytic infiltration, additional scores were given. Particular attention was paid to the presence of the foamy variant of macrophages as they are the hallmark of granulomatous inflammation, and of course to granulomas. Where repair tissue was present no additional scores were allocated.

Finally, mean scores as well as standard deviations were calculated for the purposes of comparison.

RESULTS

As there was no obvious difference in lesions found between the younger and older test dogs the results of both subgroups were added together.

Lesions produced by Preparation C

Lesions in rabbits

The injection sites in rabbits demonstrated already during macroscopic examination severe lesions. These were diffuse, had a diameter of more than 2 cm and were in 4 cases necrotic in the centre.

Also in the histological slides the central coagulative necrosis was 4 times the dominant lesion and only a small demarcation zone of proliferating fibrous tissue was present.

Lesions in dogs

The total quantity of the corresponding lesions in dogs seemed to be the same but no necrosis was recognizable in any of these injection sites. The shape of the lesions were more elongated in dogs than in rabbits.

Histologically all injection sites in dogs demonstrated a completed repair by scar tissue. Only few pseudocysts with flat epithelium varied this pattern and many residues of myofibrils were maintained in the periphery.

Lesions produced by preparation A

Lesions in rabbits

As compared with the necrosis caused by the C preparation a different aspect was seen in the rabbit muscles of the A preparation injection sites. Here we found only a few small, slightly greyish discolored strips in which a few pseudocysts could be recognized.

In the corresponding histological rabbit lesions predominated single or grouped pseudocysts scattered through the otherwise intact muscle tissue. In general the lining epithelium was flat and only in 3 cases few pseudocysts were surrounded by a greater number of macrophages. A striking feature of these macrophages was their foamy aspect and their vague cell membrane particularly at the lining of the lumen. A few eosinophilic granulocytes participated.

Lesions in dogs

The transversal cuts of intramuscular injection sites in dogs revealed in most cases a pronounced reticular but also greyish discolored pattern.

The lesions of half of the number of injection sites were also histologically comparable with those in rabbits. The others demonstrated a pronounced granulomatous inflammation and the same reticular pattern as seen during macroscopic examination. The granulomas were mainly composed of foamy macrophages, their centre was often lytic and sometimes infiltrated by a low number of granulocytes. The layer of the surrounding fibrocytes was more or less obvious and also the degree of lymphoid infiltration between the granulomas varied. Small foci of the inflammated tissue were necrotic.

GRAPH I.

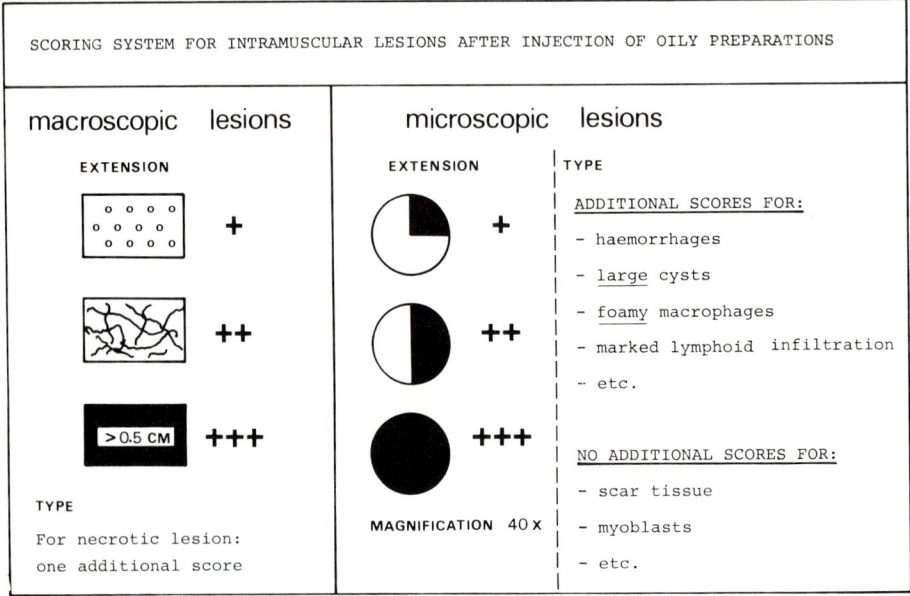

SCORING SYSTEM FOR INTRAMUSCULAR LESIONS AFTER INJECTION OF OILY PREPARATIONS

macroscopic lesions

EXTENSION

+

++

> 0.5 CM +++

TYPE

For necrotic lesion:
one additional score

microscopic lesions

EXTENSION

+

++

+++

MAGNIFICATION 40 x

TYPE

ADDITIONAL SCORES FOR:

- haemorrhages

- large cysts

- foamy macrophages

- marked lymphoid infiltration

- etc.

NO ADDITIONAL SCORES FOR:

- scar tissue

- myoblasts

- etc.

Intervet 1979

GRAPH II.

COMPARATIVE MEAN MACROSCOPIC AND MEAN MICROSCOPIC SCORES AND S.D.
      OF LESIONS CAUSED BY INTRAMUSCULAR INJECTION
   OF TWO DIFFERENT OILY PREPARATIONS IN RABBITS AND DOGS

R = rabbit

D = dog

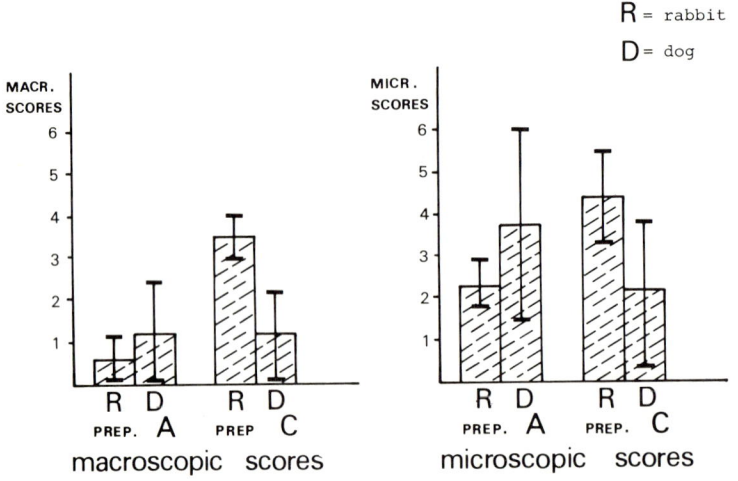

macroscopic scores

microscopic scores

Intervet 1979

The results of scoring

Preparation A lesions received higher scores during macroscopic as well as microscopic examination in dogs than in rabbits; however the reverse occurred with the C preparation lesions. The higher scores for preparation A lesions in dogs were a consequence of the more pronounced granulomatous inflammation; the lower dog scores for preparation C lesions were due to the more advanced repair. See graph 2.

DISCUSSION

Following any injection two major responses occur locally in tissues : the first is mechanical and chemical damage and the second is absorption and/or phagocytosis and/or encapsulation. The effects of preparation C were more simple than those of preparation A. The adverse effect of preparation C was one of mainly mechanical and chemical destruction. The damaging properties of preparation C was similar in both species. The period necessary for the repair was of different length in the two species. With respect to the target this seems to be of lower importance.

The preparation A lesions were more complicated and the possible consequences might be serious. When material is injected which cannot be readily absorbed or degraded it must be removed by macrophage digestion or by encapsulation. Where macrophages are unable to process engulfed material easily they may show changes such as the "foamy cytoplasm phenomenon" and/or damage. Preparation A caused such a type of foreign body reaction, but the reactions were much milder in rabbits than in dogs; they were variable in both species and a number of dogs showed severe and possibly progressive granulomatous inflammation.

Probably the scoring would have produced even more realistic figures if a differentiation would have been made between early coagulative necrosis and necrosis developed during later episodes. However, if lesions become very severe the accuracy of the scoring system is of no further relevance as the tested preparation is in this case no longer acceptable at all.

The authors are indebted to the co-workers of the histological, pharmacological as well as pharmaceutical laboratories of Intervet International B.V., for their excellent technical assistance.

REFERENCES

1. Appraisal of the safety of chemicals in foods, drugs and cosmetics, edited and published by The Editorial Committee of the Ass. of Food and Drug Officials of the U.S. p. 19 (1965).
2. Behrens, H., Matschullat, G. and Tuch, K.: Über die Verträglichkeit öliger Vitaminlösungen beim Schaf nach intramuskulärer Applikation. Dtsch. Tierärztl. Wschr. 82 (1) 27-31 (1975).
3. Benitz, K.-F., Dambach, G.: Morphologic quantification of muscular lesions after injection of aqueous solution. Arzneim.-Forsch., 16 (5) 658-661 (1966).
4. Hanson, D.J.: Local toxic effects of broad-spectrum antibiotics following injection. Antibiotics and Chemotherapy, 11 (6) 390-404 (1961).
5. Immelman, A., Botha, W.S. and Grib, D.: Muscle irritation caused by different products containing oxytetracycline. Journal of the South African Veterinary Association, 49 (2) 103-105 (1978).
6. Kazunaga Fukawa, Yoshihiko Ito, Noriyuki Misaki and Kazuyoshi Bando : A new method for the local irritation test. 1. Tissue regeneration test for intramuscular acetic acid injection. Yakugaka Zasshi 95 (11) 1307-1316 (1975).
7. Kracht, J.: Parenterale Verträglichkeitsversuche mit Miglyol 812-Neutralöl. (1963) pers. comm.
8. Rasmussen, F.: Tissue damage at the injection site after intramuscular injection of drugs. Ass. for Vet. Clinic. Pharm. 2, 51-52 (1978).
9. Shintani, S., Yamazaki, M., Nakamura, M. and Nakayama, I.: A new method to determine the irritation of drugs after intramuscular injection in rabbits. Toxicology and Applied Pharmacology 11, 293-301 (1967).

SOME BIOPHARMACEUTICAL CONSIDERATIONS OF SUBCUTANEOUS AND INTRAMUSCULAR
INJECTIONS USED IN VETERINARY MEDICINE

J.S. DOWRICK
Beecham Pharmaceuticals Research Division, Worthing, (U.K.)

ABSTRACT

The current status of biopharmaceutics in relation to parenteral dosage forms
is reviewed, pointing out the wide variety of fluid systems available and the
numerous factors which can affect the rate of drug release. Release mechanisms
in the case of aqueous and oily injectable suspensions are discussed with examples
taken from bioavailability studies with Clamoxyl (Amoxycillin) Aqueous Injectable
Suspension and an antibiotic oily injectable suspension.

It is more than 30 years since differences in physiological availability
among different dosage forms of vitamins were first demonstrated by Oser et al
(refs. 1 and 2). Since then there has been a steadily growing interest in
bioavailability, spurred on in the early 1970's when it was found that some
brands of commonly used medicines such as digoxin tablets had widely differing
therapeutic activity due to an apparently minor modification in the manufacturing
process. This emphasised only too clearly that the molecular structure of a
drug is not the sole factor involved in drug action and consideration must be
given to the 'dosage form' itself - a term taken to include the chemical nature
(salt or derivative), the crystalline state and the particle size of the drug
in the form presented to the patient.

The term 'biopharmaceutics' was coined in the early 1960's by Levy and Wagner
to define the "study of the relationship between some of those physical and
chemical properties of the drug and its dosage forms and the biological effects
observed following administration of the drug in its various dosage forms".
A large body of knowledge has now been accumulated on gastrointestinal and
percutaneous absorption of drugs but less is known about absorption from the
subcutaneous and intramuscular routes. There are two main reasons for this
apparent lack of progress.

Firstly, there are just as many, if not more different types of injection to
deal with than orally administered dosage forms. Not all drugs can be formulated
as simple aqueous solutions either because of poor solubility or instability,

therefore a common approach is to use alternative biologically acceptable solvents which may or may not be miscible with body fluids. However it is not always possible or even desirable to obtain a true solution and in such cases the drug is present as an undissolved phase. The physical nature of both this dispersed phase and the continuous phase (the vehicle) can vary considerably to give solubilised systems, colloidal dispersions, emulsions and true suspensions. In addition the vehicle can be an aqueous, oily or a non-aqueous water miscible liquid. Combinations of the above dispersed phases and vehicles can give 15 potentially different systems and even then the more recent developments such as triple phase emulsions and liposomes have been omitted. However it must be pointed out that whilst all these systems can be prepared, some are more commonly used than others; furthermore some of the systems are used far more in veterinary than in human medicine, notably suspensions and oily vehicles. Naturally, the systems of greater commercial importance have had more research devoted to them than the less usual ones.

Secondly, there are many factors affecting drug release from each type of injection when administered intramuscularly or subcutaneously. In the simplest case where an aqueous solution has been injected the drug solution is able to mix and diffuse directly into the tissue fluid then pass by various mechanisms into the lymphatic or capillary system thence into the general circulation. The biological factors involved in this process have been extensively reviewed (refs. 3 and 4) and will be discussed elsewhere. However in progressing from aqueous solution to aqueous suspension thence to oily suspension more complex stages must be written into the absorption process. (table 1)

Table 1   Stages in the absorption from aqueous and oily suspensions

STAGE	AQUEOUS SUSPENSION	OILY SUSPENSION
1	Drug particle in aqueous depot	Drug particle in oily depot
2	Drug dissolves in aqueous depot	Drug particle reaches oil/water boundary
3	-	Drug particle becomes wetted
4	Drug dissolves in tissue fluid	
5	Drug enters tissue fluid or capillaries	
6	Drug passes into blood system	

Each stage is in itself a quantifiable process which is determined by the following physico-chemical factors (refs. 5 and 6): (i) the volume of the injected formulation (ii) the concentration of the drug in the vehicle; (iii) the presence or absence of enzymes such as hyaluronidase in the formulation; (iv) the surface area of the depot; (v) the nature of the solvent or vehicle; (vi) the tonicity (vii) the viscosity (viii) the intrinsic dissolution rate of the drug in the tissue fluid; (ix) the crystalline or polymorphic form of suspended drugs; (x) average particle size and particle size distribution; (xi) the presence of any coating on the drug particles; (xii) the presence of pharmaceutical adjuvants such as suspending agents;

(xiii) the presence of vasoconstrictors; (xiv) the partition coefficient of the
drug between the vehicle and tissue fluid which is in turn dependant upon the
chemical nature of the drug itself.

If one considers these in relation to the number of different systems to which
they must be applied the complexity and magnitude of the task can be appreciated.
It is appropriate therefore to quote from Wagner's original 1961 review since it
was not only applicable in his second review in 1971 but is also equally valid today:
"One may generally summarise the above factors by saying that they are the same
factors which control the rate of dissolution of a solid and/or its transfer from
one phase to another. There are many lifetimes of useful research in just using
the above list as a guide and designing experiments in such a way that one isolates
only one variable at a time and studies its relative importance with typical types
of drugs such as neutral molecules, weak acids, weak bases and their salts. If
we had such fundamental information the formulation of a given parenteral product
would not be quite so empirical as it is at present".

To illustrate some of these points I shall briefly review the biopharmaceutics
of two types of injection commonly used in veterinary practise and also include
one or two of our own studies. Firstly, let us consider an aqueous suspension of
for example procaine penicillin G. In this case the drug is in the form of a
salt which has very low solubility in water suspended in an aqueous medium usually
containing buffers, stabilisers and suspending agents. In the enclosed environment
of the vial the system is in equilibrium; a small proportion of the drug having
dissolved in the vehicle until it is saturated. When the suspension is injected
the equilibrium becomes unbalanced and the drug crystals begin to dissolve. The
rate at which this dissolution and absorption takes place is essentially the
'positive' factor in determining the blood level profile. Superimposed on this
of course are the 'negative' factors, ie. the rate at which the drug is metabolised,
hydrolysed or excreted.

There are many ways in which the bioavailability of this type of product can be
modified by changing the physical factors to meet a specific requirement so that
with skill, a variety of products can be formulated, all derived from the same
drug molecule. Figure 1 summarises the relationship between some of these factors,
the majority of which must be decided during the design and manufacture of the
product.
It should be obvious therefore that two brands of the same drug will not
necessarily be 'bioequivalent'. Only occasionally is the user himself able to
have any control over the bioavailability - for example in the case of products
sold as a powder which require the addition of water before use. Such an example
is Clamoxyl Aqueous Injectable Suspension. This product is a sterile powder
containing amoxycillin trihydrate for reconstitution with Water for Injection to
form a stable suspension. Directions are supplied for preparing a choice of three

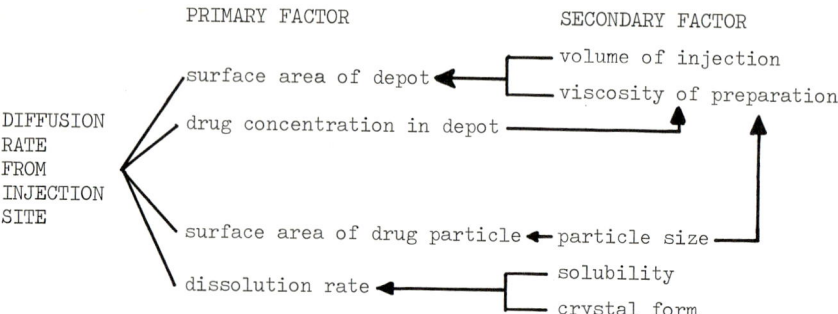

PRIMARY FACTOR   SECONDARY FACTOR

surface area of depot ◄─────┬─── volume of injection
                            └─── viscosity of preparation

DIFFUSION   drug concentration in depot ─────────┐
RATE
FROM
INJECTION
SITE
              surface area of drug particle ◄── particle size ──┐

              dissolution rate ◄─────┬─── solubility
                                     └─── crystal form

FIG. 1. : Relationship between the factors affecting the diffusion rate of a
drug in aqueous suspension from the injection site

concentrations, 50 mg/ml, 100 mg/ml and 200 mg/ml the main purpose of this
flexibility being to give convenient volumes when dosing species of widely
differing body weights. However we were interested to observe in our development
studies that different bioavailability could be obtained from using the same dose
of amoxycillin at different concentrations. As one might have predicted, the
50 mg/ml being the most dilute and having the largest volume, gave a higher peak
blood level and shorter duration than the 250 mg/ml (later modified to 200 mg/ml)
(fig. 2).

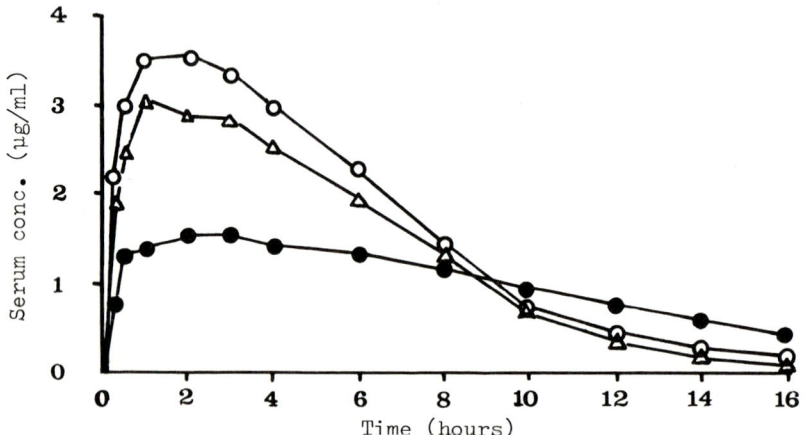

FIG. 2.   Plots of average serum amoxycillin concentration versus time after
intramuscular administration of a 7 mg/kg dose of Clamoxyl Aqueous Injectable
Suspension reconstituted at 50 mg/ml (O—O) 100 mg/ml (△—△) and 250 mg/ml (●—●)

The reasons for this can be attributed to

(a) Greater area of fluid at the injection site.

(b) Larger proportion of drug initially in solution,
     eg. administering a dose of 200 mg :-

4 ml of 50 mg/ml consists of ⎰ 184 mg in suspension
                              ⎱ 16 mg dissolved (8.7% of dose)

whereas 1 ml of 200 mg/ml consists of ⎰ 196 mg in suspension
                                      ⎱ 4 mg dissolved (2.0% of dose)

(approximate figures at 20°C)

  (c) Lower viscosity of 50 mg/ml suspension.

This viscosity effect has been observed by previous workers (ref. 7) who prepared
highly concentrated, paste like aqueous suspensions of procaine penicillin G.
These were thixotropic in nature and produced a sustained depot effect after
intramuscular injection.

   Turning our attention finally to oily suspensions we are faced with a far more
complex set of problems, the main one being how the drug moves from the oil into
the tissue fluid. There is still a great deal of fundamental work to be carried
out in this area, but in cases where the drug has negligible solubility in the
oil phase, (such as in penicillin suspensions) it is axiomatic that there should
be movement of the drug particles towards the oil/tissue fluid interface. Wetting
of the drug particle must then follow before it can dissolve in the tissue fluid.
As long ago as 1948 Buckwalter and Dickison (refs. 8 and 9) examined the
bioavailability of a series of oily penicillin suspensions and this gave some
insight to the mode of action of these formulations. Perhaps their most
significant finding was the effect of particle size. In contrast to aqueous
suspensions where the smaller particle size and concomitant increased surface
area gives a fast release, in most oily suspensions the converse was true.
Furthermore the rate of drug release (and hence the rate of appearance in the
blood stream) depended very much on the nature of the oily vehicle, ie. its
hydrophobic nature and its viscosity. Several hypotheses have been postulated
for these phenomena, for example it has been suggested that the particles gravitate
through the vehicle to the tissue fluid interface. If, therefore, the particles
are very small, simple physical laws tell us that this movement will be slow,
indeed if the vehicle has a gel structure with a finite 'yield value' then such
movement is considerably retarded (ref. 10). However evidence from some of our
own studies suggests that other processes could also be involved:

(i) Oily suspensions of similar particle size and density but with different
crystalline form can release at different rates. These differences are greater
in hydrophobic vehicles than hydrophilic ones. This would imply that the rate
at which the particles are wetted can be an important factor; furthermore if the
surface of the drug particle is large or porous it will take longer for the oil

to be displaced from a given amount of drug.

(ii) In a recent study we compared the bioavailability of two batches of an
experimental antibiotic oily suspension of similar particle size but with
different rheological properties. When administered by the intramuscular route
in a controlled crossover study, statistically significant differences in
bioavailability were observed (fig. 3), the formulation with the lower viscosity as
might be expected, released slightly faster resulting in a higher peak blood
level. However when the test was repeated by the subcutaneous route the difference
was much smaller. (fig. 4) This would suggest that the rheological properties of

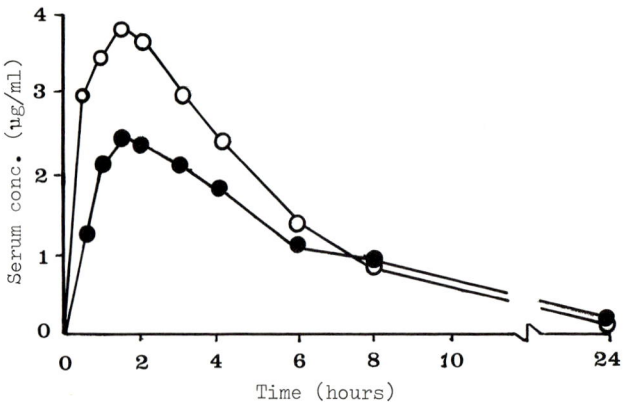

FIG. 3. Plots of average serum antibiotic concentration versus time after
intramuscular injection of a 7 mg/kg dose of an oily suspension with low (O—O)
and high (●—●) viscosity.

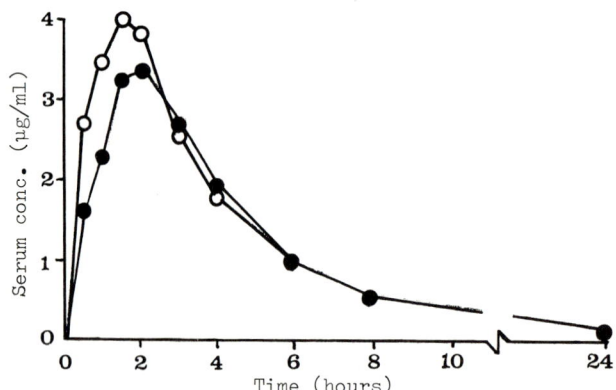

FIG. 4. Plots of average serum antibiotic concentration versus time after
subcutaneous injection of a 7 mg/kg dose of an oily suspension with low (O—O)
and high (●—●) viscosity.

the suspension, together with the motility of the tissue into which it is
injected can play an important part in distributing the injected material and

increasing the rate at which drug particles are brought into contact with the tissue fluid.

It has been said in the past that 'any science with more than seven variables is an art'. Certainly it has been the case that in the past many of the dosage forms to which I have been referring have been designed largely on an empirical basis. However, as the amount of basic pharmaceutical research in this area increases, formulators will be better able to predict and control the bioavailability of their products and thereby maximise the biological effect from the drug.

Acknowledgements

Blood level studies were carried out by Mr. J.F. Buswell, Mrs. S.J. Lay and Mr. G.H. Palmer. The author thanks Mrs. J.M. Kerr for assistance in preparing the manuscript.

References

1. D. Melnick, M. Hochberg, and B.L. Oser, J.Nutr. 30, 67 (1945)
2. B.L. Oser, D. Melnick, and M. Hochberg, Ind. Eng. Chem., Anal. Ed. 17, 401 (1945)
3. J. Schou, Pharmacol. Rev., 13, 441 (1961)
4. B.E. Ballard, J.Pharm. Sci., 57, 357 (1968)
5. J.G. Wagner, J. Pharm. Sci., 50, 359 (1961)
6. J.G. Wagner, 'Drug Design' (E.J. Ariens ed.), Vol.1, p.466. Academic Press 1971
7. S.S. Ober et al, J.Amer. Pharm. Assoc. Sci., Ed., 47, 667 (1958)
8. F.H. Buckwalter and H.L. Dickison, J.Amer. Pharm. Assoc. Sci., Ed. 37, 472 (1948)
9. F.H. Buckwalter and H.L. Dickison, J.Amer. Pharm. Assoc. 47, 661 (1958)
10. E.L. Parrot, 'Pharmaceutical Technology' Burgess 1970

INJECTION SITES AND DRUG BIOAVAILABILITY

A.B. MARSHALL and G.H. PALMER
Beecham Pharmaceuticals Research Division, Animal Health Research Centre,
Tadworth, Surrey, England.

ABSTRACT

The established dogma that intramuscular absorption is better than subcutaneous is no longer tenable in man and our preliminary work suggests it is not tenable in animals.

Drug absorption from extravascular parenteral sites is a complex process with many biological variables.

The region of the body injected is at least as important as the route involved.

The Gluteus medius site is suggested for obtaining reproducible intramuscular injections in calves. The rationale for using a deep intramuscular injection is questioned.

There has been little work in the veterinary field to examine the effect that different sites of injection exert on drug bioavailability. In this paper we wish to review briefly the factors known to affect bioavailability in man and laboratory animals, to report our findings concerning antibiotic absorption in the domestic species and to outline a procedure for defining reproducible injection techniques.

The injection site dogma

There has been a widely held belief in both human and veterinary medicine that the effect of injection site on bioavailability can be largely summarised as in Fig.1, i.e. intramuscular injections show a bioavailability intermediate between intravenous and subcutaneous.

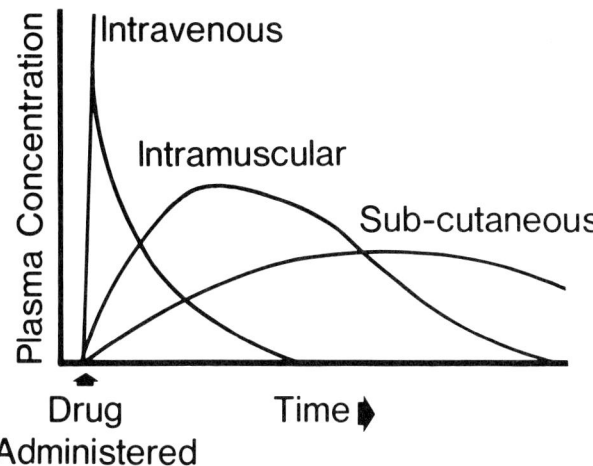

Fig.1 The injection site dogma

The dogma questioned

This concept has been fundamentally questioned by Nora et al (1964) as a result of their studies with insulin. In diabetic children they injected radio-active insulin into 4 sites and measured the half life of the radioactivity. Their results are summarised in Table 1.

Table 1. Half life (minutes) of radioactivity from two intramuscular sites in children and their overlying subcutaneous sites following injection of labelled insulin (Nora et al, 1964)

	Quadriceps Femoris	Deltoid
Intramuscular	314	224
Subcutaneous	310	232

Nora et al have clearly demonstrated that the region of the body rather than the tissue involved is the prime determinant for insulin absorption in diabetic children.

Implications for veterinary medicine

We consider it important to examine critically the effect of different injection sites on bioavailability in domestic animals for 3 main reasons:

1) A better understanding of the biological factors affecting bioavailability may lead to therapeutic advantages.

2) With a choice of sites of equivalent bioavailability we can select:

    a) Those avoiding valuable meat cuts.

    b) Those that minimise tissue residue problems.

    c) Those that minimise pain and inconvenience, especially in amenity animals.

    Subcutaneous sites may fulfil these requirements.

3) It should lead to a better standardisation of experimental pharmacological work between different research establishments.

Biological factors affecting drug bioavailability

The main biological factors will be briefly summarised under 6 headings:
1) Route 2) Disease 3) Physical activity 4) Region of the body (a) in man
(b) in animals 5) Age/weight 6) Species/weight.

1) <u>Route</u>. There are large differences in bioavailability depending on whether the drug is given orally, intravenously or by other parenteral routes.

Intravenous administration gives very rapid and complete bioavailability. The oral route provides excellent absorption for some products (e.g. amoxycillin) and very poor absorption for others(e.g. neomycin, phthalylsulphathiazole). Subcutaneous and intramuscular routes bypass any barrier offered by oral administration (i.e. acid instability, significant metabolism on first pass).

2) <u>Disease</u>. Renal, hepatic, cardiac and thyroid disease can all have major effects on serum concentration/time curves. This may be by interference with blood circulation or, as in renal and hepatic disease, by interfering with drug metabolism and excretion.

3) <u>Physical activity</u>. In an extensive review Ballard (1968) noted that absorption may be via capillaries or lymphatics. Both are plentiful subcutaneously and in fascial planes but lymphatics are rare in muscle tissue proper. Large molecular weight substances (MW >10,000) are absorbed primarily via lymphatics. Increased activity of the injection site (e.g. exercise) will lead to increased lymph and blood flow and this will lead to more rapid absorption. Barnes & Trueta (1941) injected black tiger snake venom subcutaneously into the leg of rabbits. If the leg was immobilised in a plaster cast the animals survived for more than 8 hours, when the leg was unrestrained death occurred in less than 2 hours.

4) <u>Region of the body</u>

    a) Findings in man

The work of Nora <u>et al</u> (1964) with insulin (MW 6,000) has already been summarised. A review by Reeves (1975) indicates that in general the findings of Nora <u>et al</u> have been confirmed and extended to include; lidocaine (MW 234), gamma globulin (MW 150,000), cephacetrile (MW 361) and possibly gentamycin (MW 463) and cephaloridine (MW 416).

Korttila & Linnoila (1975) have shown that diazepam (MW 285) is better absorbed after intramuscular injection into the deltoid as compared with the thigh.

The general observation is that absorption from the deltoid may be 20-25% better than from the gluteal group. A possible explanation for these observations that is consistent with the effects of cardiac disease and limb immobilisation is provided by the work of Bederka et al (1971) and Evans et al (1975).

Bederka et al injected several compounds into rats. They found the absorption rate was affected by vasoactive compounds and suggested that blood flow was the rate limiting step.

Evans et al assessed the resting muscle blood flow in man by measuring the rate of disappearance of radioactive Xenon injected into the muscles. They found deltoid blood flow to be 19% greater than gluteal flow, with the quadriceps group intermediate.

b) Findings in domestic animals

We are not aware of any systematic investigation of the effects of injection site on bioavailability in domestic animals.

We have recently examined several sites in calves using a 15% oily suspension of ampicillin trihydrate (Penbritin Injectable Suspension - Beecham, England) and a 10% aqueous suspension of amoxycillin trihydrate (Clamoxyl Aqueous Injectable Suspension - Beecham, England). The details are summarised below.

i) Ampicillin

37 kg calves were injected with ampicillin at 10 mg/kg into four sites:

- intramuscularly (IM) into the Gluteus medius
- IM into the rump (centre of gluteal fossa - largely intermuscular)
- subcutaneously (SC) into the rump
- SC over the ribs behind the shoulder

The mean peak serum level and mean percentage area under the curve (AUC) are given in Table 2.

Table 2. Peak serum level and % AUC for ampicillin in calves after injection at 4 different sites

Injection site	No. of calves	Peak mcg/ml	% AUC (0-24 hr)
IM Gluteus medius	12	3.9	119
IM rump	4	4.6	125
SC rump	8	3.3	100*
SC ribs	12	4.6	130

*$P < 0.05$

Two conclusions can be drawn. Firstly, there are differences of 30% between subcutaneous sites in different regions of the body. Secondly bioavailability from subcutaneous sites cannot be ranked as consistently lower than intramuscular sites.

ii) Amoxycillin

40 kg calves were injected with amoxycillin at 7 mg/kg into four sites:
- SC neck - IM neck - IM rump - SC rump
The mean peak serum level and mean percentage AUC are given in Table 3.

Table 3.   Peak serum level and % AUC for amoxycillin in calves after
injection at 4 different sites

Injection site	No. of calves	Peak mcg/ml	% AUC (0-24 hr)
SC neck	6	2.8	104
IM neck	6	3.8	129*
IM rump	6	3.0	100
SC rump	6	2.8	106

*P<0.05

This data indicates that bioavailability may differ by 29% between IM
injections in different regions of the body.

At this early stage we cannot draw firm general conclusions about the effects
of injection site on bioavailability. However it does not appear that subcutaneous injections are consistently of lower bioavailability compared with
intramuscular as implied by the classical dogma. Rather there appears to be a
range of intramuscular bioavailability for different regions of the body and a
range for subcutaneous sites.

5) Age/weight

There appears to be a factor of age or weight affecting bioavailability since
calves of different weights injected at the same dose rate do not show the same
serum concentration-time curves. Figure 2 gives the serum profiles obtained
after IM injection of 3 groups of calves with 10% amoxycillin aqueous suspension
at 7 mg/kg bodyweight.

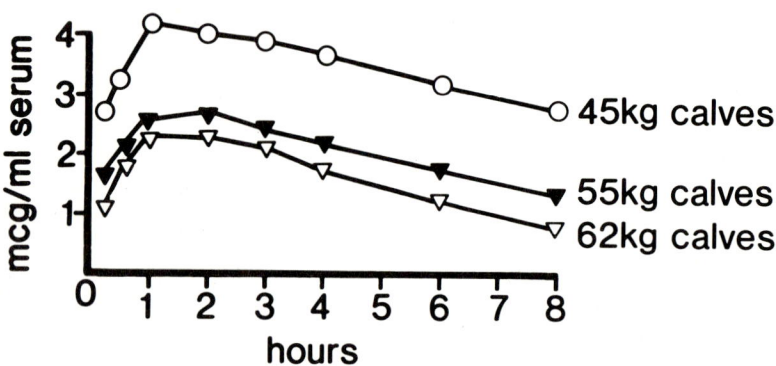

Fig.2   Effects of age/weight on bioavailability of amoxycillin in calves
after IM injection

6) Species/weight

As a variation of the age/weight phenomenon just described we find even
greater variations between species. In Fig.3 are shown the serum concentration
time curves for 5 species all injected intramuscularly, all with 10% amoxycillin
aqueous suspension and all at 7 mg/kg (with the exception of cats given 50 mg/cat,
equivalent to perhaps 10-12 mg/kg).

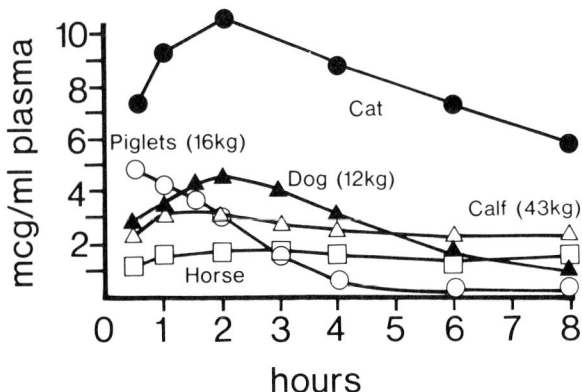

Fig.3 Effect of species/weight on bioavailability.

The trend is for physically small individuals (piglets, dog, cat) to have
an early high peak followed by a rapid decline, whilst physically large individuals
(calves, horses) show a lower, constant plateau of antibiotic in the blood.

Standardising injection techniques

A pre-requisite for any work comparing injection sites is a reproducible
method for obtaining truly intramuscular and subcutaneous injections. We have
investigated this in recently killed calves by giving 5 ml injections of dilute
aqueous crystal violet as a dye marker, followed by dissection and photography.

The slides (not reproduced here) show that the common injection site in the
centre of the gluteal fossa gives a predominantly intermuscular injection often
around the sciatic nerve, with the attendant risk of nerve damage if the injected
solution is irritant. Because of the broad thin muscle sheets in this region it
is difficult to give truly intramuscular injections.

An intramuscular injection can be obtained by injecting at the midpoint
between the Tuber ilium and the Trochanter major of the femur into the belly of
the Gluteus medius. This corresponds to the site recommended in man (Zelman 1961).

Injections in the neck are usually predominantly intermuscular because of the numerous small muscle fascicles. In many cases the injected solution lies next to the ligamentum nuchae.

In the posterior thigh it was difficult to find reference points to allow consistently intramuscular injections. The injection was often intermuscular commonly close to the sciatic nerve with the risk of nerve irritation.

It is our impression that the often repeated instruction to use a _deep_ intramuscular injection, serves only to increase the risk of nerve irritation. It will disguise rather than reduce any tissue reaction and does not appear to offer any advantages in respect of bioavailability.

REFERENCES

Ballard, B.E. 1968 J. Pharm Sci 57, p.357-378
Barnes, J.M. & Trueta, J. 1941 Lancet 1 p.623-626
Bederka, J. Jr. et al 1971 European J. Pharmacol. 15 p.132-136
Evans, E.F. et al 1975 Clin. Pharm. Ther. 17 p.44-47
Korttila, K. & Linnoila, M. 1975 Br. J. Anaesth. 47 p.857-862
Nora, J.J. et al 1964 J. Pediatrics 64 p.547-551
Reeves, D.S. 1975 J. Antimicrobial Chemother 1 p.350-353
Zelman, S. 1961 Amer. J. Med. Sci 241 p.563-574

INTRODUCTION OF FEVER MODELS

A.S.J.P.A.M. VAN MIERT

Department of Veterinary Pharmacology and Toxicology, Utrecht University, Utrecht (The Netherlands).

ABSTRACT

Febrile reactions are associated with other symptoms such as shivering, inhibition of gastric secretion and motility, and changes in heart rate and cardiac output. Therefore, fever possess potential therapeutic problems if fever alters the pharmacokinetic behaviour of drugs being administered to treat these conditions.

Fever models have been developed which allowed a more profound analysis of the mechanisms underlying the febrile reactions. Furthermore, these models are very useful: (1) as screening models to find new substances with antipyretic activity, and (2) to study the mode of action of these agents. A variety of fever models are shortly described and discussed. We have utilized the goat as a model; the results of studies with various exogenous pyrogens in this species are reviewed. Some evidence is presented, which suggests that these models are useful to study the effect of fever upon the pharmacokinetic behaviour of drugs.

INTRODUCTION

Fever is one of the most common and well-known manifestations of disease. Yet clinical information about the pathogenesis of fever remains meagre (2). Fever is the rise in deep body temperature which occurs following infection and inflammation, and may be produced by a wide variety of organisms including both Gram-negative and Gram positive bacteria, viruses, fungi, yeasts and protozoa, and by many inflammatory and related reactions such as tissue damage and necrosis, malignancy, antigen-antibody reactions and tissue graft rejection (3,26). Fever differs from hyperthermia associated, for example, with exposure to toxic doses of uncouplers of oxidative phosphorylation (67). Hyperthermia is brought about as a result of the inability of the body to balance heat loss with heat gain; in fever in contrast the balance is maintained at a higher level than normal.

EXPERIMENTAL MODELS

Experimental models have been developed for investigating febrile reactions.

Much of the recent experimental work in the pathogenesis of fever has been
conducted with pyrogens, substances which are released following infection and
inflammation. The rabbit is most sensitive to the action of pyrogens when compared
with other species (66). Therefore, the rabbit has been the most frequently used
animal for this type of study. Further, pyrogen tests - important biological
control tests for drug preparations - are done in rabbits (46,59). Injection and
infusion fluids are the preparations most likely to be contaminated by pyrogens.
Contamination by pyrogens is particularly hazardous to a patient who is critically
ill or undergoing major surgery (19). Other species which are used in the experimental
work on fever are the cat (17,18,21), the monkey (39,41), the sheep (12,49), and
the goat (63,65), while the yeast-fevered rat is often used as a screening model
to find new substances with antipyretic activity (44,60).

PYROGENS, FEVER AND ASSOCIATED CLINICAL SYMPTOMS

Pyrogens may be differentiated into two basic categories: firstly, the exogenous
pyrogens which are produced by infectious agents (Table 1) and secondly, the
·endogenous pyrogens which are formed and released by the host. The existence of

Table 1.   E X O G E N O U S   P Y R O G E N S

Agents

Myxoviruses	Influenza, Newcastle disease	3, 26, 56, 57
Bacteria	Staphylococci, Pneumococci	3, 4, 10
Bacterial products	Lipid A	21, 50
	Endotoxins from Gram-negatives	3, 26, 65, 66, 68
	Staphylococcal enterotoxins	14, 17, 18
	Listeria monocytogenes hymolysin	55
	Streptococcal exotoxins	14, 35, 40, 54
Yeast	Saccharomyces cerevisae	44, 60
Yeast products	Sodium nucleinate	25, 68
Antigens	Tuberculin, Johnin	1, 3, 26, 36
	Serum albumin	43, 52
	Penicillin G	15
	Soluble A_g-Ab complexes	43, 52
Steroids	Etiocholanolone	33, 73
Pharmacologic substances	Poly 1: Poly C	57, 70
	Bleomycin	24

endogenous pyrogens was first demonstrated by Beeson (8) in 1948 who found that
extracts of leucocytes (polymorphonuclear neutrophils) were pyrogenic when injected
intravenously into rabbits. Endogenous pyrogens are heat-labile and evoke febrile

responses characterized by shorter latency, more rapid rise to peak height, monophasic temperature curves and more rapid fall to normal values than are produced by exogenous pyrogens (Figure 1). Moreover, endogenous pyrogens induce fever in

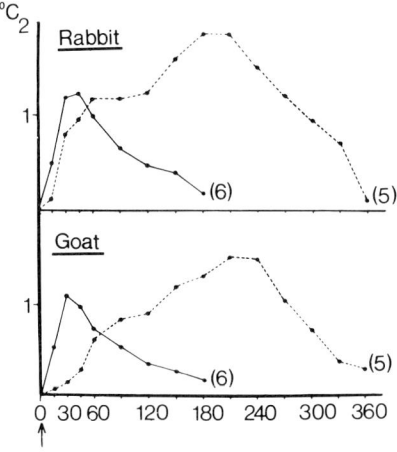

Fig. 1.
Mean febrile responses of normal recipients following intravenous injection of LPS E.coli 0.5 µg per kg body weight (●---●), and leucocytic pyrogen in LPS E.coli-tolerant recipients (●——●). Number of animals used in parentheses (After Van Miert and Atmakusuma (1970), Zbl. Vet. Med., Reihe A, 17: 174-184)

exogenous pyrogen-tolerant animals (3,26,65). Since endogenous pyrogenic material was first obtained from leucocytes, it is often referred to as leucocytic pyrogen, although it is now recognized that not only leucocytes but also monocytes, Kupffer cells, and other fixed cells of the reticular endothelial systems can produce similar substances (3). It is now generally accepted that endogenous pyrogens are the common mediators in many experimental fevers (3,42) and there is evidence that these substances act on thermoregulatory centres within the hypothalamus through the stimulation of prostaglandin synthesis (42,47,74). In accord with the results of animal experiments, Philipp-Dormston and Siegert (48) reported enhanced prostaglandin E levels in cerebrospinal fluid samples from febrile patients with meningitis, pneumonia or pyelonephritis.

Furthermore, fever models are very useful to study the mode of action of anti-pyretic drugs (16). These agents inhibit both endogenous and exogenous pyrogen-induced fever and bring down the increased prostaglandin activity in the cerebrospinal fluid. Moreover, antipyretic agents inhibit the synthesis of prostaglandins in vitro. However, these agents do not lower prostaglandin-induced fever. In addition, there is a lot of evidence from in vitro and in vivo studies which indicates that antipyretic agents have no influence upon the synthesis and release of endogenous pyrogens (16).

Many other clinical symptoms accompany clinical fever (19,23,34). These symptoms for example include depression, anorexia, increased respiration rate, inhibition of gastric secretion and motility, and changes in heart rate and cardiac output. The pathogenesis of these symptoms is not yet understood. However, there

is some evidence which indicates that the effects of exogenous pyrogens on
thermoregulation and on the stomach seem to be due to different mechanisms (Van
Miert, section 7, this congress). These various clinical symptoms may have serious
consequences in some patients. For example, the diminished forestomach motility
during clinical fever inhibits the microbial degradation of the ingested feed and
the elimination of fermentation gases in ruminants. Moreover, the clinical pattern
of fever - accompanied by other symptoms - possess potential therapeutic problems
if fever alters the absorption, distribution, biotransformation and/or excretion
of drugs being administered to treat these conditions. The aim of drug administration
is to induce a desired therapeutic effect, which most likely will obtained by
establishing and maintaining, for a certain period of time, an effective concentration
of the agent at its site of action. The size of the dose, route of administration,
and bioavailability of the drug formulation determine the amount of active ingredient
entering the bloodstream. For most drugs, there exists a range of plasma concentrations at which effects of therapeutic intensity are achieved. An understanding
of the influence of disease states such as fever on the absorption, distribution,
biotransformation and excretion of therapeutic agents is presently being sought.
Therefore it is an advantage to have experimental fever models for investigating
the effects of fever upon these processes.

THE GOAT MODEL

We have utilized the goat as a model for analysing the mechanisms underlying
the actions of pyrogens, especially with relation to the inhibition of the forestomach
contractions. In summary, there are differences in latency time and febrile response
after intravenous injection of exogenous pyrogens (Table 2). These results confirm
those of Atkins and colleagues who did the same type of experiments with rabbits (3)

Exogenous pyrogens differ markedly with regard to their chemical properties
(Table 1). Moreover, most exogenous pyrogens do not gain access to the hypothalamus
from the systemic circulation, because of their molecular size. It is now generally
accepted that the cells capable of producing endogenous pyrogen are activated by
exogenous pyrogens, and it is this circulating material which is the common
mediator of fever (3,26). In goats, the presence of circulating endogenous pyrogens
during endotoxin-induced fever could be demonstrated (65).

We could not find a correlation between the changes in heart rate and the rise
in body temperature during exogenous pyrogen-induced fevers (69,70). However,
inhibition of forestomach motility was observed in each fever model. This is in
agreement with the observations made in febrile patients. It seems unlikely that
endogenous pyrogens have a direct effect on rumen motility (64).

Most studies of pyrogen-induced associated clinical symptoms will also result
from extravascular injections but the responses are less consistent (8,26) and
larger doses are required (Figure 2). Endotoxins are macromolecular complexes with

a molecular weight of about 10^6. Nothing is known about the bioavailability of pyrogens after extravascular administration. Moreover, there is the problem of a proper injection technique. Using a dye tracer method Evans and colleagues (7) found that intRAmuscular injections were often intERmuscular.

TABLE 2.   FEVER INDUCED BY INTRAVENOUS INJECTION OF PYROGENS IN CONSCIOUS GOATS

Pyrogen	Dose per kg i.v.	Shivering (biphasic)		Temperature Reaction (biphasic)		N
		Latency time	Duration	Time of peaks	Mean of peaks (°C)	
Newcastle disease virus*	0.7 ml	39(18- 53)	26(17- 33)	220(165-255)	1.96(1.4 -2.35)	7
Johnin°	5 µg	61(46- 79) 135(114-140)	41(26- 57) ± 70	113(90-135) 306(270-345)	1.05(0.45-1.7) 2.08(1.25-2.45)	8
Poly 1:Poly C	15 µg	61(43- 58) 124(111-142)	25(21- 30) 35(15- 46)	86(75- 90) 177(150-195)	0.69(0.1 -1.4) 0.98(0.7 -1.2)	5
	30 µg	45(32- 64) 125(115-142)	27(15- 36) 29(18- 33)	75(60- 90) 177(150-195)	0.25(0.0 -0.75) 1.25(0.6 -2.6)	5
Sodium Nucleinate from yeast	5 mg	34(25- 49) 112(101-124)	32(26- 39) 34(19- 54)	74(60- 75) 165(135-195)	0.94(0.85-1.0) 1.03(0.35-1.55)	6
	10 mg	23(19- 25) 118(82-135)	36(23- 59) 32(15- 40)	69(60- 90) 174(135-195)	0.81(0.55-1.15) 1.37(1.0 -1.85)	7
LPS E.coli	0.01µg	43(31- 51) 121(111-131)	30(22- 43) 25(15- 39)	79(75- 90) 180(180-210)	0.82(0.55-1.5) 1.15(0.7 -1.9)	7
	0.1 µg	26(21- 42) 120(112-130)	27(12- 39) 47(38- 65)	82(75- 90) 215(180-240)	0.82(0.3 -1.45) 1.62(1.2 -2.2)	5
LPS S.typhi-murium	0.2 µg	22(17- 46) 102(84-119)	40(31- 53) 89(60-103)	84(75- 90) 225(165-270)	0.70(0.15-1.1) 1.75(0.9 -2.2)	8
Endogenous Pyrogen•	2.10^8 cells	9(7- 12)	14(8- 22)	43(35- 50)	1.15(0.6 -1.45)	6

N number of goats per group
* NDV La Sota haemagglutination titre 1:240
o in previously vaccinated animals (with a killed culture of M.johnei)
• obtained from peritoneal exudate cells

66

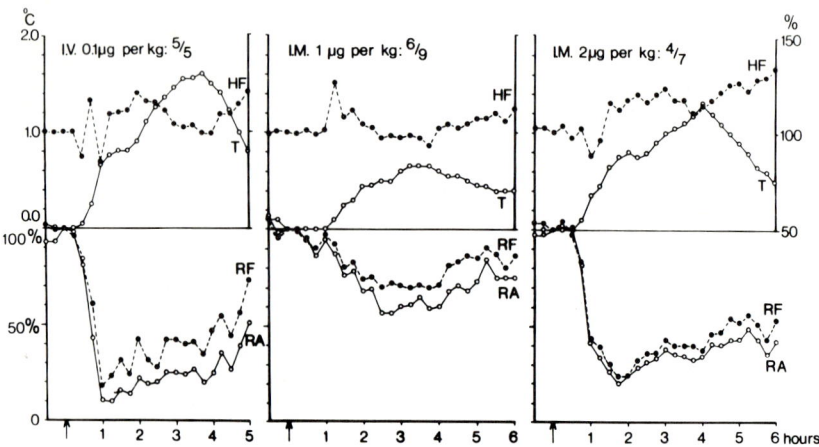

Fig. 2. Changes in rumen motility (RF and RA), body temperature (T) and heart
rate (HF) after LPS E.coli administration (= ↑). RF = frequency of rumen
contractions per 15 min expressed in % of the initial value; RA = summation
derived from 15 min intervals of amplitude expressed in % of the initial
value. Mean values are shown. Left panel: 0.1 µg per kg intravenously;
all goats responded. Panel in the middle: 1 µg per kg intramuscularly;
responses were observed in 6 of the 9 animals tested. Right panel: 2 µg
per kg intramuscularly; responses were seen in 4 of the 7 goats tested.

Effects of pyrogen-induced fever upon pharmacokinetics of drugs

Fever produced by pyrogens has considerable primary and secondary effects in
the circulation (5,19,22). Sudden flooding of the circulation with endotoxin can
lead to responses which vary from an ordinary high fever to what is frequently
called endotoxin shock (32,61). During endotoxin shock, the blood flow to many
organs, such as the kidneys and liver, is reduced. Exceptions are the brain and
the heart which consequently receive an increased fraction of the dose, especially
in the early moments after intravenous drug administration (51). In this condition
the clearance of the drug is inhibited and the plasma level remains almost constant.
Dr. van Gogh and I observed this once in one accidental case (72). Under such
circumstances the volume of distribution of a drug can also be reduced (9). On
the other hand, Dr. Ladefoged has shown that in endotoxin treated animals a reduction
of plasma protein binding can occur (28,38) which promotes tissue penetration by
the drug. Dr. Baggot reported an increased distribution volume for penicillin G
in beagles during the acute stage, based on the febrile response, of an induced
generalized streptococcal infection (6).

Bradley and Conan (13) have shown increases in hepatic and total splanchnic
blood flow during fever. In normal volunteers, changes in drug metabolism during
pyrogen induced fever have been reported (11,27,58). In one of our experiments

with goats, the pattern of urinary metabolites of sulphafurazole was altered during *Salmonella typhimurium* endotoxin-induced fever (72). Bacterial endotoxins exert many effects, direct and indirect, on the liver (62). At present time, sufficient data are not available to permit a clear understanding of how fever affects drug metabolism.

After intravenous injection of most exogenous pyrogens, two shivering episodes could be observed (Table 2). After a certain latency time some muscle twitching - especially in the hind legs - could be seen, immediately followed by a period of intense shivering. Increased absorption after muscle exercise has been noted with several drugs, including antibiotic agents (31,53). We therefore carried out an experiment to compare the absorption of ampicillin from shivering and non-shivering muscles. During shivering, the rate of absorption from the buttock site was faster, resulting in significantly higher serum levels of ampicillin when compared to the values from the control experiment (29).

Although the stomach is not itself an important site of drug absorption (45), the rate of gastric emptying can markedly influence the rate of intestinal absorption It is therefore likely that disease processes which influence gastric emptying will also affect the absorption rate of orally administered drugs. Groothuis has utilized the calf as a model for studying the effect of fever on drug absorption after oral administration (30). In this section, he will give us more information about this pharmacokinetic aspect.

Dr. Ladefoged has used rabbits and pigs as experimental subjects to study the effects of pyrogen-induced fever upon pharmacokinetics (28,37,38). In one of his latest papers (28) he reported that the renal clearance of sulphathiazole in pigs was markedly decreased during *E.coli* endotoxin-induced fever, while the inulin clearance was unaffected. Several investigators have shown that there is a rise in the effective renal plasma flow during fever and that this change in kidney blood flow is not dependent on body temperature (19,20). Cooper reported an increase in urine flow during the renal vasodilatation after administration of endotoxin. Therefore I find the interesting observations made by Dr. Ladefoged difficult to understand. In his contribution this afternoon, he hopefully will give us an explanation for this inhibited clearance rate.

REFERENCES

1. Allen, W.M., Berrett, S. and Patterson, D.S.P. (1970), J. Comp. Path., 80: 267-27
2. Atkins, E. and Bodel, P. (1979), Fed. Proc., 38: 57-63
3. Atkins, E. and Bodel, P. (1974) in: The inflammatory process.vol.3 ed. B.W. Zweifach, L. Grant and R.T. McCluskey, Academic Press New York-London, 467-513
4. Atkins, E. and Freedman, L.E. (1963), Yale J. Biol. Med., 35: 451-471
5. Armin, J. and Grant, R.T. (1957), J. Physiol., 138: 417-433
6. Baggot, J.D. (1977), Principles of drug disposition in domestic animals. W.B. Saunders Company, Philadelphia-London, 180-185
7. Baxter, J.S. and Evans, J.M. (1973), J. Sm. Animal Proc., 14: 297-302
8. Bennett, I.L. and Cluff, L.E. (1957), Pharmacol. Rev., 9: 427-479

9. Benowitz, N.L. and Meister, W. (1976), Clin. Pharmacol., 1: 389-405
10. Berlin, R.D. and Wood, W.B. (1964), J. Exp. Med., 119: 715-726
11. Blaschke, T.F., Elin, R.T., Berk, P.D., Song, C.S. and Wolff, S.M. (1973), Ann. intern. Med., 78: 221-226
12. Bligh, J. (1972) in: Essays on temperature regulation. ed. J. Bligh and R.E. Moore, North-Holland, Amsterdam, 105-120
13. Bradley, S.E. and Conan, N.J. (1947), J. Clin. Invest., 26: 1175-1183
14. Brunson, K.W. and Watson, D.W. (1974), Infect. Immun., 10: 347-351
15. Chusid, M.J. and Atkins, E. (1972), J. Exp. Med., 136: 227-240
16. Clark, W.G. (1979), Gen. Pharmac., 10: 71-77
17. Clark, W.G. and Borison, H.L. (1963), J. Pharmacol. Exp. Ther., 142: 237-241
18. Clark, W.G. and Page, J.S. (1968), J. Bacteriol., 96: 1940-1946
19. Cooper, K.E. (1971) in: Pyrogens and Fever, ed. G.E.W. Wolstenhome and J. Birch, Churchill-Livingstone, Edinburgh-London, 5-21
20. Cranston, W.I., Vial, S.V. and Wheeler, H.O. (1959), Clin. Sci., 18: 579-587
21. Dey, P.K., Feldberg, W., Gupta, K.P. and Wendlandt, S. (1975), J. Physiol. 253: 103-119
22. Dhondt, G., Burvenich, C. and Peeters, G. (1977), J. Dairy Res., 44: 433-440
23. Diernhofer, K. (1959), Dtsch. tierärztl. Wschr., 66: 141-149
24. Dinarello, C.A., Ward, S.B. and Wolff, S.M. (1973), Cancer Chemother- Rep., 57: 393-398
25. Dressel, H. and Jacker, H.J. (1972), Acta Pharm. Jugoslav., 22: 137-144
26. Eichenberger, E. (1966) in: Handbook of experimental Pharmacology. vol. 15, ed. O. Eichler, Springer Verlag, Berlin-New York, 215-378
27. Elin, R.J., Vesell, E.S. and Wolff, S.M. (1975), Clin. Pharmacol. Ther., 17: 447-457
28. Friis, Ch. and Ladefoged, O. (1979), Zbl. Vet. Med. Reihe A, 26: 146-151
29. Groothuis, D.G., Werdler, M.E.B., van Miert, A.S.J.P.A.M. and van Duin, C.Th.M. (1979), Res. Vet. Sci. in press
30. Groothuis, D.G., van Miert, A.S.J.P.A.M., Ziv, G. and Nouws, J.F.M. (1978), J. Vet. Pharmacol. Therap., 1: 81-84
31. Harding, S.M., Eilon, L.A. and Harris, A.M. (1979), J. Antimicrobial Chemother., 5: 87-93
32. Hinshaw, L.B. (1964) in: Bacterial Endotoxins, ed. M. Landy and W. Braun, Rutgers The State University, 118-125
33. Kappas, A., and Ratkovits, B. (1960), J. Clin, Endocrinol. Metab., 29: 898-900
34. Keutsch, G.T. (1976), N.Y. State J. Med., 76: 1998-2001
35. Kim, Y.B. and Watson, D.W. (1972) in: Streptococci and streptococcal diseases, ed. L.W. Wannamaker and J.M. Matsen, Academic Press, New York, 33-50
36. Kopecky, K.E. and Larsen, A.B. (1975), Am. J. Vet. Res., 36: 1727-1729
37. Ladefoged, O. (1977), Acta Pharmacol. et Toxicol., 41: 507-514
38. Ladefoged, O. (1978), Acta Vet. Scand., 19: 479-486
39. Lipton, J.M. and Fossler, D.E. (1974), Am. J. Physiol., 226: 1022-1027
40. Masek, K., Raskova, H. and Rotta, J. (1972), Naunyn-Schmiedeberg's Arch. Pharmacol., 274: 138-145
41. Myers, R.D., Rudy, T.A. and Yaksh, T.L. (1974), J. Physiol., 243: 167-193
42. Milton, A.S. (1976), J. Pharm. Pharmac., 28: 393-399
43. Mott, P.D. and Wolff, S.M. (1966), J. Clin. Invest., 45: 372-379
44. Niemegeers, C.J.E., Lenaerts, F.M., and Janssen, P.A.I. (1975), Arzneim. Forsch. Drug Res., 25: 1519-1524
45. Nimmo, W.S. (1976), Clin. Pharmacokinetics, 1: 189-203
46. Pharmacopoeia of the U.S.A. (1965) 17th edition, Mack Publ. Company, Easton PA
47. Philipp-Dormston, W.K. and Siegert, R. (1974), Med. Microbiol. Immunol., 159: 279-284
48. Philipp-Dormston, W.K. and Siegert, R. (1975), Klin. Wschr., 53: 1167-1168
49. Pittman, Q.J., Cooper, K.E., Veale, W.L., and van Petten, G.R. (1974), Clin. Sci. Mol. Med., 46: 591-602
50. Rietschel, E.Th. (1975), Naunyn-Schmiedeberg's Arch. Pharmacol. 286: 73-84
51. Roland, M. (1975), Triangle, Sandoz, J. Med. Sci., 14: 109-116
52. Root, R.K. and Wolff, S.M. (1968), J. Exp. Med., 128: 309-323
53. Schmidt, H. and Roholt, K. (1966), Acta Pathol. Microbiol. Scand., 68: 396-400

54. Schuh, V., Hribalova, V. and Atkins, E. (1970), Yale J. Biol. Med., 43: 31-42
55. Siddique, I.H., Ying, L.C. and Robinson, B.B. (1969), Can. J. Comp. Med., 33: 292-296
56. Siegert, R. (1967), Zbl. Bakt. 205: 110-121
57. Siegert, R., Philipp-Dormston, W.K., Radsak, K. and Menzel, H. (1976), Infect. Immun., 14: 1130-1137
58. Song, C.S., Gelb, N.A. and Wolff, S.M. (1972), J. Clin. Invest. 51: 2959-2966
59. Todd, R.G. (1967), Extra Pharmacopoeia Martindale, 25th edition, The Pharmaceutical Press, London
60. Turner, R.A. (1965), Screening Methods in Pharmacology. Academic Press, New York-London, 298-299
61. Urbaschek, B. and Urbaschek, R. (1979) in: Microcirculation in inflammation. ed. G. Hanck and J.W. Irwin, S. Karger, Basel, 74-104
62. Utili, R., Abernathy, C.O. and Zimmerman, H.J. (1977), Life Sci., 20: 553-568
63. Van Miert, A.S.J.P.A.M. (1973), Zbl. Vet. Med. Reihe A, 20: 614-623
64. Van Miert, A.S.J.P.A.M. (1979) in: Fever. Proc. Int. Symposion on Fever. Dallas, Texas, USA, April 10-11, ed. J.M. Lipton, Raven Press, New York
65. Van Miert, A.S.J.P.A.M. and Atmakusuma, A. (1970), Zbl. Vet. Med. Reihe A, 17: 174-184
66. Van Miert, A.S.J.P.A.M. and Frens, J. (1978), Zbl. Vet. Med. Reihe A, 15: 532-543
67. Van Miert, A.S.J.P.A.M. and Groeneveld, H.W. (1969), Eur. J. Pharmacol., 8: 385-388
68. Van Miert, A.S.J.P.A.M., van der Laar, J.A.J. and van Duin, C.Th.M. (1976), Zbl. Vet. Med. Reihe A, 23: 697-705
69. Van Miert, A.S.J.P.A.M. and van Duin, C.Th.M. (1974), Zbl. Vet. Med. Reihe A, 23: 697-705
70. Van Miert, A.S.J.P.A.M. and van Duin, C.Th.M. (1979), J. Vet. Pharmacol. Therap., 2: 69-79
71. Van Miert, A.S.J.P.A.M. and van Duin, C.Th.M. (1978), Arzneim. Forsch. - Drug Res., 28: 2246-2251
72. Van Miert, A.S.J.P.A.M., van Gogh, H. and Wit, J.G. (1976), Vet. Rec., 99: 480-481
73. Wolff, S.M., Kimball, H.R., Perry, S., Root, R. and Kappas, A. (1967), Ann. Intern. Med., 67: 1268-1295
74. Ziel, R. and Krupp, P. (1976), Experientia, 32: 1451-1452

THE EFFECT OF ENDOTOXIN-INDUCED FEVER ON THE PHARMACOKINETICS OF DRUGS IN
RABBITS AND PIGS

O. LADEFOGED
Department of Pharmacology and Toxicology, Royal Veterinary and Agricultural
University, Copenhagen (Denmark)

ABSTRACT

The effects of endotoxin-induced fever on the pharmacokinetics of 6 different drugs were investigated in 5 endotoxin-models in rabbits and/or pigs.
It was shown that the effect of endotoxin on pharmacokinetic parameters depends on the animal species and the test drugs applied. The pharmacokinetic
model used to describe the plasma concentration versus time data in normal
animals could not in all cases be used satisfactorily in febrile animals.
The clinical implications of the findings are mentioned and the need for more
clinical pharmacokinetic investigations in the veterinary clinic is stressed.

INTRODUCTION

The effects of pathological and pathophysiological states on the pharmacokinetics of drugs are reported for several disorders in man. Clinical pharmacokinetic studies in the veterinary clinic have attracted less attention,
but it is obvious that optimal pharmacotherapy, based on pharmacokinetic
science can only be implemented if more information on the effects of disease
states on the pharmacokinetics of drugs in domestic animals becomes available.
Great difficulties arise in this context since it may be impossible to have
access to sufficient numbers of animals with well defined and characterized
diseases for experimental purposes. Therefore disease models may be preferred
in some cases to gain more knowledge of the influence of disease states on
the pharmacokinetics of drugs in domestic animals.

As fever is an important symptom in several infectious diseases in domestic animals, it is of interest to study the influence of fever on the pharmacokinetics of drugs. The endotoxin-fever models were used to investigate
the effect of E. coli endotoxin-induced fever on drug absorption, distribution and elimination in rabbits and pigs.

RESULTS AND DISCUSSION

Fever was induced by intravenous injections of lipopolysaccharide from
E. coli (Serotype 0127:B8, Sigma®). Doses between 0.1 - 0.5 µg/kg b.wt. were
used in rabbits whereas pigs were given between 1.5 µg and 2.5 µg/kg b.wt.
(intravenously). Different time schedules for injection of endotoxin and drugs
were used as shown schematically by the five models in Fig. 1 and 2.

The drugs applied as test substances were selected on basis of their elimination pathways and protein bindings. Dose of drug, route of administration
and endotoxin-model are shown in Table 1.

Table 1. Summary of the drugs, the species, the route of administration and
the endotoxin-model used in the investigations.

Drug	Species	Dose mg/kg b.wt.	Route of admini- stration	Endotoxin model	Pharmacokinetic parameter investigated
Antipyrine	rabbit	100	i.v.	A,C	V_d, k_e
	rabbit	150	p.o.	A	k_a, V_d, k_e
	pig	150	p.o.	A	k_a, V_d, k_e
Phenobarbital	pig	25	i.v.	B	β
Sulphadime- thoxine	rabbit	20	i.v.	A	V_d, k_e
	pig	20	i.v.	D	V_d, k_e
Sulphathiazole	pig	60 mg/kg (prime) 0.3 mg/kg/min (maintainance)	i.v.	E	
Trimethoprim	rabbit	40	i.v.	A	V_d, k_e
	rabbit	80	i.v.	A	k_a, V_d, k_e
	pig	20	p.o.	A	k_a, V_d, k_e
Warfarin	rabbit	3	i.v.	A	V_d, k_e
	pig	1-3	i.v.	B	β

The details of the experiments are reported elsewhere (ref. 1-7).

Nonlinear curve fitting computer programs were used to calculate the pharmacokinetic parameters according to the one- or two-compartment models. Some
of the calculations were performed by means of the AUTOAN program (ref. 8).
The program includes determination of elimination kinetics, exponential
stripping, pharmacokinetic model selection and initial estimation of model
parameters.

The results of the experiments with endotoxin-model A,in which endotoxin was injected 1 hour before the drug,are listed in Table 2. The absorption rate of the drugs decreased, the distribution volume tended to increase and the elimination rate constant decreased or was unchanged in endotoxin pre-treated animals.

Table 2. The effect of endotoxin pretreatment on the pharmacokinetic parameters of drugs. Endotoxin 0.1 - 0.5 µg/ml (rabbit) and 1.5 µg/kg
(pig) was injected 1 hour before the drug administration.

Drug	Species	k_a min^{-1}	k_e min^{-1}	Changes in parameter V_d, $V_{d\,area}$ or $V_{d\,ss}$ l/kg
Antipyrine	rabbit	decrease	decrease	increase
	pig	decrease	decrease	increase
Sulphadimethoxine	rabbit		unchanged	increase
Trimethoprim	rabbit	decrease	unchanged	increase
	pig	decrease	decrease	increase
Warfarin	rabbit (shock)	-	-	decrease

The dose of endotoxin used in the warfarin experiments in rabbits caused shock and it was not possible to calculate the pharmacokinetic parameters because the kinetics of warfarin could not be satisfactorily described by the one- or two-compartment model. A remarkable increase in the measured plasma concentration in shocked rabbits during the experiment suggests that a significant reduction in the volume of distribution of warfarin took place.

The AUTOAN-calculations of the data from the experiments after oral admi-nistration of drugs disclosed that most of the plasma concentration versus time curves from the febrile animals could be better described by pharmaco-kinetic models with more than two exponential functions - indicating a change of the absorption process from first order to nonlinear kinetics.

The experiments with endotoxin - model B,which were performed in pigs,did n reveal any significant influence of endotoxin injection on the β-slope (Fig. 1 in 4 experiments with warfarin and 7 with phenobarbital. The result of one of the warfarin experiments is shown in Fig. 3. The β-slope was not signifi-cantly changed, but shortly after the injection of endotoxin some fluctuations in the plasma concentration of the drug were seen. This phenomenon was also m or less apparent in all the other experiments.

The effects of repeated endotoxin injections on the pharmacokinetics of antipyrine were investigated by means of endotoxin - model A and C. The results are shown in Table 3. Pretreatment with endotoxin 1 hour before an-

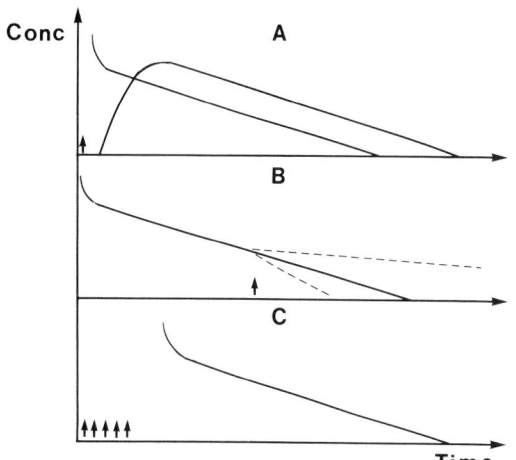

Fig. 1.
Schematic representation of
the endotoxin model A, B and
C. The arrow indicate the
injection of endotoxin in
relation to plasma concentration
versus time curve of the drug
after oral or intravenous
injection. The dotted line
(model B) indicates the possible
changes in the β-slope after
endotoxin injection.

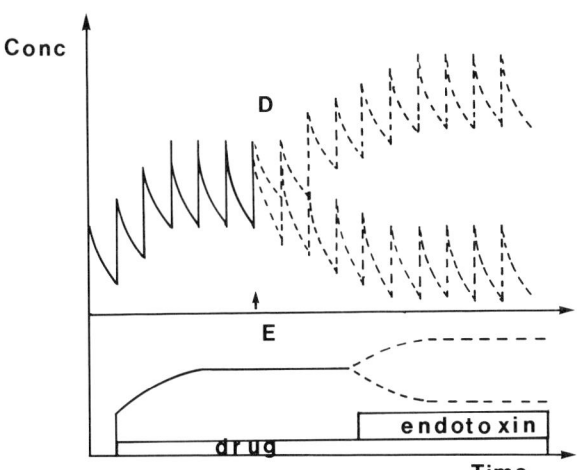

Fig. 2.
Schematic representation of
endotoxin models D and E.
In the upper part the arrow
indicates the injection of
endotoxin in relation to the
plasma concentration versus
time curve after intravenous
injection of the drug. The
dotted lines indicate the possible
changes in plasma concentrations
after endotoxin injection. The
boxes (lower part) indicate
constant rate infusion of drug
and endotoxin.

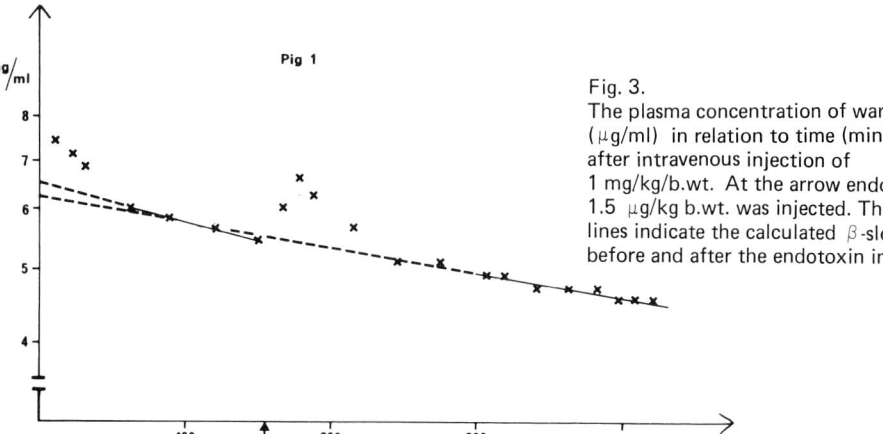

Fig. 3.
The plasma concentration of warfarin
(μg/ml) in relation to time (min)
after intravenous injection of
1 mg/kg/b.wt. At the arrow endotoxin
1.5 μg/kg b.wt. was injected. The
lines indicate the calculated β-slopes
before and after the endotoxin injection.

tipyrine injection resulted in an increase in volume of distribution and a
decrease in elimination rate of antipyrine, when the parameters were compared
to the control values. One day after 5 daily injections of endotoxin (0.1 μg/
kg b.wt.) the volume of distribution and the half-life of antipyrine were not
different from the control values, but 4 days later, i.e. 5 days after the
last endotoxin injection, there was a statistically significant shorter half-
-life as compared with the half-life in the control experiment. Ten days
after the last endotoxin injection both pharmacokinetic parameters were again
at the control level.

Table 3. The effect of endotoxin - pretreatment on the mean $\pm$ S.E.M. of
the half-life and the volume of distribution of antipyrine
(100 mg/kg b.wt. i.v. in rabbits (n = 8-15).

Group of rabbits	$T\frac{1}{2}_{el}$ min	V_d l/kg	P-values differences from control	
			$T\frac{1}{2}_{el}$	V_d
Control	129 $\pm$ 10	0.60 $\pm$ 0.03	-	-
1 hour after endotoxin inj.	150 $\pm$ 9	0.75 $\pm$ 0.01	0.05	0.05
1 day after 5 daily inj. of endotoxin	112 $\pm$ 10	0.63 $\pm$ 0.01	NS	NS
5 days after 5 daily inj. of endotoxin	102 $\pm$ 10	0.59 $\pm$ 0.03	0.05	NS
10 days after 5 daily inj. of endotoxin	118 $\pm$ 8	0.59 $\pm$ 0.01	NS	NS

Sulphadimethoxine 20 mg/kg b.wt. was injected to pigs each day for eleven
days in experiments with endotoxin (model D). From day 6 to the end of the
experiment endotoxin 1.5 μg/kg b.wt. was injected at 9 a.m. and 3 p.m. The
"steady state" concentration of the sulphonamide was reached after about 3
injections and this steady state concentration was not significantly changed
by the endotoxin injections.

In the final type of endotoxin-experiments (model E), sulphathiazole was
injected together with inulin to pigs by constant rate infusions. At steady
state the renal clearance of both compounds was measured in 3-4 clearance
periods. Later on endotoxin was injected by constant rate infusion and another
3-4 clearance periods were measured. The endotoxin infusion had no influence
on clearance of inulin while clearance of sulphathiazole was markedly reduced
from 19.7 ml/min/10 kg b.wt. to 10.5 ml/min/10 kg b.wt.

As seen from the reported results, the effect of experimentally induced fever on the pharmacokinetic parameters depend on the animal species used in the experiment and the drug investigated.

The absorption rate of the investigated drugs was reduced in the febrile animal and this effect is probably caused by changes in gastric emptying function. A change in gastric emptying rate after endotoxin injections might also explain the change in the absorption process from first-order to nonlinear kinetics in the febrile animals.

In the experiments with trimethoprim it was shown that the volume of distribution was greater in the febrile than in the normal animals. The increase in volume of distribution in the febrile animals could partly be explained by changes in the perfusion of tissues since it was the peripheral compartment which was altered, but changes in tissue and protein binding of drugs during fever might also play a role. If the dose of endotoxin injected caused shock a marked reduction in the volume of distribution of warfarin appeared. This reduction can probably be explained by a simultaneous contraction of the plasma volume.

The elimination rate constant of antipyrine is reduced in febrile rabbits and pigs. Since the elimination rate of antipyrine is strongly correlated with its metabolism by the mixed function oxidase system in the liver during normal blood flow conditions, the decrease in elimination rate in febrile rabbits and pigs may be due to a decrease in the activity of the enzyme system. However, the experiments with repeated injections of endotoxin indicate, that the liver microsomal enzyme activity in rabbits increases 5 days after 5 daily injections of endotoxin. This increase might be explained by enzyme induction, but from the present experiment it is not possible to elucidated whether this enzyme induction is caused by endotoxin as such or due to endogenous substances released or produced during fever.

The renal elimination of sulphathiazole, but not of sulphadimethoxine was decreased during the endotoxin injections. This discrepance in results may be explained by the different ways the two sulphonamides are handled by the kidney. Sulphathiazole is eliminated by active tubular secretion while sulphadimethoxine is mainly excreted by passive filtration in the glomeruli.

CONCLUSION

Provided that the endotoxin-fever-model reflects the kinetics of drugs in disease states with fever the results show that for some types of drugs the dosage regimen ought to be changed if optimal therapy is to be instituted. The clinical implication of the presented finding have to await clarification and verification in investigations performed in "real" febrile animals. However, in conclusion it can be stated:

1. that the effect of endotoxin-induced fever on the pharmacokinetics
   of drugs depends on the animal species and the drugs investigated

2. that there may be a change of the pharmacokinetic compartment model
   which best describe the plasma concentration versus time data when
   the animals become febrile

3. and that a possible induction of the mixed function oxidase enzyme
   system may take place after periods with endotoxin-induced fever.

REFERENCES

1. Friis, C. and Ladefoged, O., 1979. Renal clearance of sulfathiazole in
   pigs with Escherichia coli endotoxemia. Zbl. Vet. Med. A 26: 146-151.
2. Ladefoged, O., 1977. Pharmacokinetics of trimethoprim (TMP) in normal
   and febrile rabbits. Acta pharmacol. et toxicol., 41: 507-511.
3. Ladefoged, O., 1978. The effect of Escherichia coli endotoxin on the
   gastrointestinal absorption of antipyrine in rabbits. Proc. XIII
   Nord. Vet. Congr. Åbo, p. 363.
4. Ladefoged, O., 1978. Endotoxin induced changes in the pharmacokinetics
   of warfarin in rabbits. Acta vet. scand., 19: 479-486.
5. Ladefoged, O., 1979. The absorption half-life, the volume of distribution
   and the elimination half-life of trimethoprim after peroral administration to febrile rabbits. Zbl. Vet. Med. A, In press.
6. Ladefoged, O., 1979. Plasma concentration of sulphadimethoxine in pigs
   after multiple dosing and during injections of Escherichia coli endotoxin. Vet. Sci. Com., 3: 73-77.
7. Ladefoged, O., 1979. Pharmacokinetics of antipyrine and trimethoprim
   in pigs with endotoxin-induced fever. To be published.
8. Sedman, A.J. and Wagner, J.G., 1976. AUTOAN. A decision-making pharmacokinetic computer program. Publication Distribution Service. Ann
   Arbor, Michigan.

THE EFFECT OF E.COLI ENDOTOXIN INDUCED FEVER ON THE BLOODLEVELS OF ANTIMICROBIAL
DRUGS AFTER INTRAVENOUS AND INTRAMUSCULAR ADMINISTRATION IN VEAL CALVES.

D.G.GROOTHUIS, H.VAN GOGH and A.S.J.P.A.M.VAN MIERT
Department of Bacteriology, Pharmaceutical department and department of Pharmaco-
logy and Toxicology, Faculty of Veterinary Medicine, University of Utrecht,
Biltstraat 172, 3572 BP Utrecht.

ABSTRACT

The influence of E.coli endotoxin induced fever on the pharmacokinetic behaviour
of amoxycillin, ampicillin, trimethoprim and chloramphenicol was investigated after
intravenous, intramuscular and oral administration.

The half-life ($t\frac{1}{2}$) of trimethoprim after i.v. injection was longer and the volume
of distribution (Vd) greater in febrile calves. There were no detectable changes
after i.v. injection of amoxycillin and chloramphenicol.

During the period the body-temperature was rising, lower bloodlevels of chloramphenicol, ampicillin and amoxycillin after i.m. and oral administration were present.

INTRODUCTION

Despite the fact, that most antimicrobial drugs are administered by the oral or
intramuscular route, little is known of the effect that febrile diseases may have
on the pharmacokinetic behaviour of drugs, used in these conditions. Fever very
often is attended by clinical symptoms such as dullness, headaches and shivering
(13). Furthermore disturbances of gastric motility and the secretion of gastric
juice has been long recognized in monogastric as well as in polygastric animals
(5,15). Circulatory changes also occur: the heart-rate and cardiac output are increased and cutaneous peripheral vasoconstriction is present and the bloodflow
through liver and kidney is increased. There are some indications, that during the
fever periods in infective diseases the pharmacokinetics of drugs are changed (11,
22,30,31). The symptoms of illness associated with fever can be induced by intravenous injection of exogenous pyrogens, such as the endotoxin of E.coli (19,20,21).
When these symptoms are elicited by i.v. injection of endotoxin, it is likely that
the kinetics of drugs during the pyrexic periods will be changed, so enabling a
better analysis of the processes involved. Little is known about pyrogenic doses
of endotoxin in the calf, therefore an attempt was made to develop a calf-fever-model

and investigate the influence that fever may have on the pharmacokinetics of ampicillin, amoxycillin, chloramphenicol and trimethoprim.

MATERIALS AND METHODS

Animals

Three to four weeks old Friesian calves were used in all the experiments. Their average body-weight was 46 kg and ranged from 40 to 50 kg. They were fed twice daily with a milkreplacer only.

Drugs

Ampicillin and amoxycillin, both as trihydrate were used in the oral and intramuscular experiments and as sodium-salt in the intravenous experiments at a dose of 1 gram per calf.

Chloramphenicol powder was used orally at a dose of 5 g per calf and chloramphenicol dissolved in methylpyrrolidone was used at a dose of 2.5 g per calf by intramuscular injection. One liter of a 2.5%o aqueous solution of chloramphenicol was used for i.v. adminstration.

Trimethoprim (110 mg/calf) dissolved in 20 ml distilled water, to which lactic acid was added (1 ml lactic acid/g TMP), was injected intravenously.

Endotoxin dissolved in pyrogen free physiological saline, was injected intravenously at a dose of 5 mcg per calf.

Assays

Assays for ampicillin and amoxycillin were carried out as described by van Galesloot (9), for trimethoprim as described by Allen and Nimmo-Smith (1) and for chloramphenicol as described by Groothuis (11).

Experimental procedure

Groups of calves were injected intravenously with amoxycillin, trimethoprim and chloramphenicol to study the influence of endotoxin induced fever on the distribution and elimination of these drugs. The influence of endotoxin on the rate of absorbtion of ampicillin, amoxycillin and chloramphenicol after intramuscular injection in the neck and after oral adminstration were investigated.

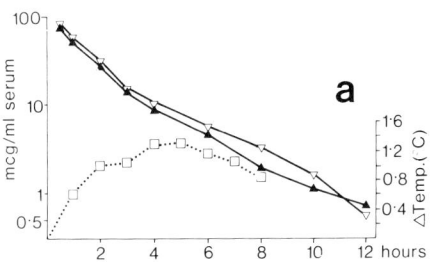 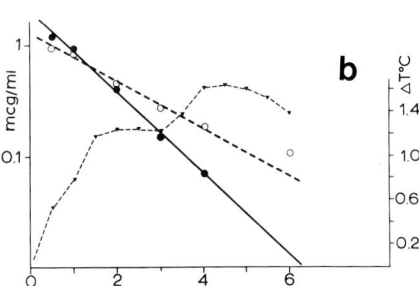

Figure 1. The effect of endotoxin induced fever on the serumconcentrations of amoxycillin (a) and trimethoprim (b) after i.v. injection. Serumconcentrations of amoxycillin, ▲————▲ without endotoxin and △————△ with endotoxin. ☐----☐ rise in body-temperatur (n=6). Serumconcentrations of trimethoprim, ●————● without endotoxin and ○————○ with endotoxin. △-----△ rise in body-temperature (n=4). Doses were: amoxycillin 1g per calf, trimethoprim 110 mg per calf and endotoxin 5 mcg per calf.

Table 1. The effect of E.coli endotoxin induced fever on the pharmacokinetic parameters of amoxycillin, trimethoprim and chloramphenicol after i.v. injection

drug	dose	Cpo	AUC	t½	Vd	Clearance
amox.')						
+	22.7		194	2.5	0.27	0.128
−	22.7		184	2.9	0.28	0.129
P			0.93	0.16	0.65	0.89
TMP'')						
+	1.87	1.36	2.76	1.45	1.40	0.80
−	2.05	2.20	2.50	0.87	1.03	0.85
P			0.41	0.001	0.10	0.59
chlor''')						
+	44	53.0	330	8.1	1.3	0.12
−	44	64.8	320	7.5	1.3	0.13
P		n.d.	n.d.	n.d.	n.d.	n.d.

Drugs were injected concurrently with the endotoxin intravenously; ') amoxycillin 1g per calf; '') trimethoprim 0.1 g per calf; ''') chloramphenicol 2.1 g per calf; + parameters with endotoxin; − parameters without endotoxin; P level of significance at which the compared parameters are different (Student's paired t-test).

RESULTS

The endotoxin fever model

After injection of endotoxon the clinical symptoms exhibited by the calves were variable. A rise in body-temperature of less than 0.6°C was considered not to be a feverish response.

Reactions were classified as follows:

1) no reaction
2) good reaction, i.e. biphasic rise in body-temperature, depression, increased rate of respiration, occasional coughing, production of some loose faeces and shivering.
3) pre-shock; the animals became recumbant, dyspnoeic, sunken eyed and the body-temperature tended to fall. After the critical period the animals recovered and belonged to group 2.
4) shock, this phenomenon occurred 15 minutes or about one hour after the injection of endotoxin. The most dramatic symptoms were: a sudden onset of respiratory distress, choking and death. Shortly before death, or soon thereafter a blood tinged foam was present at the nostrils.

Drug bloodlevels after intravenous injection

The mean serum amoxycillin concentrations after i.v. injection of amoxycillin-sodium are presented in Figure 1. The body-temperature rose to a maximum of about 1.2°C. The serum drugconcentration time curves, with and without endotoxin, are almost identical. Also the pharmacokinetic parameters, calculated with the FARMFIT-computer programme, presented in Table 2, are almost identical, which is illustrated by the high "P-values".

The same situation was found after i.v. injection of chloramphenicol. From Table 2 it can be concluded that the serumcontrations and the pharmacokinetic parameters are not changed by endotoxin induced fever. An average maximum rise in temperature was achieved 4 hours after endotoxin injection.

The calculated serum concentration time curve of trimethoprim, with concurrent endotoxin injection, is less steep and starts at a lower concentration compared to the curve achieved with no endotoxin (Figure 1). No detectable levels of trimetho-prim were present in the healthy calves, but were evident in the endotoxin treated group, 6 hours after dosing. Four hours after endotoxin injection reached the average rise in body-temperature its maximum of $+1.7^{\circ}$C.

The injection of endotoxin caused a significantly ($P < 0.001$) longer elimination half-life ($t\frac{1}{2}$) and a substantially greater volume of distribution (Vd) of trimethopr

after i.v. injection. The area under the serumconcentration time curve (AUC) and
the total body clearance (Cl) are unchanged.

Drug bloodlevels after oral administration

Due to the nature of the changes caused by endotoxin induced fever, the results
of the studies with the three drugs, ampicillin, amoxycillin and chloramphenicol
are discussed simultaneously.

As in the i.v. experiments the endotoxin was injected directly after the drug
administration. As before, the endotoxin caused a biphasic rise in temperature with
an average maximum increase of $0.9^{\circ}C$.

During fever the absorption of the three drugs was delayed, which shifted the
curves to the right (Figure 2a). This change was most pronounced during the time
the body-temperature was rising. The area's under the curve, which are shown in
Table 2, indicate the amount of drug absorbed. Two to four hours after injection
of endotoxin, a sharp increase in fever index (FI) occurred and coincided with the
biggest differences between the absorbed amounts of drugs compared with the
healthy group. It can be noted that with increasing FI-values the "P-level",
indicating the level at which the absorbed amounts of drugs are different, decreases.
In the chloramphenicol and the amoxycillin experiments these differences are
significant ($P < 0.05$).

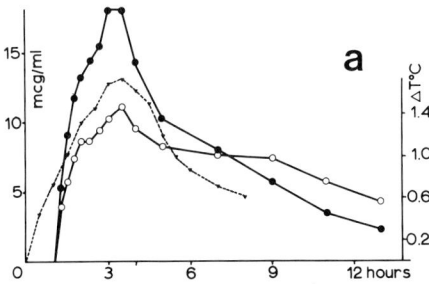 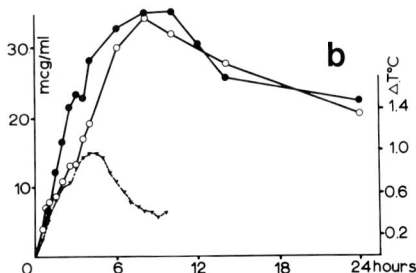

Figure 2. The effect of E.coli endotoxin induced fever on the serumconcentrations
of amoxycillin (a) and chloramphenicol (b) after i.m. and oral administration
respectively. Serumconcentrations of antibiotics,●————● without and O————O
with endotoxin; ▼------▼ rise in body-temperature. Doses were: amoxycillin 1 g
per calf, chloramphenicol 5 g per calf and endotoxin 5 mcg per calf.

Table 2. The effect of E.coli endotoxin induced fever on the rate of absorption of ampicillin, amoxycillin and chloramphenicol after oral administration.

time hours	ampicillin				amoxycillin				chloramphenicol			
	−	+	P	FI	−	+	P	FI	−	+	P	FI
0-1	0.3	0.4	.29	0.15					3	4	.18	0.21
1-2	1.0	1.0	.84	0.45					12	10	.54	0.60
0-2					3.2	2.4	.12	0.84				
2-3	1.7	1.1	.28	0.50					21	12	.01	0.61
3-4	1.7	1.3	.22	0.63					26	16	.04	0.85
2-4					12.5	6.3	.00	1.82				
4-5	1.5	1.5	.97	0.74								
4-6					16.8	12.3	.06	1.48	62	49	.83	
5-6	1.3	1.5	.88	0.57								0.92
6-7				0.49								0.73
6-8	1.7	2.5	.97		16.8	17.6	.83	0.68	68	64	.45	
total 36h.	11.7	12.7	.38		49.3	38.6	.11		816	746	.26	

Table 3. The effect of E.coli endotoxin induced fever on the rate of absorption of ampicillin, amoxycillin and chloramphenicol after i.m. administration.

time hours	ampicillin				amoxycillin				chloramphenicol			
	−	+	P	FI	−	+	P	FI	−	+	P	FI
0-1								0.42				0.40
1-2					8	5	.09	1.04	4	6	.23	0.82
0-2				0.52								
2-3					15	9	.75	1.56	17	14	.04	1.14
3-4					18	11	.01	1.68	20	17	.72	1.32
2-4	23	11	.001	1.43								
4-5					13	9	.01	1.46	21	17	.15	1.05
5-6								1.00				0.59
4-6	20	13	.005	1.16					41	36	.23	
5-7					18	15	.53					
6-7								0.82				0.21
6-8	14	9	.02	0.37					38	36	.92	
total 36h.	66	40	.001		95	138	.11		300	305	.26	

Legends table 2 & 3. Ampcillin and amoxycillin 1 g per calf. Chloramphenicol oral 5 g per calf and i.m. 2.5 g per calf. Endotoxin was injected concurrently with the oral dosing, 1 hour before the i.m. injection of amoxycillin and chloramphenicol and 2 hours before ampcillin administration. + serum drug concentration indices(mcg.hour/ml) with endotoxin;−serum drug concentration indices (mcg.hour/ml) without endotoxin; P level of significance at which the serum drug concentration indices with and without endotoxin were different (Student's paired t test); FI fever index indicating for the rise in body-temperature at time-intervals (hour. $\Delta T^{o}C$)

Drug bloodlevels after intramuscular administration.

The average rise in bodytemperature ranged from 0.9°C to 1.6°C in the three groups. As in the oral experiments, the injection of endotoxin, which was administered one hour before the intramuscular administration of chloramphenicol and amoxycillin, and two hours before the ampicillin injection, had a decreasing effect on the rate of absorption of these drugs (Figure 2b). Whereas the maximum serum concentrations after oral administration were almost equal in the endotoxin treated and healthy groups, the level was lower in the corresponding groups treated by intramuscular injection. Table 3 shows the same relationship between rise in body-temperature and amount of drug absorbed. While the FI is clearly decreasing, differences between absorbed amounts of drug are still apparent.

DISCUSSION

The reaction to an endotoxin injection is considered to be substantially an immunological response. Pittman (1974) showed that in newborn lambs the first injection of endotoxin failed to produce fever, but a second challenge in the same lambs 60 hours old caused fever. Control lambs, also 60 hours old did not respond to a first challenge either (24). There was an indication that this phenomenon was still present 12 days after birth. The calves used in the present experiments came from different sources, and were probably not uniformly exposed to "endotoxins". This might explain the diversity in reaction. Some calves were extremely sensitive to endotoxin (3), while others did not respond to the same dose. The same findings are reported by others (29). Kids born in one herd of goats responded more homogenously to a single endotoxin injection (10). Fed with milk replacer only, kids from this herd might be a better endotoxin fever-model for the veal-calf than the veal-calf itself.

The pharmacokinetics of drugs regularly appears as the subject of several symposia and review-articles. Despite the continual use of antimicrobial drugs in animals, suffering from febrile diseases, little is known of the effect of fever on the pharmacokinetics behaviour of these drugs. A greater volume of distribution of penicillin was observed during the febrile episodes in experiments with streptococci infected dogs. (2). Lower bloodlevels of quinine were observed during febrile episodes in malaria. A less evident lowering of bloodlevels of the same drug could be induced by artificial induced fever with etiocholanolone (27). In dogs with fever, induced either by experimental pneumonia with Pseudomonas aeruginosa or by intravenous injection of E.coli endotoxin, and in man with etiocholanolone induced fever, significant lower bloodconcentrations of gentamycin were observed after i.v. injection of gentamycin sulfate (23). It is very likely, that these lower bloodlevels were caused by a greater volume of distribution of the drugs. A greater volume of distribution of warfarin and trimethoprim in rabbits was observed during endotoxin induced fever (8,14). As the clearance is unchanged (table 2) and ln2 is a constant, the longer half-life ($t_{\frac{1}{2}}$) and the greater volume of distribution (Vd) are connected by the formula: $Cl = \dfrac{Vd \times ln2}{t_{\frac{1}{2}}}$. Given the unchanged Cl after i.v. injection it seems obvious that the changes in the pharmacokinetics are principally determined by a changed Vd. Shifts of the pH in certain compartments and/or se- en ex-creta could be an explanation. A lower serum-protein-binding of the drug could also account for a greater Vd(14). In pigs bloodconcentrations of sulphathiazole are higher during endotoxin induced fever, while in contradiction those of trimethoprim are lowered. Sulphathiazole is a weak acid (pKa 7.12) and trimethoprim a weak base (pKa 7.6). Small pH-shifts can induce substantial changes in the degree of ionosation of both drugs. The unchanged distribution and elimination of amoxycillin and chloramphenicol fit in this explanation, since amoxycillin is an acid (pKa 2.4) and chloramphenicol is alkaline nor acid.

The stomach itself is not an important site of absorption, but its emptying rate can markedly influence the absorption from the small intestine (4). E.coli endotoxin is a strong inhibitor of gastric motility in monogastric and polygastric animals. (17,18). Since the elimination and distribution of amoxycillin and chloramphenicol are unchanged,the changed bloodlevels, after oral and intramuscular administration of the drugs during endotoxin induced fever, must be caused by a changed rate of absorption. This is most pronounced during the time the body-temperature is rising, as indicated by the lowest P-values. The unchanged total amount absorbed indicates that the absorption is only delayed and the endotoxin-effect short lasting. Clinical fever in general lasts longer and therefore might show a more clear effect on the pharmacokinetics (20).

The lower bloodlevels observed during fever after intramuscular injection into the neck muscles appears to be a more complex phenomenon. Not only the volume of injection, but also the site of injection in the body, determine the rate of absorption from the injection site (25). Furthermore, exercise and local circumstances such as inflammation caused by previous injections or by the injection itself, do change the rate of absorption (26,28). Hypothetically it is possible, that during fever there is a reduced bloodsupply to the non-shivering muscles, i.c. neck-muscles, in favour of the shivering ones, or that the total peripheral circulation is reduced. Both hypotheses can be possible, since very sick animals, which do not shiver and have a reduced peripheral circulation, show a decreased rate of absorption.

CONCLUSIONS
1) The calf endotoxin-fever-model is, in contrast to similar models where other species of mammals are used, less useful, because of the variation in reaction to a standard dose of endotoxin.
2) The pharmacokinetics of i.v. injected amoxycillin and chloramphenicol are not changed by endotoxin induced fever.

3) The pharmacokinetics of i.v. injected trimethoprim are changed during fever, as shown by a longer $t\frac{1}{2}$ and a greater Vd.

4) During fever, the rate of absorption of ampicillin, amoxycillin and chloramphenicol, administered orally or intramuscularly, is reduced.

REFERENCES

1. Allen, J.G. and Nimmo - Smith, R.H. (1978) Trimethoprim. In Laboratory methods in antimicrobial chemotherapy. Published by: Churchill Livingstone, Edinburgh, London and New York. 227 - 231.

2) Baggot, J.D. (1977) Principles of drug disposition in domestic animals: the basis of veterinary clinical pharmacology. W.B. Sanders company, 184-185.

3) Berczi, J., Bertok, L., Bereznai, T. (1966) Can.J.Microbiol., 12: 1070-1071.

4) Bischop, C.R., Janzen, R.E., Landals, D.C., Manns, B.D., McCartney, D.J., Morgan, G.A., Pawlyshyn, V.P., Schienbein, A.J., Scigliano, B.W. and Taylor, K.L. (1973) Can.Vet.Journ., 14: 269-271.

5) Brunaud, M. (1954) Rev.Med.Vet., 105: 535-580.

6) Burgess, G.W. (1971) Vet.Bull., 41: 887-895.

7) Cooper, K.E. (1971) Some physiological and clinical aspects of pyrogens. In Pyrogens and fever. Published by: Churchill Livingstone, Edinburgh and London.

8) Friis, Ch. and Ladefoged, O. (1979) Zbl.Vet.Med.Reihe A, 26: 146-151.

9) Galesloot, Th.E. and Hassing, F.(1962) Neth.Milk and Dairy J., 16: 89-95.

10) Gogh van, H. and Miert van, A.S.J.P.A.M. (1977) Zbl.Vet.Med.Reihe A, 24: 503-510.

11) Groothuis, D.G., Miert van, A.S.J.P.A.M., Ziv, G. and Nouws, J.F.M. (1978) J.Vet.Pharm.Ther.,1: 81-84.

12) Groothuis, D.G (1980) The pharmcokinetic behaviour of antimicrobial drugs in veal calves and their antibacterial activity in relation to salmonellosis (S.dublin). Ph.D.Thesis, University of Utrecht.

13) Keusch, G.T. (1976) N.Y.State J.Med.,76: 1998-2001.

14) Ladefoged, O. (1978) Acta Vet.Scand.,19: 479-486.

15) Leek, B.F. and Miert van, A.S.J.P.A.M. (1971) J.Physiol., 215: 28-29.

16) Meyer, J. and Carlson, A.J. (1917) Amer.J.Physiol.,44: 222-233.

17) Miert van, A.S.J.P.A.M. and de la Parra, D.H. (1970) Arch.Int.Pharmacodyn.Ther., 184: 27-33.

18) Miert van, A.S.J.P.A.M. and Duin, C.Th.M. (1974) Zbl.Vet.Med.Reihe A,21: 692-702.

19) Miert van, A.S.J.P.A.M. (1973) Zbl.Vet.Med.Reihe A, 20: 614-623.

20) Musa, B.E., Conner, G.H., Carter, G.R., Gupta, B.N. and Keaky, K.K. (1972) Am.J.Vet.Res., 33: 911-916.

21) Urbaschek, B. (1976) Zbl.Bakt.Hyg., I Abt.,Orig.A, 235: 26-35.

22) Nimmo, W.S. (1976) Clin.Pharmacokin., 1: 189-203.

23) Pennington, J.E., Dale, D.C., Reynolds, H.Y. and MacLowery, J.D. (1975) J.Inf.Dis., 132: 270-275.

24) Pittman, Q.J., Cooper, K.E., Veale, W.L. and Van Petten, G.R. (1974) Clin.Sci. Mol.Med., 46: 591-602.

25) Reeves, D.S., Bywater, M.J. and Wise, R. (1974) The Lancet i.i., 1421-1422.

26) Schmidt, H. and Roholt, K. (1966) Acta Path.Microbiol.Scand. 68: 396-400.

27) Trenholme, G.M., Williams, R.L., Rieckmann, K.H., Frischer, H. and Carson, P.E. (1976) Clin.Pharm.Ther., 19: 459-467.

28) Winters, R.E., Litwack, K.D. and Hewitt, W.C. (1971) J.Inf.Dis.,124: S90-S95.

29) Wray, C. and Tomlinson, J.R. (1972) Res.Vet.Sc., 13: 546-553.

30) White, G. (1976) Personal communication.

31) Young, J.K. (1973) Mod.Vet.Pract., 54: 21-22.

CHEMICALLY INDUCED MODULATION OF THE IMMUNE RESPONSE

J.G.Vos

National Institute of Public Health, P.O.Box 1, 3720 BA Bilthoven, The
Netherlands

INTRODUCTION

Interest in the influence of toxic chemicals on the immune system has increased
markedly in recent years. Most attention has been given to chemicals of environmental concern that decrease the immunological responsiveness or increase the susceptibility to infection; less data are available on compounds that enhance immune
functions. The present article summarizes methods used in our Institute to detect
immune modulation in toxicity testing. Detailed information is given elsewhere (Vos,
1977; Faith et al, 1979; Vos, 1980). First, parameters will be discussed to screen
chemicals for possible effects on the immune system. Next, different function tests
are given to assess in the rat the cellular immunity, the humoral immunity and the
phagocytosis by macrophages.

SCREENING TESTS TO DETECT IMMUNOTOXICITY

It is well established that the most profound effects of compounds which interfere with the immune response occur when the animal is confronted with the compound
during the ontogenesis of the lymphoid system. A sensitive system to detect effects
on the immune system is, therefore, a reproduction study which includes a thorough
evaluation of the lymphoid system. However, this does not imply that studies to
detect such effects should always be conducted in animals during the developmental
phase of the immune system. For practical reasons, initial assessment could be done
in a 3-week range-finding study or in a 3-months semichronic toxicity study.

During these experiments body weight gain and food intake are recorded. At the
termination of the toxicity study, thymus, spleen, lymph nodes (popliteal and mesen-
teric nodes) are grossly examined, weighed and processed for histopathological examination. For the determination of peripheral lymphocyte and monocyte numbers (as
precursors of macrophages) total and differential leucocyte counts are carried out.
Concentrations of main serum immunoglobulin classes (e.g. IgM and IgG) can be measured by single radial immunodiffusion or by the enzyme-linked immunosorbent assay
(ELISA). The latter assay is routinely used in our Institute in the screening program for immunitoxicity and is described elsewhere (Vos et al., 1979[a]).

From these different parameters (weight gain, food intake, weight and histology of lymphoid organs, peripheral blood counts, serum IgM and IgG levels) a conclusion may be reached whether the chemical has an effect on the immune system. Such an effect can be direct or indirect (secondary to an effect elsewhere, e.g. caused by malnutrition or an altered endocrine balance). Especially an interaction of the chemical with the endocrine system which indirectly can cause an effect on the immune system should be considered, as various hormones (in particular glucocorticosteroids) do modify the immunological responsiveness (White and Goldstein, 1972; see also Vos, 1977). For this reason, pituitary gland, thyroid, adrenals, testes, ovaries are also weighed and microscopically examined in our screening program. When the effect on the immune system can not be attributed to an indirect effect of which the functional significance is known, and the effect is a sensitive parameter, functional studies should be carried out.

FUNCTION TESTS ON THE IMMUNE SYSTEM

Function studies (Table I) of the immune system are necessary in order to evaluate the functional significance of the chemically induced effect on the lymphoid system found in a routine study, and to gain insight into the mode of the action of the chemical.

TABLE I

In vivo and in vitro function tests of the immune system

Cell-mediated immunity

    In vivo
    - Resistance to Listeria monocytogenes infection
    - Rejection of skin transplants
    - Delayed-type hypersensitivity to tuberculin or ovalbumin
    In vitro
    - Transformation of lymphocytes by PHA and Con A

Humoral immunity

    In vivo
    - Thymus-dependent antibody synthesis to tetanus toxoid or ovalbumin
    - Thymus-independent antibody synthesis to E.coli lipopolysaccharide (LPS)
    In vitro
    - Transformation of lymphocytes by LPS

Phagocytosis by macrophages

    In vivo
    - Clearance of carbon particles (phagocytosis)
    - Clearance of Listeria monocytogenes (phagocytosis and killing)
    In vitro
    - Determination of phagocytosis and intracellular killing of Listeria monocytogenes

The choice of function tests depends mainly on the effects seen in the routine toxicity study: when thymus atrophy is the main characteristic, the cell-mediated response should be studied first. In cases when the effect is primary on serum immunoglobulins, one should test the capacity of the animal to generate a humoral immune response. Before starting function tests that allow a separate study of the different phases of the immune response, one should obtain insight into whether the overall response is impaired. For this purpose it is particularly useful to measure if the resistance to infection is impaired by the chemical.

As already discussed in the previous section, subtle effects on the immunological responsiveness will be more easily detected when the animal is confronted with the chemical during the developmental phase of the lymphoid organs. If the chemical passes the placenta and is excreted in the milk, e.g. 2,3,7,8-tetrachlorodibenzo-p-dioxin (Vos, 1977; Faith et al., 1979) and hexachlorobenzene (Vos et al., 1979[b]), pre- and postnatal maternal treatment is probably the most sensitive test system to detect an altered immune response. For chemicals which do not readily pass the placenta and are not readily excreted in the milk, e.g. di-n-butyltindichloride (Seinen and Penninks, 1979) pups can be treated postnatally by oral intubation. Function studies of the pups could be performed at the time of weaning or later.

In conclusion, the present available data clearly show that the developing organism is more at risk to the immunomodulating effects of different chemicals than the corresponding adult. As a consequence of this, functional assessment of effects of chemicals on the immune system should preferably be carried out after combined pre- and postnatal exposure.

REFERENCES

Faith, R.E., Luster, M.I. and Vos, J.G., 1979. Effects on immunocompetence by chemicals of environmental concern. Reviews in Biochemical Toxicology. In press.
Seinen, W. and Penninks, A., 1979. Immune suppression as a consequence of a selective cytotoxic activity of certain organometallic compounds on thymus and thymus-dependent lymphocytes. Ann. N. Y. Acad. Sci., 320: 499-517.
Vos, J.G., 1977. Immune suppression as related to toxicology. CRC Crit. Rev. Toxicol., 5: 67-101.
Vos,J.G., 1980. Immunotoxicity assessment: screening and function studies. Arch. Toxicol. In press.
Vos, J.G., Buys, J., Beekhof, P. and Hagenaars, A.M., 1979[a]. Quantification of total IgM and IgG and specific IgM and IgG to a thymus-independent (LPS) and a thymus-dependent (tetanus toxoid) antigen in the rat by enzyme-linked immunosorbent assay (ELISA). Ann. N. Y. Acad. Sci., 320: 518-534.
Vos, J.G., van Logten, M.J., Kreeftenberg, J.G., Steerenberg, P.A. and Kruizinga, W., 1979[b]. Effect of hexachlorobenzene on the immune system of rats following combined pre- and postnatal exposure. Drug Chem. Toxicol., 2: 61-76.
White, A. and Goldstein, A.L., 1972. Hormonal regulation of host immunity. In: F.Borek (editor), Immunogenicity, Frontiers of Biology Vol. 25. North-Holland Publishing Company, Amsterdam pp. 334-364.

POTENTIAL AND LIMITATIONS OF IMMUNOTHERAPY.
Lessons from a eight-year experience with levamisole.

J. SYMOENS
Janssen Pharmaceutica, B-2340 Beerse (Belgium).

Biologic or synthetic compounds that enhance host defense mechanisms have received considerable interest during the last ten years. One of them, levamisole, is a simple chemical extensively used as an anthelmintic in animals and man (fig. 1). Levamisole is probably the most extensively studied of all immunotherapeutic agents. Its immunologic and clinical effects are described in more than 1500 reports or publications.

The first hints of a possible effect on immunity came in the late sixties, when an increased resistance to infection was observed in cattle, pigs, dogs and sheep dewormed with levamisole (ref. 1). In 1971, Renoux wrote that levamisole augmented the response of mice to a Brucella vaccine (ref. 2). Today, its immunological spectrum can be summarized as follows.

Levamisole induces maturation of T-lymphocytes in immunologically immature animals such as thymus-less mice. It also restores the various effector functions of T-lymphocytes, polymorphonuclear neutrophils and mononuclear phagocytes in compromised hosts. It seems not to influence B-lymphocytes directly. Levamisole thus selectively influences cell mediated immune functions and has little or no effect on humoral immunity. At therapeutic dose levels, levamisole does not stimulate immune responses above normal physiological level.

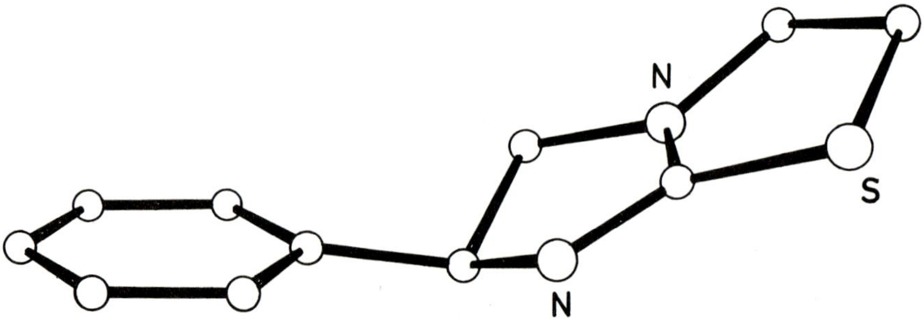

Figure 1

The effects of levamisole on the immune system are virtually identical to those of the thymic hormones. There are good reasons to think that levamisole is a thymomimetic agent (for reviews, see ref. 3, 4).

CLINICAL EXPERIENCE IN MAN

In 1973, the clinical usefulness of levamisole as an immunotherapeutic agent started to be explored in man. The drug is now available in several countries for the treatment of chronic or recurrent diseases, with infection predominating in some and lymphoid infiltration in others.

1. Children with primary immune deficiency disorders, i.e. with a deficit of T-cells, B-cells or phagocytes, are highly susceptible to infections by viruses, bacteria, fungi or protozoa, including organisms normally of low virulence. These patients frequently have recurring or chronic infections of the skin, the lungs, the upper respiratory tract or other organs from early life on. Levamisole reduces the frequency and severity of infectious episodes and restores immune functions in patients with a defect of T-cells or phagocytes. Levamisole does not substitute for antibiotics or gammaglobulin treatment, but it does reduce the need for such treatment probably by stimulating host defense mechanisms against infection.

2. Levamisole also reduces the frequency, severity and duration of episodes of recurrent bacterial or viral infections in adults in whom no overt immune defect is found with the available immunological techniques. It shortens the anergic period which follows certain viral infections such as acute hepatitis and influenza and hastens recovery of these diseases. Patients with chronic pyogenic skin infections or chronic brucellosis also usually benefit from long-term treatment with levamisole (for review, see ref. 5).

3. Extensive controlled studies in patients with rheumatoid arthritis revealed that levamisole tempers the progression of the disease and causes clinical improvement in approximately two-thirds of the patients. Levamisole seems to have a similar tempering effect in other chronic inflammatory diseases but controlled studies are needed to substantiate these findings (for review, see ref. 6).

4. Finally, controlled studies in animals and in over one thousand patients with various types of cancer have shown that levamisole can increase the duration of remission and survival following adequate cytoreductive therapy. Levamisole is an adjunct to such treatment, not a replacement. The potential of levamisole to prolong survival is directly related to the thoroughness with which the tumor mass is removed by cytoreductive treatment (for review, see ref. 7, 8).

CLINICAL EXPERIENCE IN ANIMALS

The clinical experience with levamisole in veterinary medicine is much more limited. Initial attempts to increase antibody production after vaccination failed, for obvious reasons. Preliminary data suggest that levamisole is beneficial in pyodermic infections of dogs (ref. 9), in rodent ulcers of cats (ref. 9), in actinomycosis of cattle (ref. 10) and sows (ref. 11), in aleutian disease of mink (ref. 12), in systemic lupus erythematosus in dogs (ref. 13) and in cancer of dogs (ref. 14) and cats (ref. 15). The largest and most convincing experience, however, is in the prevention of calf mortality by pre-treatment of pregnant cows with levamisole.

It is well known that certain farms each year again have to deal with neo-natal calf disease, the main problem being diarrhea. In spite of therapy with electrolytes and antibiotics, this may lead to an abnormally high mortality rate.

The suggestion was made that immunotherapy of the cow during the dry-off period could result in the birth of a calf with a stronger immunocompetence, so that its resistance against bacterial or viral infection would be enhanced.

The first experiments in this respect were done in Israel. In a problem herd, Tamarin treated 40 cows on a blind basis, either with levamisole or with placebo. The animals received an injection once a week during 4 weeks before delivery. Four of 20 control calves died; all 20 calves from levami-sole-treated cows survived. Similar experiments by other investigators all showed a similar trend, with an overall death rate of 5.8% in control calves and 1.7% in calves from levamisole-treated cows (table 1).

These experiments also showed that pretreatment of cows during the dry-off period reduces the morbidity in neonatal calves. In a recent trial performed by Marsboom in Belgium, 50.9% of control calves were ill during one or more days compared to 32.2% in calves from treated cows (table 2). Analyzed in function of the duration of illness, the number of calves that are sick for one or two days is similar between both groups but the number of animals that are sick for three days or more is significantly higher in the control group (table 3).

In conclusion, treatment of cows with levamisole during the dry-off period results in less dead and less diseased calves. If, in spite of this treatment, there is an outbreak of disease, its duration is shorter than in the non-treated animals.

Table 1:
Prevention of calf mortality by pretreatment of pregnant cows with levamisole[*]

Investigator	Treatment	Calves born	died	
Tamarin (ref. 16)	control	20	4	
	levamisole	20	0	
Flesh (ref. 17)	control	32	8	
	levamisole	16	0	
Marsboom (ref. 18)	control	117	7	
	levamisole	104	2	
Marsboom (ref. 19)	control	369	8	
	levamisole	323	2	
Antoine (ref. 20)	control	70	8	
	levamisole	69	5	
Total	control	608	35	5.8%
	levamisole	532	9	1.7%

* 2.5 or 5 mg/kg intramuscularly or by application on the skin (poor-on method) once weekly on four consecutive weeks before farrowing.

Table 2:
Prevention of calf mortality by pretreatment of pregnant cows with levamisole.[*]
Number of diseased calves (ref. 19).

Cow treatment	Total number of calves	Number of diseased calves	%	P-value[**]
Placebo	369	188	50.9	0.001
Levamisole	323	104	32.2	

* 5 mg/kg, poor-on;
** X^2 test for two independent samples (Siegel, S.: Nonparametric Statistics, McGraw-Hill Book Co., New York, 1956, pp. 104-111).

Table 3:
Prevention of calf morbidity by pretreatment of pregnant cows with levamisole.[*]
Duration of disease (ref. 19).

Days of disease	Control (188 calves) number of calves	%	Levamisole (104 calves) number of calves	%	P-value[**]
1	51	27.1	38	36.5	n.s.
2	40	21.3	30	28.8	n.s.
>2	97	51.6	36	34.6	0.007

* 5 mg/kg, poor-on;
** X^2 test for two independent samples (Siegel, S.: ibidem table 2).

IMMUNOTHERAPY: LESSONS FROM THE LEVAMISOLE EXPERIENCE

The clinical research with levamisole as an immunotherapeutic agent in animals and man, though not yet completed, has shown at least some of the potential and limitations of immunotherapy. The conclusions reached with levamisole are probably valid for other compounds such as the thymic hormones that act on the immune system in a similar way. Immunotherapy is potentially useful in at least three different fields.

1. Immunotherapy improves host defenses to invasion by infectious agents or tumoral cells. As a result, the abnormally prolonged healing time after certain infections is shortened and tumor patients are less likely to relapse after adequate cytoreductive treatment.

2. Immunotherapy can restore the immune balance in chronic inflammatory diseases and in autoimmune diseases. It tempers the progression of the disease, as shown in NZB/NZW mice and in patients with rheumatoid arthritis. Total remission, however, is rare.

3. Immunotherapy can enhance the immune response in immatures and in the aged. Studies are ongoing to evaluate whether this enhances the resistance to infection in immatures and whether this reduces the incidence of cancer in the aged.

Some of the limitations of immunotherapy can be summarized as follows :

1. Host defenses are not increased above normal level with a levamisole-like drug. The host thus remains susceptible to invasion by virulent agents.

2. Drugs like levamisole that selectively act on the cellular arm of the immune response do not increase humoral immune responses. All attempts to potentiate B-cell dependent vaccines have failed.

3. The effects observed with levamisole are reproducible only if populations of patients are studied. Individual patients sometimes fail to respond to treatment with levamisole. Usually, there is no correlation between clinical improvement and restoration of immune functions by the parameters currently measured. There is no immunologic predictor for clinical responsiveness. Immunotherapy thus remains empirical to a large extent. Some of its indications are reminiscent to those of the prewar so-called unspecific stimulation therapy.

4. Some patients receiving immunotherapy have shown unwanted immunologic reactions such as agammaglobulinemia or agranulocytosis. These reactions, which are probably an expression of immunologic overshoot, are rare and apparently occur in genetically predisposed patients. One may expect that

such reactions will be more frequent with drugs that indiscriminitely stimulate humoral and cellular immunity above normal level, than with drugs that selectively restore cellular immune functions to normal.

In conclusion, immunotherapy, as we know it today, is a useful adjunct to anti-infectious, anti-tumoral, anti-inflammatory and corticosteroid therapy in a still limited number of diseases. It is not a replacement. The list of indications will undoubtedly expand as the results of ongoing controlled studies become available.

Other drugs than levamisole will soon come. BCG and C. parvum are being tested in cancer treatment, the thymic hormones are being tested in primary immune deficiency diseases, in rheumatoid arthritis and cancer. There is room also for drugs which selectively modulate subsets of immunologically competent cells such as suppressor T-cells or helper T-cells.

It is a feature of current research to properly define the role of immunotherapy in the therapeutic armamentarium.

REFERENCES

1. Janssen, P.A.J.:
   The Levamisole Story.
   In: Progress Research, 20, ed. E. Jucker, Birkhäuser Verlag, Basel und Stuttgart, 347-383, 1976.

2. Renoux, G. and Renoux, M.:
   Effet immunostimulant d'un imidothiazole dans l'immunisation des souris contre l'infection par Brucella abortus.
   C.R. Acad. Sci. Paris, 272, 349-350, 1971.

3. Symoens, J. and Rosenthal, M.:
   Levamisole in the modulation of the immune response: the current experimental and clinical state. A review.
   J. Reticuloendothel. Soc., 21, 175-221, 1977.

4. Symoens, J., Rosenthal, M., De Brabander, M. and Goldstein, G.:
   Immunoregulation with levamisole.
   Springer Semin. Immunopathol., 2, 49-68, 1979.

5. Symoens, J., De Cree, J., Van Bever, W. and Janssen, P.A.J.:
   Levamisole.
   In: Pharmacological and Biochemical Properties of Drug Substances, 2, ed. M.E. Goldberg, American Pharmaceutical Association, Academy of Pharmaceutical Sciences, Washington, 407-464, 1979.

6. Symoens, J. and Schuermans, Y.:
   Levamisole, a basic antirheumatic drug.
   Clin. Rheum. Dis., 5, 603-629, 1979.

7. Amery, W.K. and Chirigos, M.A.:
   Studies of levamisole in experimental tumor systems.
   In: Advances in Pharmacology and Therapeutics, 4, Prostaglandins - Immunopharmacology, ed. B.B. Vargaftig, Paris, 169-176, 1978.

8. Amery, W.K. and Verhaegen, H.:
   Effects of levamisole treatment in cancer patients.
   J. Rheumatol., 5, 123-134, 1978.

9. MacEwen, E.G.:
   General concepts of immunotherapy of tumors.
   J. Am. Anim. Hosp. Assoc., 12, 363-373, 1976.

10. Rosenberger, G.:
    Klinische Prüfung von Levamisol bei der Aktinomykose.
    Unpublished Report, June 1976.

11. Becker, H.:
    Vorversuch zur konservativen Behandlung der Gesäugeaktinomykose der
    Sau mit Levamisol.
    Unpublished data, November 1976.

12. Kenyon, A.J.:
    Treatment of Aleutian mink disease with levamisole.
    Curr. Chemother., 357-358, 1978.

13. Monier, J.C., Lapras, H. and Fleury, C.:
    Effect of levamisole on the lupus-like syndrome of mice and dogs.
    Dev. Comp. Immunol., 2, 361-366, 1978.

14. MacEwen, E.G., Withrow, S.J. and Patnaik, A.K.:
    Nasal tumors in the dog: retrospective evaluation of diagnosis, prognosis
    and treatment.
    J. Am. Vet. Med. Assoc., 170, 45-48, 1977.

15. MacEwen, E.G., Hayes, A., Harvey, H.J., Mooney, S., Hardy, W.D.
    and McClelland, A.J.:
    Levamisole progress report from the Veterinary Cancer Unit.
    Unpublished report, December 1976.

16. Tamarin:
    Unpublished data, 1976.

17. Flesh, J., Ovadia, H. and Nelken, D.:
    Prevention of calf mortality by pretreatment of pregnant cows with leva-
    misole.
    Refuah Veterinarit, 34, 97-98, 1977.

18. Marsboom, R.:
    Unpublished data, 1978.

19. Marsboom, R.:
    Unpublished data, 1979.

20. Antoine, H. and Symoens, J.:
    Unpublished data, 1979.

THE USE AND EVALUATION OF BACTERIAL VACCINES IN IMMUNOTHERAPY OF CANCER

E.J.RUITENBERG, J.L. SIRKS, J.G.KREEFTENBERG and P.A. STEERENBERG

National Institute of Public Health, P.O. Box 1, 3720 BA Bilthoven,The Netherlands

ABSTRACT

The use of bacterial vaccines for cancertherapy by immunostimulation raised the need for methods to check their suitability for this purpose.

A provisional scheme for the quality control of the two bacterial vaccines concerned, viz. living Bacillus Calmette Guérin (BCG) and killed Corynebacterium parvum is presented.

Control methods for this type of vaccines include tests on identity, absence of contaminating microorganisms and safety which are required for any vaccine.

In addition for the control of vaccines for immunostimulation in cancertherapy some special methods for safety and potency testing are required. Some assays are proposed:

1) In vivo macrophage dependent-spleen clearance of Listeria monocytogenes.
2) An in vivo test for measuring the reaction of the draining lymph node and an in vitro test based on the stimulation of lymphocytes by concanavalin A.
3) A chemically induced fibrosarcoma in mice. Optimal doses, route and time interval were established both in prophylactic and therapeutic situations, including intratumoral application.

These models yield information on some effects of bacterial vaccines for immunostimulation. They are suitable for comparison of various types of vaccines. Whether these results have any relevance to the anti-tumor effect in the clinical situation is not clear.

INTRODUCTION

The use of bacterial vaccines for cancer therapy by immunostimulation raised the need for methods to check their suitability for this purpose.

We have in our Institute devised a provisional scheme for the quality control of the two bacterial vaccines concerned viz. living Bacillus Calmette Guérin (BCG) and killed Corynebacterium parvum. It includes a series of tests which can be assigned to four main groups (Table 1).

Some of them, like those mentioned under "general", the safety tests by inoculation of animals under 2.3. and the stability tests are also used for the control of the BCG vaccine for the prevention of tuberculosis (20). The guinea pig skin reactivity test (18) is mentioned under safety tests as well as under potency tests.

More relevant seem,however, tests which may give information about the immuno-stimulating potency of the vaccines. They are mentioned in Table 1 under 3.3. to 3.6. and will be discussed in detail below.

It should be realized that C.parvum is always used as a killed vaccine, whereas BCG is applied as a living vaccine and produced in different ways.Consequently,some back ground information on the methods to prepare BCG vaccines is presented first.

TABLE 1 – Tests for control of bacterial vaccines for immunostimulation in
cancertherapy

		BCG	C.parvum
1.	General		
1.1	Identity	x	x
1.2	Absence of contaminating microorganisms	x	x [1]
1.3	Absence of tubercle bacteria	x	n.a.
1.4	Dry weight	x	x
1.5	Number of culturable particles	x	n.a.
1.6	O_2 uptake rate	x	n.a.
2.	Safety		
2.1	Pyrogenicity	x	x
2.2	Histamine sensitizing factor (HSF)	n.a.	x
2.3	General safety test in animals	x	x
2.4	Guinea pig skin reactivity test	x	n.a.
3.	Potency		
3.1	Guinea pig skin reactivity test	x	n.a.
3.2	Spleen weight test	x	x
3.3	Listeria clearance in vivo	x	x
3.4	Lymph node stimulation in vivo	x	x
3.5	Lymphocyte stimulation in vitro	x	x
3.6	Tumor model in vivo	x	x
4.	Stability		
4.1	Spleen weight test	x	x
4.2	Culturable particles	x	n.a.
4.3	O_2 uptake rate	x	n.a.

[1] n.a. = not applicable

MATERIALS AND METHODS

Method for the preparation of BCG vaccine

The method in most BCG production laboratories is based on the original method
of Calmette. It consists of growing the BCG bacteria as a veil on the surface of
a liquid Sauton medium harvesting them by filtration or centrifugation and bringing
them into a homogeneous suspension by means of a ball mill containing steel balls.
During this process part of the bacteria is damaged and soluble antigens are released
into the resuspension fluid. This may have a negative effect on the immunostimulating
properties of the vaccine (9).

A second method has been developed by Ungar et al. (19). It consists of dispersing
the BCG bacteria already during growth by adding a wetting agent such as Tween 80
or Triton WR 1339 to the liquid culture medium. This method eliminated the necessity
of grinding the bacterial mass in a ball mill.

A third method, developed by Van Hemert (5) gives an even better dispersed and
homogeneous growth of the bacteria by using instead of a number of flasks one large
vessel containing a liquid medium with Tween 80 which is constantly stirred. This
method is used in our Institute for the production of BCG vaccines for immuno-

stimulation. It obviates like the second method the necessity of homogenising in a ball mill. If subsequently the vaccine is freeze dried in a suitable way (17) the product will contain mainly living bacteria and a minimal amount of soluble antigens.

One should take into consideration the possibility that these differences in production methods might influence the therapeutic potency of the vaccine used for immunostimulation in cancertherapy.

RESULTS

Effect of BCG and C.parvum on in vivo Listeria clearance

To study the effect of BCG-RIV (homogeneous culture) and C.parvum (Wellcome) on the induction of anti-Listeria resistance, mice were immunized intravenously (i.v.) with BCG at day -21 or with C.parvum at day -3. Intravenous challenge with 6×10^5 L.monocytogenes was performed at day 0. The choice of the immunization-challenge intervals for BCG and C.parvum was based on previous experience (14,15). Autopsies were performed at various days after Listeria challenge. The spleens were removed aseptically and Listeria bacteriae were enumerated according to previously described procedures (14).

In Fig. 1 the effect of pretreatment of BCG and C.parvum on the Listeria clearance is shown. At day 1 post infection (p.i.) there is a significant decrease in Listeria spleen counts in the BCG and C.parvum pretreated animals. This is in keeping with previously published findings by others and ourselves (13,14,15). Increased spleen counts in C.parvum pretreated mice on day 8 are compatible with the inhibitory effect of C.parvum on T cell function when this agent is given i.v. prior to antigenic stimulation as was observed previously in other systems (16).

It is known that specific T cell dependent immunity against Listeria involving the co-operation of sensitized T cells and activated macrophages is operating from day 2 p.i. onwards (7,8). For studying the stimulatory effect of BCG and C.parvum on macrophage function by means of this Listeria clearance model enumeration of Listeria bacteria in the spleen should, therefore, be performed on day 1-2 p.i. since at that time only the non-specific macrophage-mediated effect is present and no side effects of C.parvum are as yet detectable.

Effect of BCG vaccines on lymph node stimulation in vivo

Mackaness et al. (9) desribed an in vivo assay to differentiate between the immunopotentation of different strains and preparations of BCG vaccines. In brief: BCG is injected subcutaneously in the foot pad of mice. The cellular response in the draining i.e. the popliteal, lymph node is measured by incorporation of ^{3}H thymidine at different intervals after inoculation.

Fig. 2 shows the results of a typical experiment. BCG grown as a surface pellicle and ground in a ball mill and lyophilized shows an early peak at day 3 and a second

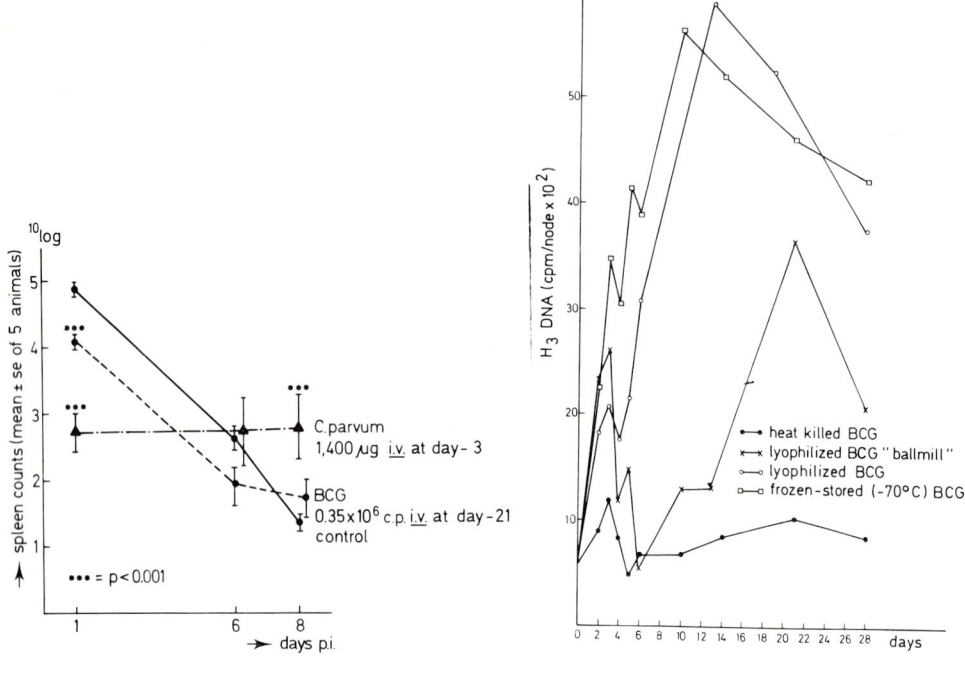

Fig.1.
Effect of BCG or C.parvum on Listeria
in $B_{10}LP$ +/nu mice.

Fig.2.
Measurement of the cellular response
by incorporation of ^3H thymidine, in
the popliteal lymph nodes of Swiss
mice at different intervals after
inoculation of the footpad with
BCG preparations.

one at day 21. BCG vaccines grown in dispersed homogeneous culture show both when
lyophilized or after storage at $-70^{\circ}C$ a continuous increase of ^3H-thymidine incorporation until 10 - 14 days after inoculation, after which a gradual decline was
observed. When this type of BCG vaccine was heat killed only a small peak at 3 days
was seen (3).

From these data it was concluded that the use of a ball mill in the vaccine
production had a different effect on lymph node stimulation.

By histological studies of lymph nodes stimulated with BCG activation of both
the T and B areas was demonstrated (12). This could be confirmed by us using
BCG-RIV (unpublished results). The increase in total amount of cells in the lymph
node can be caused by cell proliferation in the lymph node, but attraction of
lymphocytes from the periphery can also play a role (21).

Effect of BCG vaccines on in vitro stimulation of lymphocytes

Previously we described a lymphocyte transformation test which measures the synergistic activity of BCG on mitogen stimulation (4).

In brief: suspensions of mouse spleen cells or human lymphocytes were prepared and cultured in microtiter trays. Different amounts of BCG vaccine and a constant amount of a suboptimal concentration of concanavalin A (Con A) were added. Tritiated thymidine was added, the cells were harvested and the radioactivity measured. Results are expressed as means of triplicate cultures in counts per minute (cpm).

In Fig. 3 the results of the stimulation of the mouse spleen cells by different BCG vaccines in combination with Con A is shown.

BCG-RIV P 22 and P 44 vaccines were lyophilized, grown in a homogeneously dispersed culture. Lyophilized BCG B and C were obtained from different producers. In contrast to the RIV product these BCG preparations were grown as a surface pellicle and ground in a ball mill.

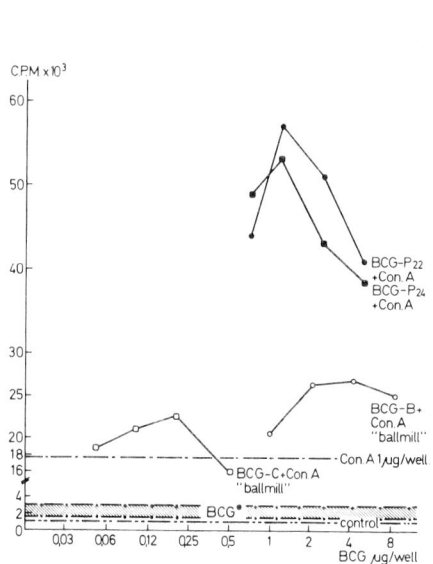

Fig. 3.
In vitro stimulation of mouse spleen cells by different BCG vaccines in combination with Con.A.

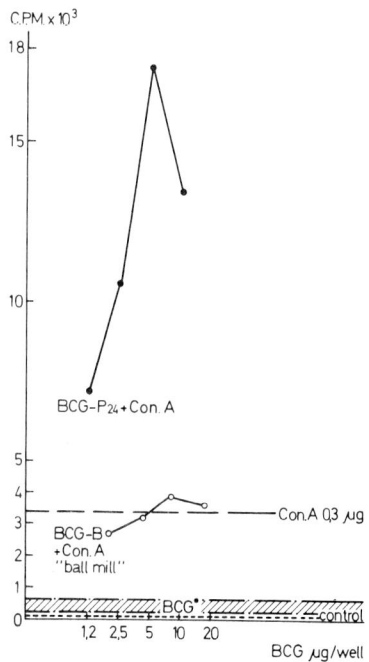

Fig. 4.
In vitro stimulation of human lympho-cytes from a mantoux negative donor, by BCG and the combination of BCG+Con.A in a 3 days culture.

The response of mouse spleen cells cultured together with different amounts of BCG was independent of the type of BCG used. Stimulation was usally not more than about 2 - 8 times the medium control culture.

Stimulation of spleen cells with Con A, together with BCG-RIV P 22 or P 24 showed a synergistic action. BCG preparations which has been ground in a ball mill lacked this property.

As BCG is used in man, we examined if the above mentioned effect would also happen when human lymphocytes were tested. The results were comparable with those obtained with mouse spleen cells. Again a difference in synergistic activity between BCG-RIV P 24 and the ball mill vaccine B could be demonstrated (Fig. 4).

The strongest synergy was observed with the BCG-RIV vaccines. These vaccines are prepared from homogeneously dispersed cultures. The other tested BCG preparation are from cultures grown as a surface pellicle and homogenized in a ball mill which results in many dead bacteria and soluble antigenic material (9).

An explanation for the difference in synergistic activity of these vaccines together with Con A, could be the amount of soluble antigen present in the ball mill vaccines. In recent experiments it could be demonstrated that a part of the synergistic activity could be ascribed to some of the stabilizers present in BCG vaccines. However, this could not explain completely the differences observed between the BCG preparations.

Whether this property of BCG is important for the immunostimulating potency of BCG in man remains obscure.

Effect of BCG and C.parvum on a chemically induces fibrosarcoma

By means of 20-methylcholanthrene a fibrosarcoma was induced chemically in Balb/c mice. Studies were performed on the basis of injection of 5×10^5 tumor cells in the hind foot and tumor growth was evaluated by measuring foot thickness at various days post inoculation. The characteristics of this tumor model are: a) a chemically induced, b) mesenchymal, c) solid, d) non-metastasizing, e) non-antigenic tumor.

Treatment schedules included :
1) prophylactic model i.v. administration of vaccine prior to tumor cell inoculation,
2) prophylactic model (combination of tumor cells with agent on day 0 via subcutaneous administration),
3) therapeutic model (intratumoral - i.t. - administration),
4) therapeutic model (i.v. - administration).

All data obtained are summarized in Table 2.

TABLE 2 – Summary of results of various treatment schedules (mouse-fibrosarcoma model)

Vaccine	Dose	Route	Days -21	-3	0[1]	+3	+7
BCG	0.35×10^5 c.p.[2]	i.v.	+[3]				0
	0.35×10^6 c.p.	s.c.				-	
		i.t.					0
	1.75×10^7 c.p.	i.v.					+
	3.5×10^6 c.p.	s.c.				-	
		i.t.					0
C.parvum	70 µg	i.t.				0	+
	700 µg	s.c.			+		
		i.t.				-	0
	1,400 µg	i.v.		0		+	+

[1] = day 0 is inoculation with tumor cells
[2] = c.p. = culturable particles
[3] = + = inhibition; 0 = no effect; - = enhancement

By using different treatment schedules (dose, route and time interval) different effects of the agent studied could be established. Since with one and the same agent both inhibition, no effect and tumor enhancement could be observed, it is difficult to generalize the results obtained. However, since an optimal inhibitory effect can be established by selecting a certain combination of the three variables (dose, route and time interval) the model can be used to evaluate the potency of the immunopotentiating agents studied.

The following conclusion is therefore justified: the model yields information on certain effects of bacterial vaccines used for immunostimulation, but statements on the effectiveness of any product should be based on careful studies including all variables.

DISCUSSION

The anti-tumor effect of immunostimulatory agents for cancer immunotherapy can only be evaluated in patients with malignancy. However, it is desirable that knowledge about some characteristics of the agents is collected in preclinical studies.

To this end the protocol presented in this paper was developed. The assays mentioned are not only relevant to compare vaccines based on different principles, like BCG and C.parvum, but also to study a possible difference between various methods of preparation as is the case for BCG. Furthermore, batch to batch variation can be examined.

Using the protocol it is possible to characterize a vaccine in descriptive terms. Whether such a characterization has any relevance for the anti-tumor effect in patients with malignancy is not clear at all. Therefore, it is highly desirable that the tumor models used should be relevant to the situation in man (1).

Consequently, the use of more realistic animal tumor models, as the squamous cell eye carcinoma in cattle (6) or mammary carcinoma in dogs, as guides for human cancertherapy should be expanded.

Many clinical trials in man using bacterial vaccines as anti-tumor agents have been conducted after the first encouraging results of Mathé and co-workers (10).

However, apart from some incidental observations (11) no clear evidence came forward to suggest that this form of immunotherapy had any positive effect on remission and survival time.

Why is the clinical picture so different from the results obtained from the animal tumor studies in which in general BCG and C.parvum induced a marked inhibition of tumor growth? Two considerations should be taken into account. First, immunotherapy is applied in general after other forms of therapy (surgery, chemotherapy and radiotherapy). It is possible that the removal of the primary tumor mass inhibits the development of an adequate increased anti-tumor resistance when this is based on a specific anti-tumor immunity. In this context, it is worth mentioning that the ultimate goal in most tumor diseases is the prevention, arrest or regression of metastases. Therefore, theoretically it is conceivable that immunotherapy should precede conventional therapy in order to prevent distal spread.

Next, the immunogenicity of the tumor might be relevant to its response to immunotherapy.Most animal studies are conducted with immunogenic tumors. Therefore, it might be important to increase the immunogenicity of the human tumors to render them more vulnerable to immunotherapy. In this connection it is important to mention the promising results obtained with the enzyme neuraminidase both in experimental models and in human malignancies (2). By neuraminidase treatment surface antigens on tumor cells are demasked and the cells are consequently more immunogenic. In combination with non-specific BCG or C.parvum immunostimulation this procedure might yield better results.

In conclusion, on one hand preclinical experiments should be guided by models closely resembling the human situation, but on the other hand one should try to translate data from experimental models to clinically relevant procedures.

REFERENCES

1. Bast,Jr.R.C., Bast, B.S., Rapp, H.J., 1977. Ann.New York Ac. Science, 277: 60-93
2. Bekesi, J.G., Roboz, J.P., Holland, J.F., 1976. Ann.New York Ac. Science, 277: 313-331
3. Bruynzeel, D.P., Ettekhoven, H., Kreeftenberg, J.G., 1977. Development in Biological Standardization, 38: 91-96
4. Bruynzeel, D.P., Ettekhoven, H., Kreeftenberg, J.G., 1978. Cancer Immunol. and Immunotherapy, 3: 253-258
5. Hemert, P.A. van., 1973. Thesis, Delft
6. Kleinschuster, S.J., Rapp, H.J., Leuker, D.C., Kainer, R.A., 1977. J. Nat. Cancer Inst. 58: 1807-1814
7. Lane, F.C., Unanue, E.R., 1972. J.exp. Med. 135: 1104-1112

8. Mackaness, G.B., 1969. J.exp. Med. 129: 973-992
9. Mackaness, G.B., Auclair, D.J., Lagrange, P.H., 1973. J.Nat.Cancer Inst. 51: 1655-1667
10. Mathé, G., Amiel, J.L., Schwarzenberg, L., Schneider, M., Cattan, A., Schlumberger, J.R., Hayat, M., De Vassal, F., 1969. Lancet, 1: 697-699
11. McKneally, M.F., Maver, C., Kausel, H.W., 1976. Lancet, 1: 377-379
12. Rappaport, H., Khalil, A., 1976. Cancer Immunol. Immunother. 1: 45-49
13. Ratzan, K.R., Musher, D.M., Keusch, G.T., Weinstein, L., 1972. Infect. Immunity, 5: 499-504
14. Ruitenberg, E.J., van Noorle Jansen, L.M., 1975. Zbl.Bakt.Hyg.,I.Abt.Orig.A. 231: 197-205
15. Ruitenberg, E.J., van Noorle Jansen, L.M., Kruizinga, W., Steerenberg, P.A., 1976. Br.J.Exp. Path. 57: 310-315
16. Scott, M.T., 1974. Cell. Immunology, 13: 251-263
17. Sirks, J.L., Cohen, H., Smith, L., 1971. Symposium Series in Immunobiological Stand., 17: 163-168
18. Sirks, J.L., Smith, L., Sekhuis, V.M. Cohen, H., 1974. J.Biol.Stand. 2:159-168
19. Ungar, J., Muggleton, P.W., Dudley, J.A.R., Griffiths, M.I., 1962. Brit.Med. J. II: 1086-1089
20. WHO Export Committee on Biological Standardization. WHO Technical Report Series, No. 329, Annex. 1, 25-51, 1966.
21. Zatz, M.M., 1976. J.Immunol. 116: 1587-1591

INTRAVENOUS BCG THERAPY OF CANINE TUMOURS

N.T. GORMAN and G.R. BETTON
Division of Immunology, Addenbrooke's Hospital, Hills Road, Cambridge, England and
I.C.I. Pharmaceuticals Division, Mereside, Alderley Park, Macclesfield, Cheshire,
England.

ABSTRACT

Intravenous BCG has been found to significantly delay the appearance of pulmonary
metastases in canine osteosarcoma and mammary carcinoma. The possible effector
mechanisms operative in this therapy are discussed with particular reference to NK
cell activity and alveolar macrophage cytotoxicity.

INTRODUCTION

The concept that the immune response can be manipulated to specifically augment an
ongoing anti-tumour response is an attractive one. The core of this concept is based
upon the principle that unique neo-antigens are expressed on the surface of neoplastic
cells. There is indeed unquestionable evidence that neoantigens are expressed on the
cell surface of viral (1) and carcinogen(2) induced tumours in both inbred and out-
bred species (3). It is, however, unfortunate that in the spontaneous human and canine
neoplasias there is neither conclusive evidence that specific neoantigens exist nor
that there is an active immune response directed against these antigens (3, 4).
This may in reality prove to be a technical rather than a conceptual inadequacy.
Therefore the initial basis for the use of immune stimulants such as BCG C. parvum
in the therapy of spontaneous neoplasia has recently become tenuous. This, however,
does not deteract, from the reported efficacy of BCG therapy in some limited clinical
situations although in general the reports have been conflicting (5-8). The purpose
of this paper is to discuss the clinical use of intravenous BCG in the therapy of
canine neoplasia and the possible mode of action.

Intravenous BCG therapy of canine neoplasias

Owen and Bostock (9) first reported that in canine osteosarcoma following amputation of the affected limb a course of intravenous BCG (Glaxo Labs., Greenford, England. Percutaneous strength BCG 3mg) administered after 1 week, 2 weeks, 4 weeks and then every 8 weeks, significantly delayed the appearance of pulmonary metastases and improved post-surgical survival time, these results were subsequently extended and confirmed (10). The expansion of this work to a fully randomised clinical trial was impossible to justify because of the well documented poor prognosis following simple amputation of the affected limb. This limitation does not apply in the case of mammary carcinoma where surgical excision of the mammary tumour is the treatment of choice and the effect of subsequent intravenous BCG could be assessed. Bostock & Gorman (11) studied a series of 34 cases of histologically confirmed invasive mammary carcinoma. Previous retrospective studies had shown that 70% of bitches with this type of histological tumour died as a direct result of metastases within one year of surgery (12). These cases were randomised into 3 groups a) surgery; b) surgery plus placebo and c) surgery plus intravenous BCG (one year course on the same protocol as the osteosarcoma trial at a dose of 0.1mg BCG/Kg body weight). The median survival time for each group in this trial is shown in Table 1.

Table 1   The effect of intravenous BCG on the median survival time and death rate of bitches following excision of an invasive mammary carcinoma

Group	No. of dogs	Mean age at surgery	Median survival time(weeks)	% dead after one year	
				All causes	Tumour
Control surgery alone	11	8.5	24	64	56
Control surgery + placebo	10	9.5	24	70	60
Treated surgery + BCG	13	10.0	100	23	15

It is clear that the survival time for both control groups is similar but that the survival time of the treated group was significantly different (p<0.02). The death rate in turn in the first post-surgical year was significantly greater in the control groups (60% + 56%) than in the treated groups (15%), where only two dogs died as a direct result of the tumour. In Table 2 the findings in all those animals destroyed because of the tumour at the end of the follow-up period are summarised.

Table 2   The cause of death in dogs following surgical excision of an invasive mammary carcinoma

Group	% dead	Local recurrence	Lung metastases	Recurrence & metastases	Other causes
Controls	86	1	8	5	4
Treated	54		1	2	4

As can be seen 18 of the 21 control bitches were dead, 13 as a direct result of the tumour and 4 from other causes. In contrast, 3 of the 13 BCG treated dogs died from

the mammary carcinoma whilst 4 had succumbed to unrelated diseases. It was important
to note that local recurrences were present in 28% of the controls and 15% of the
treated animals whilst 63% of controls compared to 23% of the treated dogs developed
pulmonary metastases.

Mode of action

As previously stated in the Introduction the action of BCG therapy was thought to
be via enhancement of a specific immune response against cell surface neoantigens.
There are only a few reports on canine tumour immunity but evidence to support neo-
antigen expression has been derived from the leukocyte migration inhibition assays
(13, 14), lymphocyte blastogenesis (15), colony inhibition (16) and the chromium [51]
release assay (17). However more recent studies have failed to provide data to
demonstrate histological type specific responses, which parallels the current situation in human tumour immunology (18, 19).

Lymphocytotoxicity

Betton & Gorman (18) examined lymphocyte cytotoxicity in 43 tumour bearing dogs
against a battery of allogeneic tumour cell lines. The precise details of lymphocyte
effector cell isolation, allogeneic target cell identification and characterisation
have been thoroughly covered in previous papers (18,20). The lymphocytotoxicity of
each effector cell population was assessed using the Chromium [51] release assay.
Briefly, this was performed in round bottomed 96-well microtest plates (Nunc, Denmark)
using a 200ul inoculation volume of medium RPMI 1640 plus 10% foetal calf serum, antibiotics and 10mM Hepes buffer. Wells contained 5×10^3 ^{51}Cr labelled allogeneic
tumour target cells and an effector:target cell ratio range of 20:1 to 160:1 or 10:1
to 80:1. Details of the cytotoxicity test, analysis of log transformed means of triplicate % release values by analysis of variance and multiple range testing at the
$p < 0.05$ level are given in ref. 18 . For comparison between experiments values for
specific cytotoxicity at 80:1 effector:target cell ratios at 8 hours were considered
(specific cytotoxicity = % release by test - % spontaneous release / (100% release
- % spontaneous release)).

It can be seen from the summary of the results in Table 3 that when effector
lymphocyte cells from tumour donors were cytotoxic for tumour targets of the donor's
histologic type there was generally activity against other unrelated target cells.
Furthermore no significant difference was found between the reactivity of effector
cells from normal and tumour bearing animals for the allogeneic cell lines.
This study, however, confirmed the presence of canine natural killer cell activity
(NK-cell) in the lymphocyte effector cell population and added to the existing speci
distribution (21-25). Further studies (26) have shown that canine NK cell activity
exhibits a) considerable week to week variation within the same animal; b) is
probably a function of the T-cell lineage and therefore similar to mice and man;
c) does not exhibit target cell selectivity which differs to the reports in man;

d) DLA compatibility between effector and target cells is not obligatory; e) there is no DLA linkage.

Table 3 Correlation of histological type of effector cell donor and target cells

Condition of effector cell donor	Proportion of positive cytotoxic effector:target cell combinations for target cells		
	Melanoma	Osteosarcoma	Mammary carcinoma
Melanoma bearing	10/63 (16	9/36 (25)	5/35 (14)
Osteosarcoma bearing	2/12 (17)	7/12 (58)	1/9 (11)
Mammary carcinoma bearing	1/12 (8)	3/11 (27)	1/12 (8)
Healthy controls	4/52 (8)	17/47 (36)	2/25 (8)
Total	17/139 (12.2)	36/106 (34.0)	9/81 (11.1)

The identification of NK cell activity in both tumour bearing dogs and healthy controls has naturally raised the question of the in vivo significance of the NK cell. If the NK cells provide some form of tumour surveillance system a selective mechanism to distinguish normal from neoplastic cells is mandatory. To date no evidence for such modulation has been reported and in vitro selectivity for malignant cells has not been shown (26,27). The failure to observe increased numbers of neoplasm in athymic (nude) mice,which are known to have good NK cell activity, has for some time argued against the importance of T-cells in tumour control. The NK cell activity of these mice, however, appears to reside in "pre-T-cells" as anti-Thy 1 sera will ablate NK cell activity (28). The recently reported (29) point mutation in the mouse called beige (bg^j) has provided an in vivo system where NK cells are present, as identified by a target binding assay but are functionally deficient; this impairment appears to be centred around the lytic mechanism (30). Amongst the many potentials of this mutant are the identification of the NK cell killing mechanisms and the role of NK cells in the control of infections and neoplastic development.

It could be argued that the improved survival time observed in the BCG clinical trials in canine osteosarcoma and mammary carcinoma may in part be due to a non-specific recruitment and activation of NK cells. Indeed this has already been demonstrated in mouse (31), rat (32) and human (33) systems. To investigate this question in the dog a series of experimental animals were immunised with either intravenous or intrapleural BCG over a period of 32 weeks on the previously described clinical schedule (9-11). The results indicated that both intravenous and intrapleural BCG injections increased NK cell activity against an individual NK sensitive allogeneic osteosarcoma cell line, but there was no dramatic overall increase in NK cell activity (34). In further experiments it was shown that NK stimulation by intravenous BCG was reproducible. However specificity for neoplastic cells was not found as normal contact inhibited canine kidney cells were also lysed (26 and Betton, unpublished data). This highlighted the controversy on the importance of NK cells in the control of neoplasia and failed to provide irrefutable evidence that the efficacy of BCG therapy was mediated via an NK cell mechanism.

Alveolar macrophage cytotoxicity

Increasing attention has been afforded to the mononuclear phagocytes, firstly in tumour surveillance and secondly as a potent tumouricidal effector mechanism (35,36). The identification of serum factors in tumour patients which adversely affect macrophage activation has further focused interest on this cell type (37). In the light o the inconclusive lymphocytotoxicity results it was of paramount importance to examine the macrophage cytotoxic potential from normal and BCG stimulated dogs.

It was consistently found in both experimentally and clinically treated dogs that diffuse hepatic and pulmonary granulomata were present following intravenous BCG treatment, these comprised large accumulations of mononuclear phagocytes (9-11, 34,38 A direct postulate from these observations was that associated with the pulmonary granulomata was a pool of non-specifically activated macrophages with the potential t destroy a percentage of pulmonary metastatic cells. This mechanism would account for the described delayed appearance of pulmonary metastases in canine osteosarcoma and mammary carcinoma cases.

Alveolar macrophages were harvested by lung lavage based on the technique of Myrvi (39) and the heterogeneous cell population purified by adherence to plastic; this resulted in a 95 - 99% pure macrophage monolayer (38). Such cell populations were collected from a series of normal and BCG-stimulated dogs and used in the ^{51}Cr releas assay, previously outlined, except that effector:target cell ratios were limited to 80:1 40:1 20:1 10:1.

The results in Tables 4 and 5 clearly indicate that alveolar macrophages isolated from normal dogs did not kill the allogeneic cells whereas those from BCG stimulated lungs were highly cytolytic.

Table 4 Specific cytotoxicity of alveolar macrophages from normal and BCG stimulate dogs

| Target cell | Specific cytotoxicity. Effector:target ratio 80:1 | | | | | | | |
| | 4 hrs | | | | 8 hrs | | | |
	A77	A78	A79	A80	A77	A78	A79	A8
H72-1503 osteosarcoma	22.0	2.7	24.0	4.4	31.0	0.2	28.7	0.
RVC-347 melanoma	23.9	0.9	24.8	0.0	35.5	5.0	39.5	0.
MDCK normal kidney	12.2	1.8	17.8	0.5	19.7	4.0	25.0	0.

A77 and A79 received two intravenous BCG injections; A78 and A80 received two placeb (saline) injections. Macrophages were collected 14 days following final immunisatio

Table 5 Specific cytotoxicity of alveolar macrophages from normal and BCG-stimulated
dogs

Specific cytotoxicity 8 hrs. Effector:target ratio 80:1

Target cell	D1	D3	D5	D7	D2	D4	D6	D8
H73-2295 mammary carcinoma	38.9	35.3	58.2	44.0	3.2	3.1	0.5	1.3
MDCK normal kidney line	28.5	12.1	40.1	27.0	0.9	1.4	0.0	0.8
H71-1843 melanoma	40.9	13.9	58.5	29.0	1.7	2.9	1.4	0.0
H72-1503 osteosarcoma	50.6	24.3	58.3	27.8	3.1	2.0	0.7	2.5

D1, D3, D5 and D7 received 3 intravenous BCG injections. D2, D4, D6 and D8 received
3 intravenous saline injections. Macrophages isolated 25 days after final immunisation.

The persistence of antigen in vivo has been suggested as a pre-requisite for the
maintenance of macrophage activation (40). Whether this is a function of continual
re-stimulation of the alveolar macrophages or a function of the pool of infiltrating
monocytes associated with the turnover of macrophages within the granulomata, remains
unresolved. It was obvious that following recent injections of BCG non-specifically
activated macrophages would be demonstrated, but the data in Table 6 indicate that
in the absence of regular restimulation the cytolytic potential of alveolar macrophages
is considerably reduced or absent.

Table 6 Specific cytotoxicity of alveolar macrophages from dogs which received
multiple BCG injections

Specific cytotoxicity 8 hrs. Effector:target ratio 80:1

Target cell	Intravenous BCG		Intrapleural BCG	
	A10	A19	A14	A20
H71-1843	0.6	N.D.	0.3	N.D.
H73-2295	0.0	N.D.	1.3	N.D.
H72-1563	0.6	0	0.9	0
RVC-347	N.D.	0	N.D.	0

A10 received 6 intravenous BCG injections. Macrophages collected 14 weeks after last
injection. A14 received 6 intrapleural BCG injections. Macrophages collected 14 weeks
after last injection. A19 received 7 intravenous BCG injections. Macrophages collected 10 weeks after last injection. A20 received 7 intrapleural BCG injections.
Macrophages collected 10 weeks after last injection.

Similar increased alveolar macrophage cytolytic activity has been demonstrated
following intravenous BCG associated with alloimmunisation experiments (34) and following intravenous C.parvum (41). A critical feature of all these experiments has been
the inability to show selective killing of allogeneic tumour cell lines. This lack of
selectivity, as with NK cell killing is of obvious concern when considering the

112

importance of tumouricidal effector mechanisms. However, as the normal canine kidney line has been in culture for two decades the term "normal" may be an over-statement, though it has been shown to differ from the allogeneic neoplastic lines as defined by Con A receptor mobility (20).

CONCLUSIONS

In the described therapy system the stimulation of alveolar macrophages by BCG produced a potent cytocidal effector mechanism. It would seem appropriate to propose that the principle effector mechanism in this intravenous BCG therapy is via a pool of non-specifically activated macrophages associated with the development and main-tenance of granulomatous lesions within the lung.

This form of BCG therapy has limited application both in man and the domestic animals. It is now generally accepted that non-specific immune mechanisms rather than specific were operative in this system (42). Attempts to specifically enhance the antigenicity of very weak tumour antigens may provide some form of rational immuno-therapy protocols (43, 44). The results of clinical trials based on this principle are awaited with interest.

REFERENCES

1 Kurth R., Fenyö E.M., Klein E. & Essex M. (1979). Nature 279, 197-201.

2 Baldwin R.W. (1973). Adv. Cancer Res. 18, 1-75.

3 Hellström K.E. & Brown J.P. (1979). In The Antigens, V p.2-82. Ed. Sela M. Pub. Academic Press.

4 Herberman R.B. (1977). Biochem.Biophys. Acta 473, 93-119.

5 Bast R.L., Zbar B., Borsos T. & Rapp H.J. (1974). New Eng. J. Med. 290, 1413-1420

6 Bast R.L., Zbar B., Borsos T. & Rapp H.J. (1974). New Eng. J. Med. 290, 1458-1469

7 Laucius J.F., Bodurtha M.J., Mastrangelo M.J. & Greech R.H. (1974). J. Reticuloendoth. Soc. 14, 347-373.

8 Hesh E.M., Gutterman J.U. & Mavligit G.M. (1977). Ann. Rev. Med. 28, 489-515.

9 Owen L.N. & Bostock D.E. (1974). Europ. J. Cancer 10, 775-780.

10 Owen L.N., Bostock D.E. & Lavelle R.B. (1977). Amer. Vet. Radiol. Sco. 18, 27-29.

11 Bostock D.E. & Gorman N.T. (1978). Europ. J. Cancer 14, 879-883.

12 Bostock D.E. (1975). Europ. J. Cancer 11, 389-396.

13 Warren R.P., Tsoi M.S., Henderson B.H., Weiden P.L. & Storb R. (1975). Transpl. Proc. 7, 481-484.

14 Ulvand M.J. (1975). Acta Vet. Scand. 16, 95-114.

15 Tsoi M.S., Weiden P.L. & Storb R. (1976). J. Immunol. 116, 1134-1139.

16 Fidler I.J., Brodey R.S. & Bech-Nielsen S. (1974). J. Immunol. 3, 375-380.

17 Warren R.P., Tsoi M.S., Henderson B.H. & Storb R. (1975). Transpl. Proc. 7, 481-4

18 Betton G.R. & Gorman N.T. (1978). J. Natl. Cancer Inst. 61, 1085-1093.

19 Gorman N.T. & Betton G.R. (1978). J. Natl. Cancer Inst. 61, 1095-1100.

20 Betton G.R. (1976). Int. J. Cancer 18, 687-696.

REVIEW OF CURRENT LEGISLATION IN VETERINARY PHARMACOLOGY AND TOXICOLOGY

DECLAN S. WHITE

Veterinary Research Laboratory, Abbotstown, Castleknock, Co. Dublin (Ireland)

ABSTRACT

Current EEC legislation applying to medicines is reviewed and proposed legislation is discussed. References are made to non-Community legislation; e.g. Convention on the elaboration of a European Pharmacopoeia.

INTRODUCTION

I am very grateful to the organisers of this Congress for inviting me to present a paper on current legislation on veterinary pharmacology and toxicology. As most of the legislation with which I shall deal is international in character it is fitting that this first Congress should be held in the country which produced Hugo Grotius who is known as the Father of the Law of Nations.

I see my task today as setting the stage for the next three speakers but before getting down to the practical aspects of legislation it may be no harm to glance at the development of law in its historical context. Broadly we can divide European historical development into three main eras-the era of the Greek city states, the era of the Empire, and the era of the modern state. The somewhat short lived era of the Greek city states with their own ideas of what constituted a state is well described by Aristotle in the Politics. This early concept of the state as a compact grouping of people with certain compatibilities tended to be obliterated by the development of the idea of the empire under the Romans followed at a later date by the concept of the Holy Roman Empire after the decline of Rome. It is only in the last few hundred years that the ancient idea of the state came to the fore again and that nationality became such a dominant force.

The Romans while attempting to make their own idea of law supreme in their vast empire nevertheless recognised local law and custom and categorised law into _ius civile_ which applied to citizens of Rome and _ius gentium_ which was an amalgam of local and Roman law. To me it seems that the Community is very much in the same position as ancient Rome and in attempting to make Community law is finding the same difficulties which faced the Roman law givers.

Among international lawyers it is to some extent accepted that the Peace Treaty of Westphalia in 1648 is the first example of an international agreement, and while it might be of interest to trace the progress of both national and inter-national law since that date I can only deal with the practical aspects of such developments. The somewhat divergent growths of the legal systems in the British Isles and the Continent could, I think, have some effect on Community law. I say in the British Isles because the law as it now stands in Ireland owes very little, if anything, to the ancient Brehon laws of the Gael but is to a great extent a replica or at least a reflection of British law.

The divergence to which I refer is the twin growth in Britain of statute or coded law in concert with common law in which precedent is of the utmost importance as opposed to the more unified growth in Continental law where coded law is of the essence. However as I am dealing with coded law today there is no need to devote any time to precedent except to say that when national laws are brought into existence in concordance with Directives which are binding on all the states of the Community it could happen in either Britain or Ireland that the rules of precedent might effect the outcome of a case.

INTERPRETATION OF STATUTES

The interpretation of statutes is of extreme importance to anyone who is involved in giving advice on new legislation either nationally at home or internationally in the Community. There are two main rules which seem straightforward enough: (1) the literal rule-that is that if the meaning of the section is plain it is to be applied whatever the result. This brings to mind the old adage-when you go to law you get law but not necessarily justice!
(2) the golden rule-that the words should be given their ordinary sense unless that would lead to some absurdity or inconsistence with the rest of the instrument. These are two extremely important rules and throw a great responsibility on the legislator. Anyone who has had experience in either trying to interpret laws or help in their promulgation knows just how difficult it is to get exact meaning from or into words. The difficulties are magnified at Community level when one is dealing with translations no matter how good the translation. The nuance of a word can be of extreme importance and almost impossible to get over in a Community of varying cultural back-ground.

CURRENT LEGISLATION

The Convention for the mutual recognition of inspections in respect of the manufacture of pharmaceutical products is not a Community instrument and as far as I know it has not been signed by any of the original six only the three latter members being signatories.

It applies only to medicines for humans and the only reason for mentioning it today is that I think that both the Directive on proprietary medicines (65/65/EEC) and the proposed Directive on veterinary medicines are very weak on this important question.   There has been some discussion at Council level but I am not satisfied that any real solution has been propounded.

The Convention on the elaboration of a European Pharmacopoeia is not a Community convention but has been promulgated in the Council of Europe.   The signatories to this convention agree that the monographs of the Convention will be binding in their respective countries but I am not at all sure if the Convention applies to veterinary as well as human medicines.   The Convention uses the simple term medicines and whether this covers both veterinary and human medicines is not at all clear from any internal evidence in the document.   The proposed Directive on analytical, pharmaco-toxicological and clinical standards and protocols in respect of the testing of veterinary medicinal products says that veterinary drugs must be of the Convention standard but at Council level the French delegation questioned if this could be maintained on economic grounds for all products.

It could be argued that the three Directives on human proprietary medicines which for the sake of brevity can be termed* (65/65, 75/318, and 75/319), are not very germane to this discussion but as the proposed veterinary Directives are modelled on the human Directives and almost slavishly follow them a few words are necessary. The main reason why the proposed veterinary Directives are modelled on the human ones is for the benefit of the manufacturers who produce both human and veterinary medicines and also to make the task of the legislators easier!   These are, I must admit, reasonably cogent arguments and ones with which I could agree if the veterinary Directives were to cover only proprietary veterinary medicines.   But as the veterinary Directive is to cover all veterinary medicines I think that some of the provisions are rather Draconian.

Some of the weakest aspects of the human Directives are to be found in Chapter IV on manufacturers and imports from third countries.   I am strongly of the opinion that there should be separate chapters on imports from third countries in both Directives.

Before I get down to the Directives of purely veterinary interest I must say a few words on the Court of Justice of the European Communities case 104/76 which has become known as the Centrafarm case.   I approach this subject with some trepidation as I am not at all sure that I understand the full ramifications of it!   While the findings of the Court are not a direct attack on Directive 65/65 it reminds me somewhat of the well known Ruy Lopez opening in chess where the attack is not directly on the King but usually in the end it is the King who suffers.

---

* Full titles of all legislation are contained in the references.

Very briefly the Court found that Dutch national law was in breach of Article 30 of the Treaty of Rome and that Article 36 of the same Treaty was not a sufficient defence.   The Dutch authorities had refused to licence the import of a well known human product on the grounds that the importer did not produce a dossier in conformity with Dutch law.   This Dutch law in my opinion conformed to articles 3 and 4 of 65/65.

As a Directive is a binding instrument it would seem that Dutch national law was in conformity with the Directive as it should be.   Therefore it seems to me that the finding of the Court indirectly invalidates Articles 3 and 4 of the Directive. As I said earlier when you go to Court you get LAW so it seems that Directives may not be fully sacroscant any more than any national law which is found repugnant to a country's constitution.

And so we finally come to the current veterinary Directives - 74/63 concerning undesirable substances in feedingstuffs and 70/54 concerning feed additives.   I think it is fair to say that 74/63 is of little veterinary interest and so I will only deal with 70/524.   The veterinary importance of this Directive is that it deals with certain veterinary additives which are really medicines, although the amounts permitted are small.   I had hoped that these products would in time be transferred to the Directive on veterinary medicines as this would seem to be a logical step.   But such does not seem to be the case.   Article 1(3) of the Veterinary Directive clearly states that 70/524 is not to be interfered with. The argument is that the promulgation of 70/524 with all its successive amendments required so much work that any fundamental alterations in its structure would be a retrograde step.   Knowing the amount of work that has gone into this Directive I have some sympathy with that view.   There has been one development in this Directive over the last few years that seems to me to have posed as many problems as the ones it has solved.   I refer here to the appointment of a Scientific Committee supernumerary to the Committee of experts.   If it takes two scientific committees to service this Directive which deals with such a limited number of veterinary drugs I dread to think how many committees will be required to service the veterinary Directive when it comes into being!

An aspect of the working of this Directive which, I think, should be looked at is the means whereby a new additive is accepted into the annexes.   At present a Delegation from one of the nine countries must act as rapporteur and it seems to me that a company should have some other means of having a product submitted and processed.   If no delegation is prepared to undertake the very unenviable job of rapporteur it seems that a company has no other means of having its product examined

PROPOSED LEGISLATION

So we finally come to the three proposed Directives-veterinary medicines, norms and protocols, and medicated feedingstuffs.   Proposed seems to be the operative word! This time last year I was convinced that the first two at least would be operable within a year. But now I am not prepared to venture any date. I think that one is entitled to be a little disheartened after two years of intensive work at Council level to see the promulgation of the directives delayed for an indefinite period. However there is still a lot to be said about them and I suppose I must say it even if my enthusiasm is somewhat dimmed.

The Directives have come in for quite a lot of adverse criticism much of which I think is justified. However, I think it is necessary to consider the preamble to the Directives before being too critical because it seems to me that if one accepts the preamble then the Directives follow logically from it. The preamble clearly states that the primary purpose must be the safeguarding of public health which objective must be achieved by means which will not hinder the development of industry and trade in medicinal products. This is to me a very clear case of wishful thinking as the two purposes must by their very nature be often in opposition. I am further perturbed by the preamble as a veterinary surgeon as in its two pages there is only one reference to animal health where it is stated that marketing authorization shall be refused where a medicinal product lacks therapeutic effect.

However if one accepts that the safeguarding of public health is the raison d'etre for these Directives then I must admit that the Directives are a logical sequent whatever faults are to be found in particular articles.

Adverse criticism of the Directives comes from two main camps-practising veterinary surgeons who find certain articles too restrictive and manufacturers who find certain articles too constrictive! Veterinary surgeons were particularly perturbed by Article 2(2d) of the first Directive which stated that the Directive did not apply to veterinary medicinal products not prepared in advance and intended for ONE particular animal. This to them was a very definite restriction on the freedom to prescribe products which might be deemed essential in the treatment of a group of animals and which had to be prepared in a hurry. Fortunately after a great battle there has been some relaxation in this Article and ONE particular animal has been extended to a small group of animals. A new Article 2a is also a further advance in that Member States may permit exemptions in respect of products intended solely for aquarium fish, cage birds, homing pigeons, terrarium animals and small rodents.

I come now to what I consider is the weakest piece of legislation in the Directive, Article 3(2) which states that no product may be administered to animals unless an authorisation has been issued. This is a classical example of Montesquieu's quip, "Les lois inutiles affaiblissent les necessaire". The article is bad on two counts. From the veterinary surgeon's point of view it clearly means that he cannot use a human product unless such product is authorised under this Directive! From the point of view of the Competent Authority it is obviously unenforcable.

It would take an army of inspectors making almost continuous swoops on farms!
I would hate to be an officer of the Competent Authority in Ireland who instituted
proceedings against a farmer for giving 'Poitin' (a highly illegal home brew) to
a calf for a "chill on the stomach".   I would be laughed out of court!   A later
speaker will deal with the whole problem of the use of human products in animals.
Here it suffices for me to say that Council has finally agreed that the Article
shall not be constructed as prohibiting the prescription of human products in animal
which are not a source of food.   Council also recognises that full enforcement
by the Competent Authority is not possible.

Today I cannot deal with all the outstanding problems and have to concentrate on
the more important ones.   A major problem has been the definition of the pre-mix
and how pre-mixes are to be controlled.   This has not been solved and I think that
the solution is to transfer the pre-mix to the proposed Directive on medicated
feedingstuffs.

I have little to say about the manufacturers' criticisms not because I don't
sympathise with them but their objections are more to the Directive as a whole
rather than specific Articles.   They argue, and I think correctly, that a number
of products will disappear from the market and that some of these will indeed leave
the veterinary surgeon less competent to deal with certain disease conditions.

I have nothing worthwhile to report on the second Directive as there are no
outstanding disagreements.   This is not to say that certain aspects of the Directive
are beyond criticism.   I think that it is fair to say that the format is very poor
and that an index would be a great help.   I will myself be very interested to hear
what Professor Grunsell will have to say about Part 3 on clinical trials as
compared with the Medicines Act.

I am not going to deal with the proposed Directive on medicated feedingstuffs
for two reasons.   Firstly I don't think that there can be any developments in
it until after promulgation of the other two Directives.   Secondly the Directive
is still at Commission level and so many divergent views have already been
expressed that agreement on a draft is very much in the future.

While I have aired some of the worst aspects of the Directives I have to say in
fairness that with the brief handed to them the Commission has done a good job.
I think it is no small miracle that so much agreement has been obtained from
delegations from such varying backgrounds and who were to a great extent
constrained by their own national legislation.

To conclude I think I can say that whatever else this paper has done it has at
least exemplified the quotation from Edmund Burke- "Laws, like houses, lean on
each other".

REFERENCES

Current Legislation

Treaty establishing the European Economic Community (1957)

Convention for the mutual recognition of inspections in respect of the manufacture of pharmaceutical products (1971)

Convention on the elaboration of a European Pharmacopoeia (1964)

Council Directive on the approximation of provisions laid down by law, regulation or administrative action relating to proprietary medicinal products (65/65/EEC)

Second Council Directive on the approximation of provisions laid down by law, regulation or administrative action relating to proprietary medicinal products (75/319/EEC)

Council Directive on the approximation of the laws of Member States relating to analytical, pharmaco-toxicological and clinical standards and protocols in respect of the testing of proprietary medicinal products (75/318/EEC)

Council Directive concerning additives in feeding-stuffs (70/524/EEC)

Council Directive on the fixing of maximum permitted levels for undesirable substances and products in feedingstuffs (74/63/EEC)

Court of Justice of the European Communities; Case 104/76 (Centrafarm)

Proposed Legislation

A Directive on the approximation of the Laws of Member States on Veterinary medicinal products.

A Directive on analytical, pharmaco-toxicological and clinical standards and protocols in respect of the testing of veterinary medicinal products.

A Directive on the approximation of the laws of the Member States on medicated feedingstuffs.

RESIDUE PROBLEMS

S. BUNTENKÖTTER

Institut für Pharmakologie, Toxikologie und Pharmazie
der Tierärztlichen Hochschule Hannover, Hannover (G.F.R.)+

ABSTRACT

Legislative aspects, primary and secondary toxicity as well as
residue problems of substances and metabolites are reviewed.

The Dutch formula for evaluating residues in edible subtrates
of domestic animals, the modification of the formula and calculation
principles are discussed.

Furthermore the threshold assessment of FDA is submitted.

INTRODUCTIONARY REMARKS

Residue problems under the topic legislation are now relevant, because
many regulations in the European countries and in oversea have come
into force.

In this field legislative aspects can be distinguished generally
in different areas:

1. The European Community (EC)
2. Eastern Europe and the neutral countries
3. The United States of America
4. Developing and other countries

This paper can only deal with national conditions in the Federal
Republic of Germany by the means of presenting an example for legislation, especially basing on the guideline 65/65 and other regulation

On the other hand an attempt should be made to explain the scientific background for evaluating residues for animal-derived food
safety comparising the usual formulas with the threshold assessment
of the Food and Drug Administration (FDA) presented 1978 at the
Relay Toxicity and Residue Bioavailability Symposium in Paris (ref. 3

After realizing all guidelines of the common market EC into national legislation to day yields the following situation in Germany:

+D - 3ooo Hannover 71, Bünteweg 17

1. A decree of limits for DDT and other pesticides for animal-derived food
2. A special law for the trade with food, tobacco, cosmetics and other articles of consumption
3. A special law for feedstuffs
4. A decree for substances with special pharmacological actions
5. The law for the trade with drugs
6. Some special decrees concerning drugs used only for formulated feedstuffs.

All these regulations result on the legal conception , that an effective control of the use of drugs and feed additives has not to start only at the end of the production chaine. It has to be set up rather before the approval during the INAD = investigational new animal drug. An approval should only be given after submission and under careful evaluation of all relevant toxicological criteria to prevent misuse and potential hazards.

PRIMARY AND SECONDARY TOXICITY

Principly it has to be differentiated between primary and secondary toxicity of drugs and feed additives. Their significance in food and the production-chaine has to be eluciated.

Whereas the primary toxicity characterizes the properties of the unchanged or metabolized substance in the treated animal (target species), the secondary toxicity is directed by the evaluation of possible risks and therefore for the safety of individuals, man or animal, consuming food or feed, coming from animal production. Relay toxicity and induced toxicity are synonyms,to which certain testing systems are attributed.

The question of secondary toxicity gained interest for the first time after the publication of EICHHOLTZ (ref. 4), who focused our attention on the overall toxicological situation in the field of human nutrition. Simultaneous impulses arose from plant protection. The investigation of relay toxicity enables us to a certain degree to evaluate possible anthropotoxic effects.

This testing sytem examines the effect of residues coming from the drug itself, from not identified (or identifiable) metabolites and therefore from the entire residue pattern.

This method can be especially helpful in evaluating substances, whose residues and overall efficiency can not or only hardly be judged seperately from those of substances like hormones or related drugs. The relay toxicity is conducted in long term and sometimes

together with multigeneration trials with laboratory animals which
fulfill the function of (pseudo) consumers of residue contaminated
material, e.g. of donor animals.

The modell of relay toxicity imitates therefore the natural chaine
of contamination (ref. 12).

Medical precursors, without creating a special definition, can
be found in the works of BRÜGGEMANN and coworkers (ref. 1; ref. 2).

By FERRANDO (ref. 5) it is possible to regard the farm animal as
an active part of relaying additive to the consumer. Thereby the
passage through this relay may completely alter the fate of the
additive as a result of metabolic reactions to the ingested compound
within the relay itself.

Thus the relaying agent may accumulate, metabolize and give an
increasing effect to total metabolites and nutrient metabolite complexes which are difficult, if not impossible, to determine exactly.

Therefore it is the overall toxicity of these groups and complexes
which may be evaluated by the so-called relay toxicity method (ref. 5)

IMPACT ON LEGISLATION

The permission of drugs and feed-additives, the establishing of
withdrawal-times and tolerances in controlling both feed and food
are the predominant measures of legislations to rule the modalities
for the food-producing animals, with the aim to guarantee the human
and animal health and to ban illegal trade and application of drugs
and feed-additives.

Sometimes it looks that officialy regulators of animal drugs are
chaising single molecules of a residue compound.

PROBLEMS OF SUBSTANCES AND METABOLITES

The following factors should be emphasized for the safety evaluation
of tissues from domestic animals and other edible substrates:

1. The intact effective substance (mother substance)
2. The nonpoisonous or poisonous metabolic compounds
3. The total quantity of effective substances and metabolites
   remaining in meat or other substrates
4. The half-life of residues

Until now little attention has been given to the fact that not
only a single effective substance may be present, but a drug or a
pesticide and/or its metabolites may occur in the presence of other
substances in meat or other tissues and substrates like milk and
eggs. An animal may have been treated simultaneously with any kind

of chemicals from medication up to food additives.

A human being may consume such a residue or residue mixtures not only acute but in the case of accumulating substances and the resulting endogen reservoir an interaction of the different residues has to be considered.

There is also little knowledge available about the effects of the interaction of substances which may accidentally encounter. The difficulties in estimating the possible hazard is limited by the uncertain factors under practical conditions.

Factors of insecurities cannot be eliminated completely even with the attempt to enforce protection rules by laws. Nevertheless the goal must be to continue establishing maximum security to the consumer in protecting public health. So far, the questions dealing with the concurrence of several active substances ranging from therapeutic substances to food-preserving mixtures are completely obscure. These are the problems that ought to be given far closer attention in the future.

CRITERIA FOR RESIDUE PROBLEMS

The commonly used formula for the limitation of tolerable quantities was inaugurated by VAN GENDEREN (ref. 14) in the frame of plant protection. There are no objections for applying these formulas for residues in meat also (ref. 11), but the animal test for establishing the no-effect-level must not necessary give representative values for the human being. However, it is supported by the requirement that two animal species have to be included in these tests.

In detail the dutch formula reads:

$$\text{Permissible level} = \frac{\text{ADI} \times 70 \text{ kg} \times 1000}{400 \text{ g}} \quad (1)$$

The formula arbitrarily presupposes an average body weight of 70 kg and a food intake of 400 gs of foodstuff daily per individual.

No account is taken of the different quantities of intake and the sensitivity of some people such as children, pregnant woman and nursing mothers. In consideration these groups HÖTZEL established in 1965 (ref. 7) a so-called child protecting factor. This induced the first modification and simplification of the formula. Including the safety factor 2,5 (child protection factor) the calculation of the permissible level follows the formula:

$$\text{Permissible level} \atop (PL) = \frac{\text{ADI} \times 7o \text{ kg} \times 1ooo}{4oo \text{ g} \times 2,5} \qquad (2)$$

$$PL = \text{ADI} \times 7o \qquad (3)$$

Calculation of the permissible level using the factor for child protection permitts us to equate the numerical values for the acceptable daily intake (ADI) in mg per person with the permissible level (PL) of residues in ppm (ref. 9).

KAEMMERER (ref. 9) offered in this context a second modification to increase the safety and to enlarge the adaptability for special metabolic conditions:

Replacing the absolute body weight into the metabolic body weight (kg ^{o,75}) considers metabolic processes and gives a more adequate measurement which contains a greater range of safety.

On this way an average body weight of 7o kg is transformed to a metabolic body weight of 24 kg (7o ^{o,75} = 24,2o). (Fig. 1)

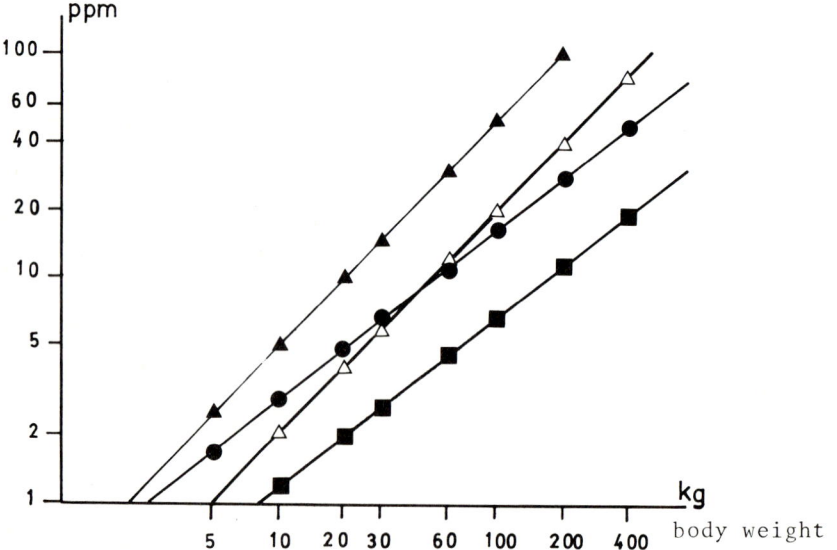

▲ = Permissible Level (PL)
△ = PL including Child Protection Factor (CPF)
● = PL metabolic
■ = PL metabolic incl. CPF

Fig. 1   Relation between Permissible Level and body weight
          (KAEMMERER, 1976) basing on an Acceptable Daily Intake
          (ADI) of o,o2 mg/kg

This replacing also permits coordination with the development of every individual person. Accordingly, the acceptable daily intake (ADI) in mg/kg bw, multiplied with the metabolic body weight yields the corresponding value for the permissible level.

Another reference system is required by KAEMMERER (ref. 9) for antibacterial substances since the tolerance formulas also take into account the acute toxicity. A permissible antibacterial level needs to be introduced stating the test strain, for example permissible antibacterial level$_{E.coli}$ in ppm.

To demontrate the relationship among the calculation values in this connection the following table is shown (cited by KAEMMERER, ref. 6 and 1oa) with a fictive no-effect-level of 1 mg/kg body weight.

$$ADI = \frac{x}{1oo} = o,o1 \text{ mg/kg body weight} = o,7o \text{ mg man}$$

$$PL = \frac{ADI \times 7o \times 1ooo}{4oo \times 2,5} = o,7o \text{ ppm}$$

effective intake (man)   = o,35 mg
effective intake (per kg man) = o,oo5 mg

$$PL_{met} = ATD \times 24 = o,24 \text{ mg/man}$$

effective intake (man)   = o,12 mg
effective intake (man per kg) = o,o17 mg

In account of cancerogenic substances the usually accepted Mantel-Bryan-factor of 2ooo has to be considered (ref. 13). Regarding the metabolic body weight one has to divide the no-effect-level:

$$\frac{\text{No-effect-level}}{2ooo} = \frac{1}{2ooo} = o,ooo5 \text{ mg/kg body weight} = o,o35 \text{ mg/man}$$

$$PL_{2ooo} = o,o35 \text{ ppm}$$

$$PL_{met_{2ooo}} = o,o121 \text{ ppm}$$

In that way, for a human being as a meat consumer the risk of residue is considerably diminished.

However, there is one restriction: all these tolerance figures are given in such a way as thought the confrontation only takes place with a single active substance. The possible interaction of different residues is thereby neglected.

The American point of view inaugurated last autumn in Paris by Mrs. CORDLE (FDA) considers the probability that a drug will yield edible tissue residues that may present a risk of human carcinogenesis (Tables 1 - 4). A function of three factors, so-called score factors, is postulated.

Score factor (1): The use of the compound as this affects the frequency to which humans may exposed to food from an animal receiving the drug.

Score factor (2): The amount of residue in the tissue to which humans will be exposed if they consume food from animal administered the drug under the proposed conditions of use.

Score factor (3): The probable biological significance of exposure as judged by an assessment of the structure of the drug and evaluation of any relevant information for predicting biological activity of the drug or its expected metabolites, including in vitro screening tests.

Three use classes are applied for score factor 1:

A: Production use and general disease prevention

B: Specific disease prevention and general therapy

C: Specific therapy

It is expected that there is at least a ten-fold difference among the classes A - C concerning the probable frequency to which the consumer will be exposed to food from animals treated with the drug. Therefore a log scale assignment of values is applied, for class A 1oo, for class B 1o and for class C 1.

The score factor 2 expresses the concentration of residue in parts per billion (ppb) and the total residue is ranged from o,1 - 1ooo ppb.

For score factor 3 one should serve three sources of information: structure and activity assessment; biological and pharmacological data and short-term screening tests for carcinogenic potential.

1, 1o and 1oo are the possible values, which grant a score range equivalent to score factor 1.

Only when the evidence from all three criteria shows no reason to suspect carcinogenic activity a score of 1 is assigned.

If an appropriate battery of screening tests for carcinogenic potential have not been conducted, and there is no basis suspecting carcinogenic activity based on the other sources of knowledge a score of 1o is assigned. Last not least a score of 1oo is determined if there is an evidence from any of the sources of information that raises a suspicion that the residues may be carcinogenic (ref. 3).

The next four tables show the threshold assessment with the different factors including the maximum residue to release drug from carcinogenicity test requirements by CORDLE (ref. 3).

In table four the multivariable interdependence is demonstrated.

Table 1   Threshold assessment (CORDLE, 1978)

Score Factor 1

Class A: Production and general
           Disease prevention

Class B: Specific disease prevention
           General therapy

Class C: Specific therapy

Table 2   Threshold assessment (CORDLE, 1978)

Factor 1 -   Frequency of human exposure
              Use classification

Factor 2 -   Amount of human exposure
              Total residue

Factor 3 -   Biological significance
              Structure assessment
              Biological activity
              In vitro test battery

Table 3   Threshold assessment - Score factor 3 (CORDLE, 1978)

Structure/ activity	Biological/ pharmacological	In vitro screening	Score value
+	(+ or -)	(+ or -)	1oo
-	+	(+ or -)	1oo
-	-	+	1oo
-	-	(no data)	1o
-	-	-	1

Table 4   Maximum residue to release drug from carcinogenicity
           test requirements

(Factor 2) Total residue ppb	(Factor 3) Structure/ biological score	Use score
1000	1	1
100	1o	1
	1	1o
1o	1oo	1
	1o	1o
	1	1oo
1	1oo	1o
	1o	1oo
o.1	1oo	1oo

FINAL REMARKS

Despite of numerous attempts of a statistical calculation based on
international established criteria, applying highly varying safety
factors, the main question of the pharmacological and toxicological
problem, which concentration of residues absolutely excludes any
harmful risk for the consumer has not been solved up to date (ref.1ob)

However, the validity of the calculation methods used so far,
cannot be denied until a really better basis for the evaluation of
the residual risk is developed.

Applying the usual and modified calculation systems one should
be conscious that the value of such calculation is restricted by
its single factor perspective.

Moreover there is to recognize that multifactorial stress situation
like a Wirkstoffrendezvous (rendez-vous of active substances, ref. 8,
ref. 11) as well as conventional coefficients and transformation
risks cannot be measured with the desired accuracy. This must be
recognized also under legislative aspects.

REFERENCES

1   BRÜGGEMANN, J. et al., 196o:
    Generationsversuche an Ratten zur Frage ernährungstoxikologi-
    scher Aspekte von Hühnerfleisch, das aus der Methylthiouracil-
    Mast stammt.
    Institutsseparatum

2   BRÜGGEMANN, J. et al., 1961:
    Arzneimittel Forschg. 11, 1o22

3   CORDLE, M.K., 1978:
When is a Residue a Residue?
Relay Toxicity and Residues Bioavailability Symposium,
Paris, October 5, 1978

4   EICHHOLTZ, F., 1956:
Die toxische Gesamtsituation auf dem Gebiete der menschlichen
Ernährung.
Springer Verlag, Heidelberg

5   FERRANDO, R., 1977:
Folia Vet. Lat. 7, 183

6   FINK, J., 1978:
Der praktische Tierarzt 59, 974

7   HÖTZEL, D., 1965:
Arzneimittel Forschg. 15, 573

8   KAEMMERER, K., 1966:
Die Bedeutung von unbekannten Metaboliten von Feed Additives
für die Gesundheit des Nutztieres und Lebensmittelverbrauchers.
Ber. Internat. Ern. Kongress Hamburg (publ. 1967)

9   KAEMMERER, K., 1976:
Dtsch. Tierärztl. Wschr. 83, 6

1oa   KAEMMERER, K., 1978:
see FINK, 1978 (ref. 6)

1ob   KAEMMERER, K., 1978:
Beiträge zur Problematik von Stoffen mit pharmakologischer
Wirkung in Nahrungs- und Futtermitteln.
DLG-Verlag, Frankfurt

11   KAEMMERER, K. and S. BUNTENKÖTTER, 1973:
The problem of residues in meat of edible domestic animals
after application or intake of organophosphate esters.
Residue Reviews 46,
Springer-Verlag, New York

12   KAEMMERER, K. and J. GROPP, 1976:
Studie zur Problematik der Durchführung chronischer Toxizitäts-
tests unter Berücksichtigung der Relais-Toxizität.
Institutsseparatum

13   MANTEL, N. and W.R. BRYAN, 1961:
J. National Cancer Inst. 27, 455

14   VAN GENDEREN, H., 1960:
Bull. Inst. Agron. Stat. Récherche Gembloux, Hors
Série 3, 1233

THE USE OF HUMAN MEDICINAL PRODUCTS IN SMALL ANIMAL VETERINARY PRACTICE IN THE U.K.

A.T. YOXALL

Department of Clinical Veterinary Medicine, University of Cambridge (U.K.)

ABSTRACT

A survey was conducted into the use of human ethical preparations by small animal practitioners in the U.K. Of 321 products used in 60 practices, the majority were topical products (especially ophthalmic products) and agents for control of gastro-intestinal function. Many of the products used were selected because they were simpler and safer than veterinary equivalent products, or because no veterinary equivalent existed for essential products such as cardiac glucosides.

INTRODUCTION

Concern has been expressed in recent years over the exposure of the public to drugs and other substances present in meat. The concept has arisen that one means of controlling such undesirable exposure would be to limit the use of medicinal substances in animals to those agents whose behaviour in particular species has been studied in some detail. Under such a scheme the use of any medicinal product for any purpose and in any fashion not detailed in the manufacturer's literature, as approved by the registration authority, would be banned.

If such a concept is to be proposed, it is important that accurate information should be available on the extent to which medicinal products are used for indications other than those for which they are registered. In the case of human ethical medicaments, which are known to be used widely in small animal practice in the U.K., it would seem additionally worthwhile to gather information on clinical usage in order to assess how such medicaments are used, what side effects have been observed, and whether any novel indications have been developed which might be worthy of further study. Accordingly, the Association for Veterinary Clinical Pharmacology and Therapeutics conducted a survey into the use of human ethical products in small animal practice in the U.K.

A pilot study in 20 practices suggested that the use of human ethical products was sufficiently widespread to justify a large scale study, and accordingly a questionnaire was circulated to 2500 members of the British Small Animal Veterinary Association.

THE SURVEY

Respondents were invited to complete a questionnaire listing all human ethical products used by them in general practice. The following information was requested for each product:

1. Proprietary name. Differences in formulation or price might affect selection of a particular product, so it was considered important to establish the proprietary brands used.

2. Form. Factors such as tablet size, availability of syrup formulation and so on, might affect selection.

3. Species in which used.

4. Indications for which used.

5. Dosage used. It was known that some products were considered useful by some practitioners and useless by others. It was thought that such discrepancies might be a function of dosage used.

6. Approximate number of cases treated.

7. Comments on efficacy, incidence of side effects and adverse reactions, problems of administration, cost.

8. Reason for first using product. Data from surveys of general medical practitioners had indicated that the suggestions of drug company representatives were the primary source of new drug information to general practitioners.

RESULTS

Of the 2500 individuals circulated, 89 returned completed questionnaires. Although this response may seem small, it should be appreciated that the number of products used by each practice was generally large, and considerable time was therefore required if the questionnaire was to be completed in full. Moreover, in many cases two or more individuals circulated would be members of the same practice, thus further reducing the total number of responses to be expected.

DAta from 60 practices has so far been evaluated, which has provided information on a total of 321 different products. Some practices record the regular use of as many as 40 different products.

REASONS FOR USE

A number of reasons for using human rather than veterinary products can be discerned:

1. Definitive drugs. Certain products are well-documented in the veterinary literature, and although the extent of veterinary, as compared with human usage is small, so that registration of these drugs for veterinary use is not economically attractive to manufacturers, their use is essential in veterinary practice. Examples include the cardiac glycosides, insulins, thyroxine and vitamin K_1 for anticoagulant poisoning.

2. "Personal influence" products. In the U.K. there are certain individual specialists, who, by virtue of their teaching of both undergraduates and participation in postgraduate courses, have had a distinct influence on therapeutic practice in their own specialties. Ophthalmic therapeutics contains many examples.

3. Generic preparations. These products (e.g. calamine preparations, magnesium sulphate poultices, tincture of chloroform and morphine) are recognised as veterinary medicaments in many cases, but may be unavailable through veterinary suppliers.

4. Preparations for novel indications or uses. In this interesting category are products that have little or no veterinary indication, in terms of published literature, but which are found to be useful in veterinary clinical practice. Examples included metoclopramide in the treatment of vomiting, diphenoxylate in diarrhoea, and bromocriptine in pseudo-pregnancy.

5. Preparations of favourable formulation. Agents may be more readily administered to small animals in the syrup formulations intended for use in infants. In other cases, tablet sizes intended for human use are apparently more useful for treating some small animal patients than the veterinary equivalent products.

6. Medical preparations cheaper than veterinary equivalents. In some cases manufacturers market apparently identical preparations on the human and veterinary markets, but with a higher price in the latter case. In other instances an agent is available in a number of proprietary preparations on the human market, one or more of which may be cheaper than the others, and cheaper than the equivalent products on the veterinary market. Generic preparations (e.g. antibiotics) are generally cheaper than proprietary products.

7. In some cases there is no apparent reason for the use of the product described in preference to a veterinary equivalent product.

CATEGORIES OF PRODUCTS USED

The products listed by respondents can be classified according to therapeutic use, which should give some indication as to the particular areas in which veterinarians find veterinary products inadequate or insufficient for their needs.

1. Topical preparations.(Skin and ear preparations).

Skin and ear preparations together constituted the largest group (49 different preparations listed). Skin and ear products are listed together, since many skin preparations are evidently used for the treatment of otitis externa. Veterinarians appear to find many of the simpler human products useful. It seems that the low-dose low-potency corticosteroid preparations, currently fashionable in human therapeutics, are being favoured by some veterinarians, in preference to the higher potency steroid creams and ointments available on the veterinary market. Simple antiseptic creams are also favoured in many instances, in preference to antibiotics, whilst corticosteroid without antibiotic preparations also are found useful. Diethyl phthallate ointment was found useful to prevent self-inflicted trauma.

2. Ophthalmic preparations (38 products listed). The most frequently-mentioned products in this category were agents for the treatment of glaucoma: demecarium bromide drops (now withdrawn); acetazolamide tablets; dichlorophenamide tablets; prostigmine drops; pilocarpine drops. Hypromellose drops were considered useful for keratoconjunctivitis sicca.

Simple products for bacterial conjunctivitis, such as sulphacetamide or penicillin eye ointment were often found useful, whilst conversely antibiotics such as gentamycin were necessary in some cases. The use of the more exotic antibiotic preparations seemed to be based largely upon culture and sensitivity test results.

3. Agents acting on the gastro-intestinal tract (29 products listed). Many respondents found diphenoxylate most useful in the control of non-specific diarrhoea, with some reservations regarding its use in cats, due to the sensitivity of this species to opiates, including diphenoxylate (Ormerod, Bogan & Lauder, 1978). Curiously, few respondents attempted to mimic the human regime in which a large dose of the drug is given initially, followed by smaller doses at 6 hourly intervals until the condition is controlled. Veterinarians appear to prefer a simple twice or three times daily dose for a predetermined period.

The control of non-specific vomiting seems to be a problem for many small animal clinicians. Metoclopramide was used by many, at doses around 1 mg/kg/day by any route. All users of this product reported a high degree of efficacy and no side-effects were mentioned. The product was reported to be useful also for oesophageal achalasia and for post-operative ileus. Other antiemetics used included prochlorperazine, which appears to produce little sedation in the dog, and perphenazine, which will give a degree of sedation which may be useful.

Faecal bulking agents, such as sterculia, ispaghula husks and methyl-cellulose were used by almost all respondents to control chronic bowel dysfunction, whether manifested as diarrhoea or as constipation.

4. Antibiotics (26 products listed). Use of human antibiotic preparations fell into two categories: (a) Use of human preparations of antibiotics commonly used in veterinary practice, when the human formulation provided a tablet size or syrup presentation convenient for animals, or when a significant cost advantage lay with a particular human formulation. (b) Use of "second-line" antibiotics such as gentamycin, flucloxacillin, carbenicillin, for specific cases, based on bacteriological culture and sensitivity testing. There was little evidence in this survey to suggest that there was any irresponsible or uncontrolled use of important

human antibiotics.

5. Agents acting on the cardiovascular system (25 products listed). Digoxin was used almost universally, although it was not always apparent that respondents appreciated the principles of digitalisation or the toxicity of the cardiac glycosides. A few respondents seemed to prefer digitoxin to digoxin, although the reason for this was not always clear. It would seem that there is still a need for further information on the use of cardiac glycosides. One or two respondents had used propranolol in a few, rather poorly-defined cases of "tachycardia", with evidently satisfactory results. Almost every available diuretic was favoured by at least one respondent, although the reasons why one diuretic was preferred over another was, in most cases, obscure. Many respondents had discovered that frusemide was much cheaper as a human generic preparation than as a veterinary proprietary preparation.

6. Others. The other agents listed fell into the following categories:

Vitamin and "tonic" products - 23 products listed. Empirical usage in most cases.

Anaesthetic and emergency drugs - 22 products listed. Including skeletal muscle relaxants, stimulants such as bemegride and nikethamide (surprisingly still widely-used), and vitamin K_1.

Analgesics and anti-inflammatory agents - 19 products listed. There is evidently still a need for an effective and safe anti-arthritic agent for dogs.

Hormones - 12 products listed. Bromocriptine for post-lactation gallactorrhoea or pseudopregnancy seems to be useful.

Urinary system - 11 agents listed. Sulphamethiazole tablets for urinary infections were popular.

Sedatives and tranquillisers - 11 products listed. Diazepam was one of the most widely-used of all products, in control of behaviour, treatment of status epilepticus and convulsive poisonings, and as a general tranquilliser.

Anti-epileptic agents - 11 products listed.

Antiparasitic agents - 9 products listed. Liquid formulations of piperazine salts are considered useful for very small animals.

Anti-tumor drugs - 9 products listed.

Antihistamines - 9 products listed. Chlorpheniramine was particularly popular.

Anti-diabetic agents - 7 products listed. Some practitioners find oral hypoglycaemic agents useful, in spite of indications in the literature that such agents are of little value in the dog.

Exocrine pancreatic replacement preparations - 6 products listed. Many human preparations cheaper than veterinary equivalents.

Respiratory system - 6 products listed.

CONCLUSION

Although this survey had several shortcomings, chiefly in that it was not possible to ensure that all respondents listed <u>all</u> the human ethical preparations commonly used by them, it would seem that a number of human products, such as the insulins and cardiac glycosides are essential to veterinary practice. Many of the other agents used are topical preparations. The evidence available does not suggest that human products are being used in an irresponsible or reckless fashion; indeed, in many cases the choice of a particular human preparation appears to be based on a desire or need to find a preparation less potent than those available on the veterinary market. It is an important point that the effect of current legislation and economic forces has been to increase the cost of registering a product for veterinary use. There is thus an understandable tendency on the part of manufacturers to register novel, potent patent-protected products that are likely to produce a satisfactory financial return. The increasing emphasis on the use of such potent products is in the interests of neither animals nor the public, and it would seem important that the veterinarian should continue to be free to use simple, safe, often generic products in preference to the more potent agents.

REFERENCE

Ormerod, E., Bogan J.A. & Lauder, I.M. (1978). Toxic Effects of Lomotil in Cats. Veterinary Record 102, 110

THE REQUIREMENTS OF THE VETERINARY PRODUCTS COMMITTEE

C.S.G. GRUNSELL

University of Bristol, Department of Veterinary Medicine, Langford House, Langford, Bristol BS18 7DU (GB)

ABSTRACT

Brief reference is made to the overall objective of the Medicines Act and the Committee structure established to implement these aims. Some account is given of the pattern of the legal requirements attaching to the application for Licences and Animal Test Certificates. There follows a more detailed description of the information and data required by the Veterinary Products Committee. Within the constraints imposed by confidentiality an attempt is made to draw on the experience of considering applications for animal tests and to identify areas of more consistent deficiency and make tentative suggestions for their correction. Following a consideration of the need for a clear statement of objective for the test, the integral parts of the planning stage are examined including some reference to controls and the importance of paying close attention to the criteria for the assessment of efficacy. This leads into comment on the analysis of the findings in the interpretation phase. An application for a hypothetical product is presented in order to illustrate some previously made points.

The Veterinary Products Committee (VPC) of which the author is currently Chairman, was established under the Medicines Act (1968) to advise the Licensing Authority on the quality, safety and efficacy of veterinary products in the UK.

There have been more than 80 meetings of the VPC since its establishment in 1971 and at every meeting the Committee has considered a number of applications for Animal Test Certificates. This has provided some background of experience for comment which follows. This would seem to fall under three headings — the aims, the planning, and assessment of results.

A. The Aims of the Trial

We are dealing here with the applicant's predictions for the product

based on the primary studies which can include the findings in laboratory animals
and in the target animal under the controlled conditions of the Company's testing
facilities. In short the question is will the product be effective in the
conditions under which it will be used in the field?

The need for precision is essential and quite simply the aim is to verify the
claim to be subsequently made. Although naturally it will be hoped by the applicant
that the product is an improvement on existing products there is no obligation so to
show.

Occasionally the licensee has been unable to resist the temptation to claim and
test for marginal possible effects and not only can this prove more expensive but
it may complicate the design of the test and make the assessment of the results
more difficult.

The Importance of the Aim

It must be on the basis of the clear statement of the hypothesis for the product
that the statistical advisor will assist in the design and planning of the test.
It will next be important for the participating practitioner in connection with the
assessment of the results he makes on a clinical basis.

The advisers to the licensing authority – the VPC – must ultimately pay great
attention to the claims proposed for the data sheet and these will arise logically
from the statement on the aims for the A.T.C.

Common Pitfalls

Difficulty can arise for example where one is dealing with a new product where
the exact mode of action is not known – this happens for instance with the agent
which can be acting effectively either as a microbiological prophylactic or as a
growth promoter.

Next problems can arise where the claim is for the treatment of a syndrome or a
symptom of multi-aetiology say gastritis or enteritis in the dog. Accurate diagnosis by the general practitioner is either impossible or only made by resource to
laboratory medicine measurements or even post-mortem confirmation.

Then we have the situation of the broad spectrum antibacterial agent
with a claim for use in respiratory disease but in which the susceptible
bacteria is usually found in a secondary role and the results of bacteriological examination of the material available in life are of doubtful
significance.

B. Planning the design of the Test

The expertise of the participants should always include the disciplines of
clinical pharmacology, statistics, epidemiology, current veterinary field
experience and with certain applications microbiology, parasitology, endocrinology and animal husbandry (including current field experience of farm livestock

production techniques). This expertise may well be available within the promoter's organisation, but the advice of the participating practitioner may be required for current veterinary experience and in some aspects of epidemiology. Some outside advice may also be required in respect of production techniques.

The planning panel will be provided with the results of the primary laboratory and pilot studies in the target species (if any) on which is founded the hypothesis to be tested. A description will be given of the clinical picture of the condition as currently seen in the field including the ease or difficulty of diagnosis and the common course of the disease with special reference to spontaneous cure.

It will be important and particularly with products for use in the companion animals, to agree the necessary criteria for animals to be acceptable for the test and conversely what will constitute grounds for exclusion.

So that appropriate modifications can be made to the design of the trial to avoid systematic and random error there must be an evaluation of the factors likely to influence the result such as age, sex, diet (including standard additives) and housing. For example environment and management could influence the severity of the clinical manifestations of respiratory disease in farm animals.

It will be particularly important for the statistician to be informed of the natural incidence of the disease in a population and its seasonal and geographic distribution. With this information together with the expected response and the likely difference between treated and control groups it will be possible for him to suggest the all important number of animals to be used.

It is obvious that the more control of bias there can be to reduce random error from variability of material and the more precise diagnosis can be, the smaller will be the test population.

The use of controls coupled with objective randomisation is an acknowledged method of avoiding systematic error. Nevertheless the provision of controls for the testing of veterinary products can represent a major difficulty for both the promoter of the product and the trialist in the field.

The techniques of matched pairs or groups, cross over trials and blind trials, are not often practicable in the veterinary field where there is no comparable facility to the NHS hospital for this purpose. The ethical objection to untreated control groups (−ive controlled trial) is recognised and may be effectively and acceptably replaced by the use of a recognised treatment in the control group (+ ive controls). However it is important to stress that acceptable efficacy of the product being tested does not depend on demonstrating its superiority to the recognised treatment.

A situation can arise in which one is virtually seeking to demonstrate the efficacy of a product in its own right and it seems as if positive controls are almost superfluous. With the testing of such a product one can safely rely on the experienced clinical trialist to give an accurate assessment of the efficacy of the product under test based on the response he would expect from the accepted product of choice. In so doing of course he must be making an estimate of what the numbers in the column headed control group would be, which cannot be acceptable to the statistician.

To achieve an optimum number of animals in the trial and to reduce the effect of individual bias on the part of the practitioner it is necessary to have a number of practices involved in the trial. Where however one is dealing with conditions of low general incidence the promoter of the product may be forced to involve a very much greater number of practices. Carried to extreme this could introduce an important variable and also make the supervision by the promoters more difficult.

C. The Assessment of the response to the product under test

The difficulties which can arise at this stage are mainly a consequence of imprecision in defining the aims, or deficient planning. The former has already been considered and the result of planning defects will be examined now under the following headings.

 1. Deficiencies in the composition of the Panel or in its deliberations.

 2. Failure to appreciate the natural history of the disease condition.

 3. Lack of on-going consultation throughout the test period.

1. Deficiencies in the Composition of the Panel or in its deliberations

Unfortunately it is often only too evident that statistical advice has not been taken at all, or it has been taken too late or that insufficient information has been provided to the statistician. Sometimes statistical analysis is at fault.

It is readily acknowledged that difficulties exist in the selection of participating practices. The practice which is over eager to participate is sometimes also most likely to 'fall out' or fail to adhere consistently to the agreed plan for the test. It may be that the promoters should carefully evaluate the practice secretarial staff before making final selection. It could be that promoters may be failing to provide sufficient financial recompense for the disruption caused in a practice engaged in a field trial.

2. Failure to appreciate the natural history of the disease

When the panel is not fully aware of the detailed epidemiology of the disease they are seeking to cure or control that insufficient attention is given to say environmental factors as important variables likely to affect the results. One has in mind here endemic conditions in farm animal populations such as respiratory disease.

The natural course of a condition must also be considered bearing in mind for example the possibility of spontaneous cure as will happen in lameness in horses.

Under this heading will come the criteria to be laid down first for inclusion in the test and equally importantly, the basis for the categorisation of response following treatment. Thus if the practitioner is to express his opinion of the result of a treatment as No Response, Poor, Satisfactory, Good or Excellent, the basis must be fully understood and agreed by the Panel. Where this is not done the final assessment may well take the predictable form of

No Response 10%: Poor 20%: Satisfactory 35%: Good 25%: Excellent 10%

It is impossible to overstress the importance of the participating practitioner's involvement in this component of the test design and of his confidence in what is agreed.

3. Lack of ongoing consultation throughout the test period

This would seem to be essential to identify any anomalies between practices in any respect and for the early recognition of unanticipated adverse side reactions. It would also be hoped there would be frequent visits by the promoter's representatives to the participating practices and periodic meetings of the whole panel to review progress.

4. The Assessment of Safety

It will be remembered that the VPC has also to advise the Licensing Authority on Safety not only to the animal and to the consumer in the case of farm animals but also to the animal owner or attendants in the application of the treatment. It remains the responsibility of the practitioner to make known any precautions to be taken whether it be in dipping sheep or in the topical applications for small animals.

5. Inherent Difficulties

It is of course of considerable value if bacteriological or post-mortem results are available to confirm clinical diagnosis but the practical difficulties of insisting on this are realised and that it is impossible to withhold treatment pending the receipt of results. Indeed in some instances they will in any case be of highly questionable significance as is the case in swabs taken from upper airways and from skin lesions.

FICTITIOUS APPLICATION FOR AN A.T.C. FOR VACCINE DSS.2

A killed vaccine prepared from Streptococcus suis, Type 2, Lancefield Group D obtained from field outbreaks of septicaemia with meningitis in pigs.

1. A PRECISE STATEMENT OF THE AIM

The object of the test is to investigate the effectiveness of the vaccine in the control of septicaemia and meningitis in pigs caused by streptococcus suis, Type 2. It is essential to define the condition precisely.

2. A CLEAR DESCRIPTION OF THE DISEASE

Characteristically pigs seen alive have marked febrile reactions and classic signs of septicaemia. Nervous signs develop quickly and pigs show opisthotonos and tetanic spasms, some show blindness adn deafness and without treatment death quickly supervenes. Often the first sign is the discovery of dead pigs. P.M. findings are those of septicaemia with congestion of the splanchnic organs. The presence of pus when the cranium is removed is a variable finding but intense congestion of the meninges is usally present. Diagnosis can only be based on bacterial culture and the recognition of characteristic histological changes.

3. SELECTION OF MATERIAL WITH EPIDEMIOLOGY IN MIND

Ten farms will be selected for the trials. These will be enterprises with breeding stock and on which pigs are reared to market weight. They will be selected on the basis of the condition having been confirmed by the bacteriological examination of material from not less than 5 post mortem examinations, and on the provision of satisfactory evidence of the condition constituting a serious problem for the enterprise. Because there can be a tendency for the infection to disappear spontaneously only farms on which the condition has been in existence for not more than a year will be used in the trial. Every attempt will be made to follow precisely the system of husbandry and management in operation at the time of the outbreak. In addition the farms selected will be those on which the sole treatment has been of affected animals and no prophylactic measures have been instigated.

4. NUMBERS RELATED TO DISEASE INCIDENCE: METHOD OF USE

It is intended to use the whole population of all six farms, dividing the stock into 2 groups of equal numbers by random selection of breeding stock in the first instance and the respective progeny will fall into the dam's group.

Use of the vaccine

All the progeny in Group A (vaccinated with DSS 2) will receive 5 ml. of the vaccine at ? weeks of age. The exact age would have been determined by preliminary work.

The Control Group will receive a placebo injection as above.

Husbandry

There will be no separation of the groups throughout and indeed steps will be taken to ensure that attendants have no knowledge of the groupings.

Duration of Test

This will be 12 months in the first instance.

5. CLEAR INSTRUCTIONS ON MONITORING THE RESULTS

Efficacy Assessment

Individual pig health records will be kept throughout, together with the results
of post-mortem examinations of _all_ pigs dying during the trial period. The
Company will employ the farmer's practitioner to examine any pig showing nervous
symptoms and make a clinical diagnosis. No pigs showing signs of meningitis
will be treated and in the event of death full p.m. examination will be carried
out including bacteriological and histological examination.

The company will fully recompense the owner for the losses arising from the
above regime.

6. FREQUENT VISITS TO CO-ORDINATE AND MAINTAIN INTEREST

The farm's Veterinary Surgeon will visit the farms at least once a month to
monitor the records etc.

The Company's veterinary representative will visit the farms with the
practitioner every other month.

7. WARNINGS ON HAZARDS

Contraindication and warnings

As Streptococcus suis Type 2 is known to cause meningitis in man, appropriate
precautions will be taken in handling dead pigs.

TEACHING OF PHARMACOLOGY

H.-H. FREY
Laboratory of Pharmacology and Toxicology, School of Veterinary
Medicine, Free University Berlin, Berlin-West (Germany)

In speaking about teaching of pharmacology and toxicology, I shall
confine myself to oral teaching and to the conditions of the Federal
Republic of Germany.

The volume of Teaching in our discipline, including drug
legislation and prescription order writing is fixed by law
(Approbationsordnung für Tierärzte of 1976) to 150 hours. Table I
shows how the obligatory lectures and courses are divided at our
4 Schools. Under the provision of 15 weeks per term, the total time
used for teaching of pharmacology and toxicology ranges from
112 - 180 hours.

In the following, I shall deal with the topics:
1. When is pharmacology taught during the curriculum
2. What should be taught in pharmacology
3. How is pharmacology taught

1. The teaching of pharmacology and toxicology is placed in the
third year of the curriculum, i.e. the first clinical year for the
veterinary student. This seems reasonable because pharmacology is a
basic discipline undispensable for the understanding of practical
therapeutics, and because physiology and biochemistry on which
pharmacology is largely based have been examined after the second
year. But the early teaching of pharmacology poses problems too:
You cannot expect knowledge and understanding of the pathophysiology
of the diseases to be treated at that level. This is especially
obvious in the case of chemotherapy: Parasitology and special
microbiology are taught in the fourth year, and so it is rather
useless to tell about the spectrum of activity of antibiotics or
anthelmintics during the third year. Thus, there is no use of
teaching a clinically orientated pharmacology and neither can
clinical understanding be tested in the examination which takes
place after the third year. You may ask understanding of general

Table I

OBLIGATORY TEACHING OF PHARMACOLOGY
(FEDERAL REPUBLIC OF GERMANY)

	Weekly hours per term		
	Winter	Summer	Total
3rd Year			
<u>Pharmacology and Toxicology</u>			
Berlin-West	3	3	6
Giessen	3	3	6
Hannover	3	3	6
Munich	4	5	9
4th Year			
<u>Prescription Order Writing</u>			
Berlin-West	2		
Giessen	1		
Hannover	1		
Munich (dispensation included)	3		
<u>Introduction into Drug Dispensation</u>			
Berlin-West	1		
<u>Course in Drug Dispensation</u>			
Berlin-West	1		
Giessen		0.5	
Hannover	1		

total: Berlin   4
Giessen 1.5
Hannover 2
Munich   3

pharmacology, but special pharmacology will be mostly confined to facts learnt by heart by the student. This situation is unsatisfactory and does not contribute to the popularity of the discipline.

Personally, I try to include clinical or applied pharmacology into the teaching of prescription order writing during the fourth year, but, as drug legislation and the formal rules of prescribing also have to be teached and exercised in this course, only about 10 hours will be available for this purpose. The ability of the student to prescribe and use drugs on a rational and intelligent basis is examined after the fourth year. The results are not very satisfactory on the average, neither regarding the ability to make use of the basic pharmacological knowledge nor regarding the health of the patients that shall be treated by the future doctors.

During the fifth and last year, professors of pharmacology

participate in the teaching of pathophysiology, at least in Berlin, and here is a last possibility to discuss some matters of functional pharmacotherapy with the students. However, there is no special examination in pathophysiology, and consequently only rather few students participate in the lectures.

2. The next problem is What to teach in pharmacology today. 50 years back, 'veterinary' pharmacology seemed self-sufficient: It had to give some basic information on the rather limited number of drugs that were available and were used by the practizing veterinary surgeon. Elder textbooks give evidence of this situation. Nowadays, things have totally changed. Especially the small animal practitioner does not hesitate to employ the most recent developments on the pharmaceutical market in his practice, usually without much knowledge about their actions and without any knowledge about their pharmacokinetics in domestic animals. But also the general practitioner has quite sophisticated drugs in his hands, drugs that should demand a thorough knowledge of pharmacology and toxicology. These conditions alone make a more scientific teaching of pharmacology mandatory. But there are other branches of our profession interested in special fields of the discipline. The problems of drug residues in food and meat hygiene, of environmental contamination by agricultural remedies or by industrial waste products must be taken into consideration. This field is clearly too big to be taught extensively in the main lectures, but at least an exemplary presentation of the complex should be given. Details may be treated in facultative lectures or, even better, be the subject of postgraduate studies.

A great number of veterinary surgeons have found and will find positions directly in the field of pharmacology and toxicology, especially in the pharmaceutical industry but also in Government Health authorities. In this sector, there is a hard competition by members of other professions: medical doctors, pharmacists, biologists, biochemists and chemists. If our profession shall keep its share in this field also in future, it is absolutely necessary to provide an education in pharmacology and toxicology that is equal or superior to that of the other professions mentioned.

Thus, we teach pharmacology and toxicology now on a broad and general scale that should not be too different from that taught at Medical Schools. We simply try to give every student the basis for his quite personal professional future, well knowing that the individual student only will need a certain sector out of the whole

complex later on. About one third of the pharmacology teaching
during the third year is devoted to general pharmacology which is
felt to be a prerequisite for a thorough understanding of drug
actions and drug therapy. During the lectures on special pharmacology
of course, attention will be paid to facts of special veterinary
interest. But at this point, the professor must very often confess
that we do not know too much about the special 'veterinary' pharmacology and toxicology of drugs used in our domestic animals. The
result is, as I have stressed before, that the veterinary practitioner
will adopt dose regimens from medicine, simply because there are no
reliable data for domestic animals. This underlines the necessity of
research in clinical pharmacology in veterinary medicine and of an
obligatory teaching of clinical pharmacology for veterinary students
at a later point of the curriculum.

In conclusion, we have to teach pharmacology and toxicology rather
early during the curriculum, in fact too early to go into details of
the practical use in veterinary therapy. The teaching of the disciplin
should then try to provide a broad and solid basis for future
application in all fields of the veterinary profession. There will
result a little more knowledge than the individual student will need
for his future activities, but this should be taken as contribution
to general education. I think it is better the veterinary student is
informed about drug dependence or anticonception in the lectures on
pharmacology than from weekly magazines. The surplus of information
will facilitate the dialogue with the medical profession and with
the natural sciences, and this should be considered as an advantage
in its own right.

3. The third complex I shall deal with is _how_ to teach pharmacolog
and toxicology. The form of teaching is in fact determined by the
numbers of students we presently have to cope with in Germany. Our
4 Schools each admit 200 - 250 first term students a year, and,
though some of them have been lost on the way, there are still
120 - 150 that actually listen or should listen to pharmacology
teaching in the third year. These numbers limit the form of teaching
to the great frontal lecture with all its advantages and disadvantages. The advantage is that pharmacology can be presented by
one or two professors as a perfect whole, at least when the teacher
has experience in the field and pedagogic skill. The disadvantage
is that the individual student remains anonymous, that a discussion
of problems in fact is impossible, that the instruction of certain

of the more static topics, as f.e. toxicology of heavy metals, disinfectants, vitamins and so on, will unavoidably be a rather monotonous display of facts, the student can only learn by heart.

The alternative would be instruction of small groups of about 10 - 15 students. This might be optimal giving room for discussion, but it meets problems both regarding the staff able to give the instruction and the localities where the groups can be instructed. For a class of 150 students, at least 10 qualified instructors and as many rooms must be available, but this is not the case at our Schools.

The frontal instruction might be accompanied by facultatory demonstrations and practical courses and this is in fact done at two of our Schools. However, the students, especially during the fourth year, have more than 40 hours of instruction a week, so the tendency to visit additional courses or demonstrations is very low. Regarding the time that is consumed in preparation and accomplishment of pharmacological demonstrations and courses, one may doubt if this rather expensive effort can pay for just a few or sometimes no students.

The outlook is rather pessimistic indeed, but we are well aware that the quality of teaching must and will decline as the numbers of students are rising.

The course in prescription order writing is held on Saturday morning at 8 o'clock, a day and a time at which only the most interested - or the most afraid - students meet. That makes it possible to give an unconventional form of instruction just sitting among the students and asking: What will you do in this situation? Are there other opinions? and why do you treat in this way?, what do you expect?, and what a dose do you give how often? Side effects and their treatment as well as therapeutical alternatives can be discussed and the auditory is suddenly awake. These are indeed the most satisfactory hours of instruction for both sides and the question arises if this kind of teaching cannot be adopted for the whole discipline. In consequence, you had to devote so and so many hours for the discussion - and not the teaching - of f.e. the pharmacology of general or local anesthesia, of circulation, chemotherapy and so on. Such a kind of instruction must be considered optimal, but it would carry most of the burden of preparation over to the student who should meet well prepared for the special topic of the day, so well prepared that he should be

able to ask intelligent questions. You will surely agree that this
is more than can be expected from students of the third year alone
on account of the heavily loaded time table they have to absolve
and the relative lack of clinical experience at that trin of
education. All in all, one more reason for special instructions
in clinical pharmacology during the last year.

What could and should then be improved of our present system of
teaching or the curriculum? I think, many of the difficulties
mentioned might be overcome by 1. introducing some clinical or
project orientated pharmacology into the last year and by 2. moving
the examinations of pharmacology/toxicology as well as of prescription order writing to the end of the 5 years curriculum. The
first point, clinical pharmacology, might be accomplished in the
frame of clinical demonstrations thus avoiding further extensions
of the time table. The student would then be well equipped and
motivated for the examinations of pharmacology and prescription
order writing at the end of the curriculum. Facts that only can be
reproduced by heart after the third year would be thoroughly
understood after the fifth year making the examination much more
comfortable for both student and examinator. To this effect,
however, the current law in the Federal Republic of Germany had
to be changed to exactly the shape it had before 1967.

PRACTICAL COURSES AND INTEGRATED TEACHING IN VETERINARY PHARMACOLOGY AND TOXICOLOGY

J. FRENS

Department of Veterinary Pharmacology and Toxicology, Utrecht University, Utrecht, (The Netherlands).

ABSTRACT

The setting up of a practical course in veterinary pharmacology is described, with advantages and drawbacks thereof. The problems and possibilities of integrating pharmacology and toxicology into the curriculum of other disciplines are discussed.

The average veterinary student views pharmacology and toxicology with some suspicion as another one of those scientific subjects like biochemistry, physiology etcetera. Obviously he or she is right. Since pharmacology is an integration of the basic sciences, with some concepts of its own added, it does have a place among these sciences.

This is both a help and a hindrance for teaching in pharmacology. It helps because it is possible to teach pharmacology/toxicology in its own right. This approach should put emphasis on the basic aspects and stress that pharmacology does not just mean the putting together of drugs for the market.

Being too "scientific" about it becomes a hindrance however, because in most veterinary curricula pharmacology/toxicology is taught in the years following the courses in basic biological sciences and prior to clinical teaching. It therefore seems to block the approach to those subjects most students have entered University for. One of the main aims a course in pharmacology/toxicology should have is to motivate the student for the subject and to make it clear that pharmacology is a basic science of importance to veterinary practice and veterinary thinking. This of course does not mean that no emphasis must be put on the actual pharmacological knowledge that is essential to the veterinarian.

It must always be remembered however that teaching veterinary pharmacology and toxicology should serve a purpose. The purpose in general is to give every graduated veterinarian a working knowledge of the subject that is adequate for the function he will have later in life. This implies that for most veterinarians not every intimate detail of pharmacology is important, but that a basis must be established on which pharmacology can function in the thoughts of the individual.

In setting up a course in veterinary pharmacology, it seems not illogical to assume the following principles:

    a. a student is basicly interested in the subjects the curriculum offers.

    b. a student must be kept interested during the course.

    c. the course should provide enough material to make it possible to reach the goals set for the course.

    d. the course should integrate pharmacology in the clinical world.

    e. the "pharmacological" way of tackling problems should be demonstrated.

Several strategies are open to achieve the effect that is wanted. So as not to interfere with others in this section, I will put emphasis on how in my view practical courses and integrated teaching can achieve something.

PRACTICAL COURSES

As pharmacology is an experimental science, it seems essential to me that some experimental work is brought into a course of the subject. This experimental work can take the form of research work or of a pre-programmed practical course. To engage all students in seemingly original research work is hard to realize, because of the number of students normally enrolled and the difficulty of providing technically feasible projects. The dilemma is that the relatively simple experiments needed for such projects obviously have been done before. On the other end of the scale it is possible to design some experiments beforehand, give the student the expected results and ask him to perform the experiment. This "cookery book" style of practical course produces results. The result is that the student sees the effect of some drugs, and learns to handle experimental animals and basic apparatus. The result most of the time is also that the student questions whether the effect is not better learned from books, whether there is a need to use experimental animals for such a purpose, whether effects cannot be better observed when demonstrated on film and in general whether he is not wasting time and animals in completing the course.

A lot can be said against these arguments, and indeed has been said during the time that we had such a course in our Institute. From the pharmacologist's point of view - and his view obviously is the most important in deciding what should be in a pharmacology course - a strong case can be made for such type of practical work. No matter how valid the arguments used are however, motivation will soon wane. The knowledge that all effects can be looked up and that if dissimilar effects are found, this can be brought back to impurities in experimental technique does not create a stimulating atmosphere. The practical course is in danger of becoming a session in which students go through the motions of working, while actually doing nothing to improve their knowledge of pharmacology. Once this stage is reached the students are wasting their time indeed, still demotivating themselves even further. It is a good teacher that can break through this and still then more effort is lost in keeping students motivated than in teaching pharmacology. The main problem in such a course is probably that the unknown is missing and the unexpected does not happen.

After working for some years with this type of course, we had the feeling in Utrecht that whatever change was made in the programme, it would be no use if the system as such was not changed. Feeling that changes were necessary, a course was introduced that had the following ingredients: It is based on a - hypothetical - clinical case. The action of drugs is broken down to different levels of integration. No information is given beforehand on the action of the drugs used, so students have to see for themselves or have to look up the effects in book that are present during the sessions. Not all students do the same thing, but they have to form teams to get the total picture.

An example of this is the following procedure in which the action of anesthetics is dealth with. Dosages and techniques are given to the student, but are left out here for the sake of brevity.

Case:

Calf with hernia umbilicalis. The calf has a hernia of respectable size. The condition of the animal is not optimal. The hernia needs surgical correction, so anesthesia is in order. Due to the condition of the animal this anesthesia should pose as little stress on the animal as possible. Anesthetics and analgetics each have their own advantages and disadvantages as to sedation, analgesic effect, side effects etcetera.

Analgesia:

The feeling of pain can be prevented by blocking painperception peripherally, blocking the pathway from painreceptor to CNS or by depressing the capability of the CNS to register pain sensation.

Check in the guinea-pig whether local injection of the following drugs blocks the reaction to local pain stimuli:

1. lidocaine
2. pentobarbital
3. propionylpromazine (Combelen[®])
4. morphine

Which of these substances reduce the feeling of pain?
To what class of drugs belong these substances?

Check in the mouse whether the feeling of pain is reduced after intraperitoneal injection of

1. lidocaine
2. pentobarbital
3. propionylpromazine

4. morphine

Which of these substances reduce the feeling of pain?

Which of these substances sedate the animal?

What reason for reduction in the feeling of pain can be given?

Sedation:

The previous experiment showed that drugs may alter the state of consciousness in the animal. Check whether sedation occurs in the rabbit on intravenous injection of

1. pentobarbital

2. propionylpromazine

3. morphine

N.B.: Check reflexes and also other symptoms like respiration, hartfrequency, pupilsize etc. All rabbits that received morphine should be treated with nalorphine at the end of the experiment.

Why is lidocaine not used in this experiment?

Which of these substances sedate the animal?

Evaluation:

All substances used have advantages and drawbacks. To make the region of the hernia in the calf analgetic and sedate the animal at the same time, several drugs may be used. The side effects are an important aspect however. Pentobarbital for instance gives a serious depression before analgesia is sufficiently pronounced. For a patient in a bad condition this may be fatal. A combination of drugs may probably reduce the side effects.

Consider what combination you would prefer and try this on a rabbit. The criteria for the combination are:

    a. the region of the navel should be analgetic

    b. the animal should be sedated

    c. the animal may show only a minor depression of respiration or other side

       effects

The result of your experiment will be observed by the staff with more or less awe.

The case goes on with the different types of tranquillizers, kataleptics etcetera and their potentiating effect on anesthesia. In this case a few things not directly to be found in books or unexpected should come to light, like the local anesthetic effect of tranquillizers of the promazine type, the species differences in reaction to morphine, the effect of an overdosage of local anesthetics.

Advantages of this type of course are that the effects found are brought home better than in the old course. The main reason for this probably is that the student has to observe all the aspects of his experimental animals and does not become fixated on the symptoms he is supposed to see. So when something shows, he will wonder if this fits in with the expected results. Some stages in the course are made so that they oppose that what is in the textbook. For instance, the normal textbook says that salivation is caused by stimulation of the para-sympathetic system. In a case that deals with cholinesterase inhibitors, the effect of several drugs on salivation is studied. When acetylcholine is injected, no salivation occurs, contrary to what the student would expect. Such instances give a good opportunity to deal with the basic principles like the halflife of a drug, bloodlevels etcetera. In the same way it shown that after injection of acetylcholine or other parasympathicomimetics there first is a rise in hart-frequency rather than a slowing down, giving a good opportunity to deal with reflex mechanisms etc.

In short, this type of practical course can be a good handle for going down to the basic principles and at the same time the relation with clinical work is not lost. Once this relation is established, there is every opportunity to go down in the level of integration, so that isolated organs and even erythrocytes are used in this course.

A problem in practical courses is the use of experimental animals. Most of the time the veterinary student has chosen the study with the ideal of treating sick animals later in life and to take care of their wellbeing. In a practical course animals are put at his disposal and are made to "suffer" for his benefit. Rightfully this leads to some initial resistance. It is the task of the teacher to take this opposition seriously. At no time students should be made to perform experiments against their will.

To deal with the problem of ethics, experiments must be designed in such a way that no real harmful effects are induced in the animals. The border between acceptable and unacceptable will be different to different people, so maybe it is a good thing to check with some colleagues before incorporating a doubtful experiment in a practical course.

Once the staff is convinced that the experiments used are appropriate and do not impose an undue stress on the animal, it should stick to this conviction. At all times it must be remembered that the issue is to a large extent emotional and not purely based on facts. If a student cannot be convinced that the benefits of the course are worth the use of animals, an alternative must be found. In our department this is done only after a serious person to person talk between teacher and student.

In the last few years we have been working with this type of course and we think that the results are beneficial in terms of enlarging the knowledge of pharmacology and in keeping the student motivated for studying the subject. This does of course not imply that our solution is the only or even the best solution.

INTEGRATED TEACHING

In the past thirty years the number of different subjects taught in the veterinary faculty of Utrecht has doubled, while the number of teachers has more than tripled. This situation is not unique for the different veterinary faculties in Europe.

The more teachers and subjects there are, the less time is available for a given subject. The less time there is available, the larger is the percentage of time that is spent on components that are essential to that subject. Added to this, the material that seems essential enlarges through the years, while contacts among teachers are less intensive than tey used to be, because of the large teaching staff.

The result is that the teaching of different subjects has become more and more self-centered and optimal coordination is lost. Poor student. He is the only one left to construct a skeleton out of the different bones that are offered him and often he can make head nor tail out of it.

Once this stage is reached, a phase in the growth curve of a faculty occurs in which the call for integration becomes louder and louder. As far as I can judge, all institutions that teach go through this phase at one time or other. This doesn't mean that integration is always a bad thing, but it is someting that should be handled with care. At worst, the integrators neglect the work to be done for integration in favor of their direct teaching obligations. Normally, one of the subjects to be integrated gets all the work that is to be done, but has to give the rewards to others and begins to feel cheated in the process. At best integration is a real joint venture of different participants.

Pharmacology and toxicology are subjects that are suitable for integration up to a point. As there are many overlapping area's with e.g. physiology at one side and with the clinics at the other side, it seems worthwhile to try and overcome the more or less strict separation between the different subjects. This also can bring pharmacology/toxicology into perspective. Provided a real integration can be achieved, a loss of identity will not occur. Especially in the field of pharmacotherapeutics and clinical pharmacology/toxicology much can be added to the vigating curriculum, once it is understood by all participants that the clinician knows more about the clinical work and the pharmacologist knows more about pharmacology.

To me it doesn't seem essential whether an integrated course goes by the name of clinical studies, pathophysiology or some other fancy name. Neither is it important which teacher actually presents the course, as long as all participants in the integration have the right to determine the contents of the course.

The hard core of pharmacology/toxicology however is best served by establishing a course in which only those aspects that are unique to pharmacology/toxicology are dealt with. This course should be under supervision of the teaching staff of the pharmacology department. With this course it can be brought to light what pharmacology/toxicology really is, while the integrated courses can show what you can do with it.

To make time available for integrated teaching, the amount of time spent on the different subjects has to decrease considerably. This has the advantage that only those things that are really essential are dealt with in the courses of the different departments. The more generalistic approach can be accomplished in the integrated veterinary studies.

In Utrecht we have started such an integrated course called "pathophysiology" a few years back. It has grown to a course that takes up a substantial amount of the time available in the third and fourth year of study. Participants in the teaching are individuals with a background in nearly all disciplines of the faculty. They form so called teaching teams for the different subjects. Such a teaching team normally has 5 to 6 participants that decide what is going to be taught and how it will be done. Much effort is given to include as much patient demonstrations in the course as possible. The subjects that we found to be very suitable for integration are the pathophysiology of renal function, digestion, metabolism, liverfunction, respiration, circulation, shock, defence mechanisms, reproduction, woundhealing and bone metabolism.

For pharmacology/toxicology this is followed by an integrated course in the fifth year called pharmacotherapeutics. In this course pharmacologists, toxicologists, pharmacists, clinicians and others deal with variable themes that may be something like urinary tract infections, clinical toxicology of different compounds, pain or any other suitable theme. In this course as well as in pathophysiology the teaching staff generally is enthousiastic about what can be achieved. As for the students, they think that it works.

AIMS AND OBJECTIVES OF TEACHING CLINICAL PHARMACOLOGY AND TOXICOLOGY

J. SANFORD

Wyeth Laboratories, Taplow, Maidenhead, Berks, Gt. Britain

ABSTRACT

Clinical pharmacology and toxicology have not been emphasised in the veterinary curriculum and have not shown the same rate of development as other clinical disciplines. The aims of teaching and the content of the syllabus are described, emphasising essential differences from experimental pharmacology on the one hand and therapeutics on the other. Arrangements for teaching these subjects by clinicians and within a clinical course are considered along with proposals for examination.

The need for postgraduate teaching is also discussed.

INTRODUCTION

Clinical pharmacology and toxicology have not, in the past, been clearly recognised as subjects in the syllabuses of most veterinary schools. This deficienc reflects the minor status assigned to veterinary pharmacology following rejection of the traditional Materia Medica some 20-30 years ago. At the same time, the rapid development of several other disciplines, such as biochemistry, virology, immunology and radiology, tended to increase the competition for limited time and facilities coupled with a misguided belief that therapeutics was a relatively unimportant part of veterinary clinical medicine. In addition, it has been suggest (ref. 1) that the development of proprietary products presented to the veterinarian ready formulated and with instructions for use, may have dissuaded clinicians from individual efforts to develop an interest in clinical pharmacology. Whatever the causes clinical pharmacology and toxicology are still in a rudimentary state in veterinary education.

AIMS

Clinical pharmacology may be defined as the science of drug action and usage in animals under clinical conditions. In this it differs from experimental pharmacology which may also involve studies of drug action in "target" species (i.e. species in which the compound will ultimately be used). Clinical pharmacolog also differs from therapeutics since the latter is concerned with the place of medicinal compounds in the management of specific diseases.

Teaching in clinical pharmacology will aim to produce a rational basis for therapeutics. It will be concerned with formulation, bio-availability, kinetics and metabolism as well as with actions and side-effects of clinical significance. It will also include factors which may modify drug action such as diet, husbandry, breed and strain differences, intercurrent disease and interactions between different therapeutic agents. The study of interactions might also be extended to include interference with diagnostic tests (ref. 2). The recognition of adverse effects must also be discussed on a logical and practical basis such as suggested by Cobb (ref. 3).

Instruction in the design execution and analysis of clinical trials is essential both to enable clinicians to organise and participate in such trials and to act as a basis for making comparative assessment of effiency, safety and economy. Current national and international requirements for the registration of medicinal products will also be considered together with those important aspects of toxicity, tissue residues and antimicrobial resistance which influence official attitudes to the use of many compounds in veterinary medicine.

Similar objectives can be identified in teaching clinical toxicology but, in this case, emphasis must be placed first on means of diagnosis, differential diagnosis and prognosis as well as on therapeutic measures. Teaching will include laboratory aids to diagnosis with the chemical analysis of appropriate samples. Since these procedures may have legal significance, the importance of confirmation of diagnosis must be stressed. The preparation and presentation of legal evidence and the functions of the veterinarian as a forensic expert must also be considered. A more detailed description of a syllabus is given in table 1.

TABLE 1

SYLLABUS

A   Clinical Pharmacology

  i)   Aspects of Drug Action   Formulation and systems of medication, mass-medication of farm animals.
       Bio-availability, kinetics and factors affecting absorption, metabolism and clearance.
       Drug disposition, tissue residues, excretion in milk.
       Adverse effects. Influence of diet and environment and interactions.

  ii) Clinical Trials   Design, conditions, numbers and type of trial.
       Preparation of a protocol.
       Selection of cases, evaluation of symptoms and response.
       Analysis of results, validation of conclusions.
       Problems of trials comparing different forms of therapy.
       Comparison of results from different trials.

158

iii) <u>Medicines Legislation</u> Requirements for clinical trial and product licences.
National and international considerations.
Significance of residues and witholding times for food products.
Use of antibiotics and resistance.

 iv) <u>Economics</u> Comparative costs of alternative forms of therapy.
Therapeutic and prophylactic medication of farm animals.
Importance of prognosis.

B   Clinical Toxicology

  i) <u>Causative agents</u> Natural poisons, plants in pastures, forage and foodstuffs.
Environmental poisons, agricultural chemicals, domestic pesticides,
disinfectants and paints.
Toxic effects of medicinal products.
Accidental or deliberate poisoning.
Industrial disasters, contamination from factories, nuclear reactors and
ineffective waste disposal.

 ii) <u>Clinical Aspects</u> Diagnosis, differential diagnosis prognosis and laboratory
tests.
Pathology, examination of specimens.
Appropriate therapy.
Kinetics of toxic agents and factors affecting.

iii) <u>Forensic Aspects</u> Collection and analysis of samples.
Presentation of evidence in a court of law.
Duties of veterinarian as a forensic expert.
Special problems of racehorses and show animals.

ORGANISATION

Having broadly defined aims and objectives, it is important to consider when
and how these topics will be taught in the undergraduate course.

Teaching of these essentially clinical subjects must be carried out in the
later part of the course when students are directly involved in clinical casework.
It should also be apparent that the teaching ought to be carried out by clinicians
having a special interest in pharmacology and toxicology. Though unusual amongst
academics in British Veterinary schools at present it must be accepted that
clinicians may develop a specialist interest in these subjects which are no
different in this respect from others such as cardiology, metabolic disease,
radiology or anaesthesia. Such clinical involvement is essential and clinical
pharmacology and toxicology cannot be taught adequately by extension of the pre-
clinical courses, taught entirely by non-clinicians who are often also not
veterinarians.

Ideally those teaching these subjects should form a separate department or
sub-department, but with the small size of many Veterinary Faculties, complete
separation from a main clinical department may not be practicable. Even if such

integration is necessary the staff responsible for teaching clinical pharmacology and toxicology should be clearly identified and have primary research interests in these subjects. A system in which one or two staff of a clinical department are assigned a few lectures in clinical pharmacology in addition to various other duties will do little to further interest in, or development of, this subject.

On the other hand, a department of clinical pharmacology might be large enough to take responsibility for teaching in both pre-clinical and clinical areas. This trend is occurring already in some British medical schools with the appointment as head of a pharmacology department of a clinical pharmacologist. If this is contemplated it is essential to ensure that the non-clinical members of the department are adequately supported and encouraged with adequate facilities and good career prospects in addition to providing proper clinical facilities for the clinicians. The ideal clinical pharmacologist/toxicologist will be a veterinarian with a degree also in pharmacology or having postgraduate training in this subject and who has, in addition, substantial postgraduate clinical training and experience.

TEACHING AND EXAMINATION

The design of suitable courses in veterinary clinical pharmacology and toxicology may take one of several forms. Although complete integration with other clinical disciplines may be ideal (ref. 4) this may not prove to be a practical solution since the content of the course may be submerged by the greater weight of other aspects of the clinical curriculum. It may be more satisfactory to organise the course into two or more short blocks of more or less formal teaching with the remainder of the available time given to integrated clinical casework. The first teaching block of some 10-20 hours would include most of the fundamentals of the subjects as described in table 1, section A (i) and (ii) and section B (i) and (ii). This first block should come early in the clinical part of the course and might logically follow the pre-clinical course in pharmacology. The second block of some 8-10 hours should come in the final year of the course and should contain the remainder of the material outlined in table 1. Clinical casework should involve, discussion of the pharmacological basis for therapy in individual cases, the opportunity to participate in clinical trials and exposure to appropriate toxicological case material as available. Teaching in preventive medicine may also include elements of pharmacology and toxicology with the prophylactic use of mass medication of farm animals, poultry and fish and the prevention of outbreaks of poisoning from contaminated food, pasture and water supplies.

Examination of students in material presented in this course is best accomplished by means of a separate examination paper, or at least by means of a separate section within a larger clinical examination. The concept of clinical pharmacology and toxicology as discrete disciplines demands an examination separate from other aspects of clinical medicine.

It would also be a function of a section or department of clinical pharmacology to run postgraduate courses. These could be both to provide specialised training leading perhaps to a further degree or could take the form of short refresher courses for practising clinicians. At all stages the aim of teaching must be to present the principles of these disciplines as a basis for clinical application rather than merely to review current therapeutic practices which may be obsolete in five or ten years time. A need for teaching in clinical pharmacology and toxicology already exists, it must now be encouraged to develop alongside other clinical specialities.

REFERENCES

1. Editorial (1978) J. Vet. Pharmacol. Therap. 1, 1-3.
2. Paul J.W. (1977) Clinical considerations regarding drug interaction in the bovine patient. Bovine Practitioner No. 12, 10-14.
3. Cobb L.M. (1979) Adverse drug reactions in Pharmacological Basis of small Animal Medicine. Eds. Yoxall A.T. & Hird J.F.R., Blackwell Oxford. Chap. 3.
4. Kaemmerer K. (1978) A Short Report on the Teaching of Veterinary Pharmacology and Toxicology in Europe. J. Vet. Pharmacol. Therap. 1, 249-250.

THE COURSE IN VETERINARY PHARMACOLOGY: CONTENT AND PLACE IN VETERINARY MEDICAL
CURRICULUM

J. DESMOND BAGGOT
School of Veterinary Studies, Murdoch University, Western Australia, 6150

ABSTRACT

The course in veterinary pharmacology should include the basic pharmacological
principles, the actions and effects of drugs on the various systems of the body,
chemical and plant toxicity, chemotherapy and clinical pharmacology. The comparative approach, with emphasis on domestic animals, distinguishes veterinary from
human pharmacology. Physiology and biochemistry provide a foundation for pharmacology while application of the discipline lies in medicine. The course appears
to be most effective when the material is presented as an independent, 'though
not isolated, discipline and is given a clinical orientation. The overall
objective of the course should be to provide a level of knowledge adequate for
making sound decisions regarding all aspects of the use of drugs in domestic
animals.

INTRODUCTION

The increased public reliance on drugs, the large number and wide range of
therapeutic agents now available, and the developments in clinical pharmacology
over the last decade have all contributed to increasing the significance of
pharmacology in veterinary medicine. The founding of the American College of
Veterinary Pharmacology and Therapeutics, the British Association for Veterinary
Clinical Pharmacology and Therapeutics and the European Association for Veterinary
Pharmacology and Toxicology indicates the willingness of individuals associated
with the discipline to share information as well as to identify and discuss drug-
related problems. The acceptance of responsibility for development, registration
and proper use of veterinary drugs can only lead to increased recognition and
support for the discipline. The Journal of Veterinary Pharmacology and Therapeutics, which represents all interests and has a world-wide circulation, is a
vital part of the discipline. In Australia and New Zealand, the veterinary
profession has shown its eagerness for further knowledge in pharmacology by
supporting the continuing education courses, the Therapeutic Jungle and More

Rational Use of Veterinary Drugs. Since the pharmacology course in the veterinary medical curriculum provides the foundation of the discipline, its content and relationship with the overall programme greatly influence the future development of veterinary pharmacology.

The course which I shall outline is based on my own experience in teaching the discipline in veterinary schools which varied both in academic programme and administrative structure. In this brief communication my aim is to establish the major components of the discipline and the topics within each component will not be discussed.

THE COURSE IN VETERINARY PHARMACOLOGY

Veterinary pharmacology deals with the action and effects of drugs in domesticated and other species of animals and compares the absorption, distribution, biotransformation and excretion processes for drugs in the different species. The discipline is also concerned with appropriate dosage of drug products, the causes, signs and reversal of drug toxicity, and with the influence of disease on disposition kinetics and dosage of drugs.

The course in veterinary pharmacology could be considered to consist of five components. A different aspect of the discipline is presented in each component, although a common underlying theme can be maintained throughout the course. For this reason it is of paramount importance that an individual who is knowledgeable in all aspects of the discipline should coordinate the entire course.

The components of the course, the number of lecture hours required for adequate presentation of each component, and the time which should be assigned to each component for activities loosely termed "practical classes" are given in Table 1.

TABLE 1. Outline of Course in Veterinary Pharmacology

Components	Assignment of Time (in hours):	
	Lectures	Practical Classes
Principles of Pharmacology and Toxicology	20	(2 x 6) = 12
Systemic Pharmacology	40	(2 x 12) = 24
Veterinary Toxicology	20	(2 x 2) = 4
Chemotherapy	26	(2 x 2) = 4
Clinical Pharmacology	14	10 to 20

PLACE IN VETERINARY MEDICAL CURRICULUM

The place in the overall veterinary medical curriculum at which veterinary pharmacology is presented can have a major influence on the theme of the course.

Perhaps at this stage it is appropriate to state that an understanding of the physiology and biochemistry of domestic animals should be considered a prerequisite for the course in veterinary pharmacology. Other disciplines may be considered desirable prerequisites for certain components of the course. Microbiology, for example, should precede chemotherapy. Mutual benefit can be derived from the concurrent presentation of the pathophysiology of conditions affecting the various systems of the body and systemic pharmacology. Introductory anaesthesia might well be integrated with the pharmacology of drugs acting on the nervous system.

In the context of a five year veterinary programme, the pharmacology course could start in the middle of the third year, continue throughout fourth year with systemic pharmacology and toxicology being presented concurrently to be followed by chemotherapy, and clinical pharmacology in the final year. Veterinary pharmacology is more effective when the course is independent of, 'though not isolated from, other disciplines. The material in the course is seen not only to be relevant but also essential when presented with a clinical orientation.

PRACTICAL CLASS ACTIVITIES

The activities associated with practical classes can usefully complement the material presented in lectures. The type of practical activity will vary with the component of the discipline. In the principles of pharmacology and toxicology component, the analysis and interpretation of biochemical and pharmacokinetic data, which are essentially mathematical exercises, might constitute the main practical activity. In systemic pharmacology, demonstrations showing the effects of drugs on normal animals can be supplemented with video-tapes. The latter are a most useful permanent record showing the results of experiments which involve surgical preparations. The effects of autonomic drugs on the various physiological parameters can be viewed and explained satisfactorily on tape. The clinical signs of drug toxicity and plant poisoning as well as the laboratory methods for drug identification can be shown on video-tapes. In the clinical pharmacology component, practical activities include discussions on the choice and dosage of drug preparations for treatment of actual cases, potential interactions and adverse effects of drugs, and also the presentation of seminar papers on species pharmacology and selected topics of clinical interest.

The exposure of students to certain service facilities in the veterinary hospital constitutes an important part of their practical training in veterinary pharmacology. Such facilities include the diagnostic toxicology and clinical pathology laboratories. In discussions with the pharmacist, the student becomes familiar with the various formulations of veterinary drugs, their storage and the legal requirements associated with narcotic and other "dangerous" drugs. Lectures in the veterinary jurisprudence course elaborate on the responsibility of the veterinarian with regard to the handling, storage and accurate keeping

of records on "dangerous" drugs as well as discussing the legal aspects of
"doping".

OBJECTIVE OF VETERINARY PHARMACOLOGY COURSE

The veterinary pharmacology course outlined in this communication is aimed at
providing a level of knowledge adequate for making sound decisions regarding all
aspects of the use of drugs in domestic animals and, to a lesser extent, in
other species. When drugs are administered irrationally or in a manner such
that they constitute environmental hazards, it reflects on the educational background of the practitioner (Davis, 1977). In my view, the ultimate responsibility
for the attitude of the veterinary medical profession towards drugs rests with
the teachers in veterinary pharmacology.

REFERENCE

Davis, L. E. (1977): Pharmacology training in schools of veterinary medicine.
Federation Proc., 36 (1): 119 - 123.

PHARMACOLOGY OF THE RUMINANT STOMACH

Y. RUCKEBUSCH and L. BUENO
Département de Physiologie, Ecole Nationale Vétérinaire, 31076 TOULOUSE Cédex, and Station de Pharmacologie-Toxicologie I.N.R.A, 31300 TOULOUSE, France.

ABSTRACT

Ruminant stomach functions involve four aspects : rumen motility, microbial metabolism, associated secretory processes and neuro-hormonal control. Difficulties in treatment of dysfunctions are due to the lack of controlled therapeutic trials as well as the use of a large extent of drugs in health animals for enhanced productivity. Two major points are emphasized: the ruminant stomach (RS) as an effector organ for drugs and their use in bloat, hypomotility states, NPN overload, vit. B_1 deficiency, lactic acidosis, abomasal ulcers...

INTRODUCTION

Adaptation to the coarse and bulky character of forage is achieved in ruminants, by regular mixing movements of the reticulo-rumen which are dependent upon the vagi nerves and are accelerated by feeding and rumination. Food conversion by microorganisms produces volatile fatty acids and gas which is expelled by eructation. Other functions of the rumen are conversion of non protein nitrogenous (NPN) substances (urea, ammonia) into microbial protein, vit. B_1-synthesis and lipid hydrogenation. The abomasal pH concentration varies from 1.05-1.32 in sucking animals where milk is directly conveyed via the reticular groove. In adults, HCO_3^- absorption from the omasum prevents undue neutralization of the gastric juice by continuous salivary secretion. Both physiological and pharmacological aspects ot these functions will be examined.

FUNCTIONAL ASPECTS of the RUMINANT STOMACH

Motility patterns

The cyclic contractions of the reticulum which occur about once per min are followed by one or two contractions of the rumen but are abolished by bilateral vagotomy and increased by 150 % after total deafferentation. The removal of extrinsic control is accompanied by stenosis of the reticulo-omasal orifice. Feeding and stretching of reflexogenic areas (cardia, reticulo-omasal orifice and rumino-reticular fold) increases the rate of rumen contractions (fig. 1). Prolonged studies on vagotomized

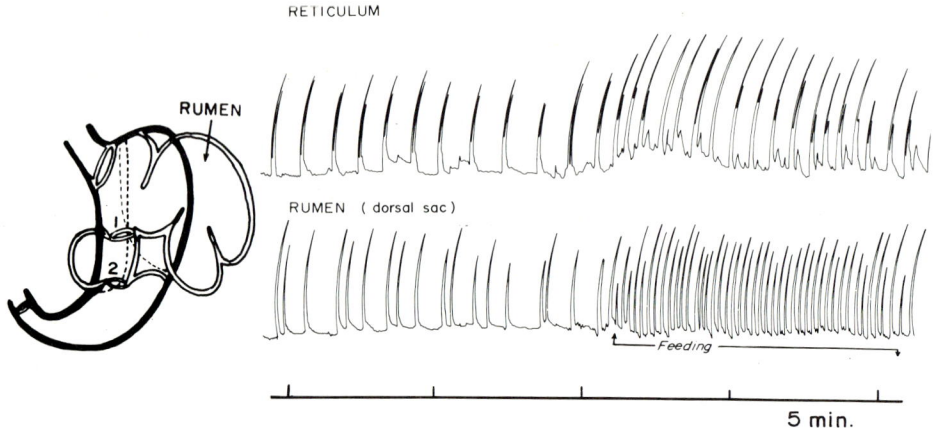

RETICULUM

RUMEN

RUMEN (dorsal sac)

Feeding

5 min.

Fig. 1. Enlargement of the reticulo-rumen from the fundic region facing the cardia and of the omasum between 1 and 2 from the lesser curvature. Increase of the frequency of reticular contractions measured by endoluminal balloons from 1.0 to 1.7 per min and of the rumen from 1.6 to 3.3 per min in a sheep receiving oats (ref. 12).

sheep showed that the resumption of a purely local activity is gradually organized into rhythmic discharges which are at a frequency range similar to the movements recorded in vitro from isolated strips of smooth muscle (14). This intrinsic activity was strongly increased by distension at 7-15 mmHg and further enhanced by direct act ing parasympathomimetic agents. As in vitro, adrenaline which is inhibitory for the rumen, has a short-lived excitatory effect on the reticular wall,(α-receptors).

Omasal motility was characterized by the relative autonomy of body contractions which persisted during local and general anesthesia. Motility was cyclic in sheep via an inhibitory setting effect of the reticulo-ruminal contractions (5). Contracti activity of the omasal leaves occurred both in vivo and in vitro at a frequency of 4 per min. This was similar to the rate of the series of closures and openings of the reticulo-omasal orifice following the second phase of reticular contractions. Omasa motility in cattle was similar to that of the sheep for the omasal canal with flow entering the omasum at each cycle. For the main body, both waves of increased press and electromyogram indicated slow contractions lasting 3-4 min, these contractions were at the origin of the slow extrusions of "lumps" of solid matter at each 3 to 4 reticular contractions (fig. 2).

The cyclical activity of the RS which develops after 4 weeks of age might be inh bited during the closure of reticular groove which may be induced in young animals by sucking from a teat and in adults when licking salt. During cephalic phases whic depend upon the degree of excitement with which the animal sucks, the intensity of reticular contractions diminishes, while after sucking, the frequency of the reticu lar contraction is reduced depending upon the degree of distension of the abomasum the milk.

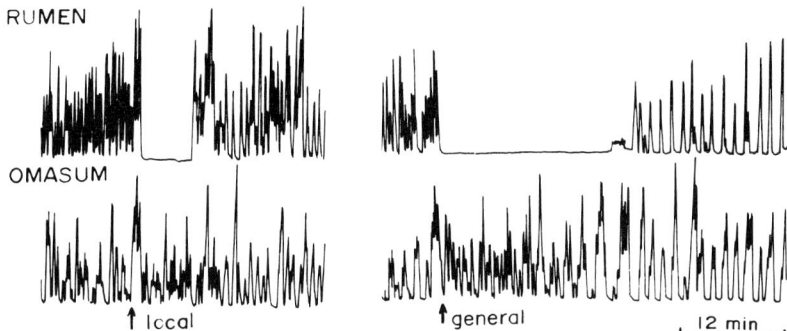

Fig. 2. *Integrated electrical activity at 6-sec intervals of the dorsal sac of the rumen and of the omasal body of sheep. The* **activity** *of the rumen is arrested without changes in the mean level of omasal activity by local anesthesia of the vagi and during general anesthesia with thiopentone (ref. 5).*

Little attention has been paid to the interactions between the activity of the different reservoirs of the RS. Distension below 8-12 cm H_2O pressure of a reservoir always increases its own intrinsic and/or extrinsic activity via the in series tension receptors. Distension of the omasum inhibited the reticulum and that of the abomasum inhibited the activity of both the reticulo-rumen and omasum (fig. 3). By contrast, acidification of the abomasum might enhance the RS activity (6).

Abomasal motility patterns are characterized in the adult by almost permanent antral activity showing only a cyclic inhibition lasting 10-15 min when the regular spiking activity phase of a myoelectric complex develops in the duodenum. During sucking, the fundic region exhibited receptive relaxation along the greater curvature despite a long-lasting increased activity of the antrum.

Secretory processes

The secretory rate of saliva varied from 0.5 to 20 ml/min per gland in sheep as a bicarbonate phosphate buffer of which HPO_4^- and HCO_3^- represented 90 per cent of the total anion content. Abundant parotid saliva secretion might be evoked by the sight

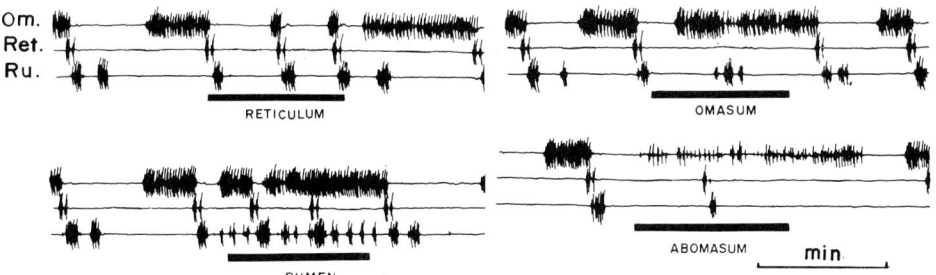

Fig. 3. *Distension of the reticulum during 70 sec increased the frequency of the reticulo-rumen contractions and that of the rumen enhanced the activity of both the reticulo-rumen and omasum. The distension of the omasum reduced the cyclic recurrence of reticular contractions while that of the abomasum had a long-lasting inhibitory effect.*

of food and feeding, and was paralleled by that of the muzzle in cattle. Urea concentration in saliva was related to rumen ammonia and blood urea content. All these phenomena were disturbed during hypomotility states.

Fundic juice secretion reached 4 to 6 litres per day in sheep fed ad lib. It is a watery fluid with a pH of 1.05-1.32. In contrast, that of the pyloric region (0.5 l per 24 h) is slightly alcaline. Sham-feeding of sheep in which the reticulo-rumen is empty does not stimulate significantly the abomasal secretion which depends largely upon the entrance of omasal contents into the abomasum, and upon the volatile fatty acids (VFA) concentration in the contents (1). Secretion of H^+ inhibited by prostaglandins E_1, E_2 and A_1 was increased by vagi nerve stimulation, by release of gastrin and via H_2 receptors (10). A specific H_2 blocker like cimetidine (400 mg) decreased by over 80 % for 5 h gastric secretion in the presence of histamine and of gastrin.

Microorganisms

The well-being and thriftiness of ruminants depend upon the maintenance of an appropriate microbial population which is in the range of 15 to 80 billions per ml and their fermentative processes, which depend on sufficient amounts of substrate, fiber, and water being supplied. The final product of carbohydrate fermentation is mixture of volatile fatty acids (VFA) at a percentage of 60-70, 15-20 and 10-15 for C_2, C_3 and C_4 acids respectively. Among the intermediary products, formic, succinic, malic acids are effective hydrogen donors for nitrate reduction ; lactic acid is commonly observed the first weeks after the animals have been placed on rations high in starch or sugars (7).

End products of proteins are ammonia, CO_2 and CH_4 as well as VFA and branched-chain C_4 and C_5 acids. Ammonia concentration is influenced by dietary protein, saliva urea content and urea diffusion (4). About 50 % of the gas mixture is inhaled into the trachea in cattle. The CO_2 evolves during fermentation of carbohydrate, deamination and neutralization of VFA by HCO_3^-. The CH_4 is formed by reduction of CO_2 via specific methanogenic bacteria. Changes due to flora are hydrogenation of unsaturated C_{18} acids which represent nearly 70 % of the total acids of food, consequently synthesis of thiamine in the rumen is markedly reduced in starch rich diets (7).

The effects of sudden changes in diets are important. In cows which receive grain instead of hay, the RS concentration of VFA may be doubled (100 mM vs. 50-60 mM), which reduces rumino-reticular motility (fig. 4). In lactic acidosis, a fall in pH from 7 to 4 represents a 1.000 fold increase in H^+ and large amounts of acid into the duodenum which in turn inhibits the RS motility (3, 16). When rumen ammonia content increases, ruminal contractions become slower and less strong. This is due to direct chemosensitivity of the rumen (6). The conversion of rumen ammonia into microbial

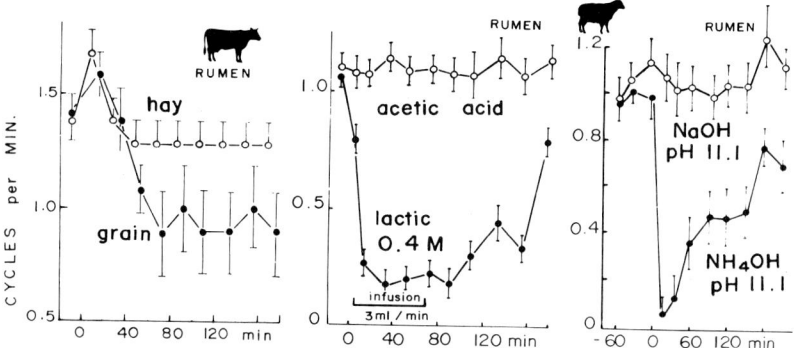

Fig. 4. Contractions of the rumen in cattle during the 3 h following a meal of 2.5 kg hay (o) versus 7.5 kg grain (●). Duodenal infusion at a rate of 3 ml/min of 0.4 M acetic acid (o) versus lactic acid (●) in sheep and intraruminal administration of NaOH, pH 11.1 (o) versus NH_4OH (●) (ref. 6).

protein is an energy consuming process provided by the VFA, the concentration of which falls after 4 h. This is accompanied by inhibition of RS motility. Increased gas tension in cardia region triggers its reflex opening, this phenomenon does not occur if the cardia is covered with fluid or foam.

Neuro-hormonal control

The periodic vagal motor discharges are dependent upon an excitatory drive from sensory inputs. Catecholamine depletion by reserpine and psychotropic drugs probably inhibits RS motility via such mechanism (12, 13). Modulating inhibitory sensory inputs arise from high-threshold tension receptors, acid receptors and pain receptors. The magnitude of vagal motor discharges may be enhanced by anti-cholinesterases (e.g. neostigmine) and abolished by drugs which block transmission either at preganglionic or postganglionic cholinergic nerve endings (e.g. tetraethylammonium, atropine) (13). The relative inefficiency of parasympathomimetic drugs in exciting the frequency of RS movements (e.g. carbachol) contrasts with their direct effects on the muscular wall which is shown by increased tone (13, 15).

RS motility is inhibited by ruminal infused or injected VFA, C_4 being more effective than C_3 or C_2 (2). Intravenous C_4 also stimulates secretion of immunoreactive insulin (IRI) and glucagon (IRG), the inhibitory effect of C_4 being absent during alloxan-induced diabetes (21). Insulin-induced hypoglycemia has been reported to increase RS motility but the effect seemed in fact restricted to the omasum and antrum as shown in fig. 5. Similar excitatory effects on the omasum and pylorus but accompanied by inhibition of the reticulo-rumen (fig. 6) have been found with the C-terminal pentapeptide Gly-Trp-Met-Asp-Phe-NH_2 (ICI 50,123 Pentagastrin) of gastrin (11) but not with other synthetic polypeptides (8), even the C-terminal octapeptide (Squibb 19,844, Kinevac) of cholecystokinin. An antigastrin-like proglumide partially prevents this effect and induces secondary contractions of the rumen (fig. 7).

170

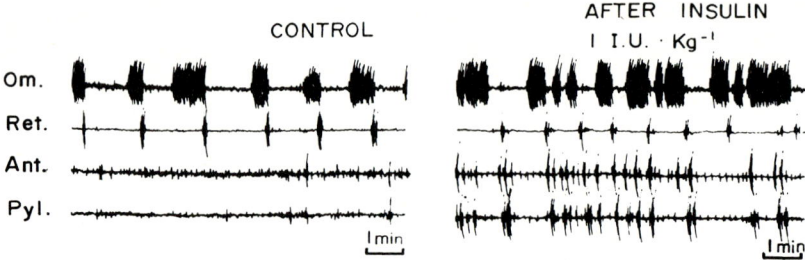

CONTROL

AFTER INSULIN
I I.U. · Kg⁻¹

Om.

Ret.

Ant.

Pyl.

Fig. 5. Omasal and antral increased electrical activities in sheep following an intravenous injection of 1 IU/kg of insulin. These changes are accompanied by an inhibition of the magnitude of the reticular (ret.) contractions and an increased frequency.

Secretin, which is released after lactic acid infusion in the duodenum inhibits reticulo-rumen activity, even if α or β adrenergic receptors sites are blocked. Tripelenamine, an antihistamine, does not prevent the secretin-induced decrease of rumen motility. Aminophylline, an inhibitor of phosphodiesterase activity, has a similar effect and consequently it has been suggested that secretin was inhibitory by an increase of CAMP (22). However, secretin could also be acting through dopamine receptor. Dopamine activites α-adrenergic receptors within the ruminal wall (19). These are blocked by metoclopramide (Primperan) which also enhanced the rate of secondary contractions of the rumen.

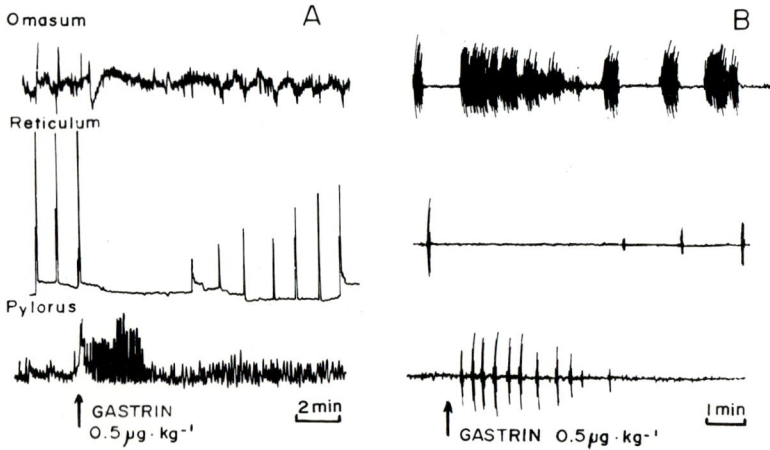

Fig. 6. Changes in the parietal pressure measured with strain gages (A) and in the electrical activity (B) of the omasum, reticulum and pylorus in sheep after an intravenous injection of gastrine. These effects persisted after atropine injection (0.4 mg/kg).

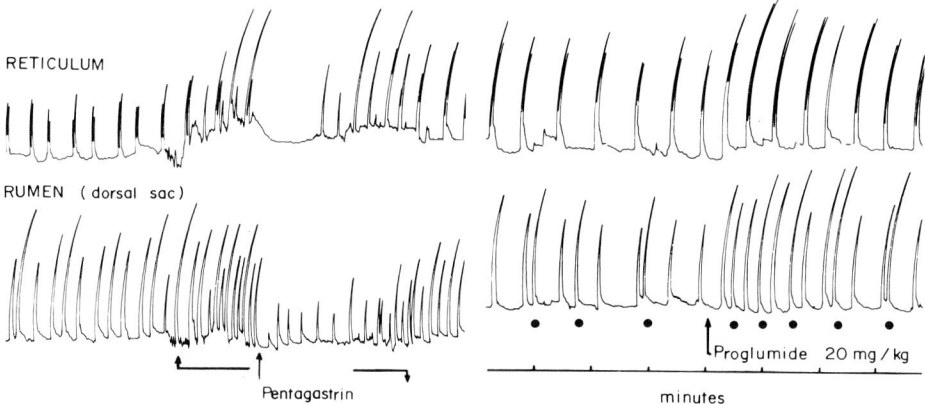

RETICULUM

RUMEN (dorsal sac)

Proglumide 20 mg / kg

Pentagastrin

minutes

Fig. 7. Left side : inhibition of reticulo-ruminal contractions by pentagastrin in sheep during feeding. Right side : increased rate of the secondary contractions of the rumen as indicated by dots following an i.v. injection of proglumide.

CLINICAL PHARMACOLOGY

Bloat

The inability to eructate gas trapped in foam of the rumen occurs with a genetic tendency in ruminants grazing on alfafa and clover (legume bloat) and is associated with rumen acidosis in feedlot bloat (grain bloat). One approach to its prevention is decreasing the ruminal protozoa by giving $CUSO_4$ (4 g/100 kg) and surfactants, e.g. prolaxalene (22 g in toto per day). None of 235 drugs screened adequately controlled grain bloat.

Hypomotility states

Gastrointestinal atony commonly occurred under intensive animal husbandry systems where excessive amounts of easily fermentable carbohydrates are supplied (16). Ruminal stasis may occur because of central nervous depression for instance during fever (18), and hence vagal discharges, subsequent acidosis and anorexia leading to a low rate of salivary secretion. Shock with release of substances like catecholamines, serotonin, prostaglandins and plasma kinines also resulted in relfex inhibition of extrinsic reticuloruminal contractions (Veenen doal, this symposium). The search for substances acting directly on the RS frequency has not proved successful (17). An harmless substance is pilocarpine (0.1-0.2 mg/kg), probably via the copious flow of salivary secretions and subsequent chewing movements (13). Another way to improve the motility is the restoration of the calcemia (12).

Non-protein nitrogen overload

Efficiency of NPN is limited by the rate at which urea is hydrolyzed. Both nitrogen assimilation and synthesis are impaired by the increased rumen pH which in turn increases free NH_3 absorption ; the subsequent peripheral blood ammonia inhibits the

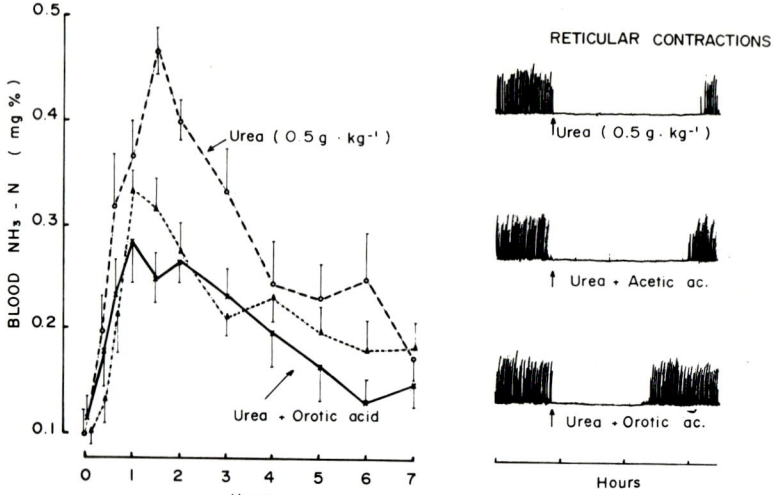

Fig. 8. Blood ammonia level and corresponding inhibition of the reticular contractions. The addition of orotic (0.2 g/kg) but not acetic acid prevented this effect (Bueno, Patent n° 77-32842).

RS motility (9) and induces anorexia (fig. 8). To limit the high rumen NH_4^+ concentrations urea hydrolysis could be reduced by physical (coating) or chemical (urease inhibitors) procedures. The rate of NPN assimilation could be increased by energy source (low weight carbohydrates) and by precursors of uridine triphosphate (UTP) such as orotic acid which incorporate free NH_3 into cytidine triphosphate (CTP)

Thiamin deficiency

Cerebrocortical necrosis reported from countries where intensive agriculture is practiced affects both sheep and cattle on a high concentrate ration. The result is an increase in, or activation of, ruminal thiaminase so that both dietary and endogenous ruminal thiamin are destroyed. Transketolases which are thiamin-dependent enzymes are inhibited and blood pyruvate levels are increased. The affected animals show various neurological manifestations that are similar in nature to thiamine deficiency syndromes in non-ruminant species. The recommended dosage of vit. B_1 in cattl is 1 g/animal and 0.2-0.5 g in sheep at 2-day intervals.

Lactic acidosis

Cellulolytic bacteria are destroyed as the pH falls from 5 to 4 due to an excess of H^+. In addition, the loss of lactate-utilizing bacteria which convert the lactic acid to the weaker VFA increases the intraruminal level of lactic acid. Most medica treatments have been shown to be unsuccessful in their objectives of decreasing moti lity and time for recovery (20). Penicillin and chlortetracycline administered with the grain prevent the onset of a lactic acid fermentation. The chances of survival with protractel recovery are improved by oral administration of alkaline salts and chloramphenicol, the latter being a strong inhibitor of liver microsomes (see fig. 9). A satisfactory treatment for severe cases is emptying the rumen surgically or by lavage in order to permit a normal fermentation to be restored by addition of ingesta from a healthy animal. High level of molasses triggers a lactic acid fermentation with proliferation of Gram (+) bacteria in the rumen and unusually high concentrations of the higher VFA, particularly butyric, valeric and caproic (7). These acids give rise to bursts of high amplitude epileptiform EEG activity accompanied by behavioural depression in sheep (fig. 9).

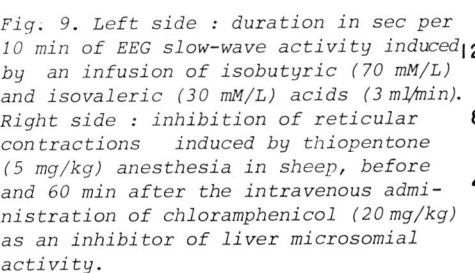 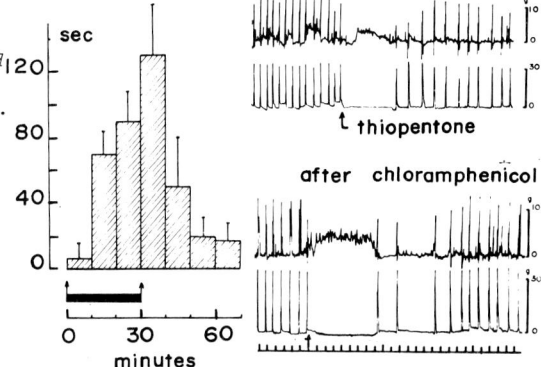

Fig. 9. Left side : duration in sec per 10 min of EEG slow-wave activity induced by an infusion of isobutyric (70 mM/L) and isovaleric (30 mM/L) acids (3 ml/min). Right side : inhibition of reticular contractions induced by thiopentone (5 mg/kg) anesthesia in sheep, before and 60 min after the intravenous administration of chloramphenicol (20 mg/kg) as an inhibitor of liver microsomial activity.

Abomasal ulcers

From 40 % to 90 % of veal calves slaughtered have ulcers apparently asymptomatic in the living animal. Outbreaks of perforating abomasal ulcers associated with abomasal atony have been observed following inclement weather. Acidosis and stress which increase gastric acid secretion might be causative factors. Impairement by H_2 blockers and/or antigastrin substances are likely.

Ion trapping

Weak organic bases are recycled from the blood to the RS by ion trapping. DDT converted to DDD only decreased the protozoal members and the total concentrations of VFA, even for 30 mg/kg per day during 6 weeks. Polyether antibiotics like monensin and lasalacid which do not alter total ruminal nitrogen, ammonia, Na^+ or total VFA concentrations decreased the molar proportion of C_2 and C_4 and increased those of C_3 and ruminal K^+. A therapeutic use is to prevent the production of 3-methyl-indole formed in the rumen from tryptophan which is involved in acute bovine pulmonary edema. Weak organic acids like sulphadiazine (pKa 6.5) are found in saliva at a high level concentrations and diffused passively across the reticulo-ruminal mucosa. However the ruminal concentration ratio to concentration free in the plasma as well as detoxification in the RS depend on the pH in the rumen contents over a range of 5.5-6.5 in health and 4.5-8.0 in disease.

To summarise, the RS pharmacology is linked to the control of the host over its

symbiotic microbial population through the quality and quantity of its food. Movement
of the forestomach compartments, buffering of VFAs by saliva and gastric emptying are
underlying factors.

REFERENCES

1. ASH R.A. - *Stimuli influencing the secretion of acid by the abomasum of sheep. J.
   Physiol., Lond., 1961, 157, 185-207.*
2. BAILE C.A., McLAUGHLIN C. - *Feed intake of goats during volatile fatty acid injections into four gastric areas. J. Dairy Sci., 1970, 53, 1058-1063.*
3. BRUCE L.A., HUBER T.L. - *Inhibitory effect of acid in the intestine on rumen motility in sheep. J. anim. Sci., 1973, 37, 164-168.*
4. BUENO L. - *Orotic acid and non-protein nitrogen overload in sheep. Ann. Rech. vét.
   1979, 10, 29-49.*
5. BUENO L., RUCKEBUSCH Y. - *The cyclic motility of the omasum and its control in
   sheep. J. Physiol., Lond., 1974, 238, 295-312.*
6. BUENO L., RUCKEBUSCH Y. - *Contrôle de l'ingestion alimentaire à partir de chémo-
   récepteurs duodénaux. C. r. Acad. Sci., 1974, 279, 409-412.*
7. DUNLOP R.H., BUENO L. - *Molasses neuro-toxicity and higher volatile fatty acids in
   sheep. Ann. Rech. Vet., 1979, 10, 462-469.*
8. FAUSTINI R., BERETTA C., CHELI R., DE GRESTI A. - *Some effects of caerulein on the
   motility of sheep forestomach and gall bladder. Pharm. Res. Comm., 1973, 5, 383.*
9. ITABISASHI T. - *Urea-ammonia poisoning and ruminal motility in goats. Nat. Inst.
   anim. Hlth Quart., 1977, 17, 128-129.*
10. OHGA A., TANEIKE K. - H_1 *and* H_2- *receptors in the smooth muscle of the ruminant
    stomach. Br. J. Pharmacol., 1978, 62, 333-337.*
11. RUCKEBUSCH Y. - *The effects of pentagastrin on the motility of the ruminant sto-
    mach. Experientia, 1971, 27, 1185-1186.*
12. RUCKEBUSCH Y., LAPLACE J.P. - *Modifications pharmacologiques du comportement ali-
    mentaire : prise de nourriture et rumination chez le mouton. Psychopharmacologia,
    1968, 12, 104-114.*
13. RUCKEBUSCH Y., FARGEAS J., BUENO L. - *Réponses pharmacologiques de la musculatu
    gastrique chez le mouton éveillé : Etude électromyographique. Ann. Rech. vét.,
    1969, 3, 131-148.*
14. RUCKEBUSCH Y., TSIAMITAS Ch., BUENO L. - *The intrinsic electrical activity of th
    ruminant stomach. Life Sci., 1972, 11, 55-64.*
15. STOYANOV L.N., LOUKANOV Y.B., VASSILEVA P.V., VASSILEV V.I. - *Comparative studie
    of the* α *and* β *adrenergic receptors in the longitudinal and circular smooth musc
    layers of the simple and complex stomach. Gen. Pharmac., 1976, 7, 399-404.*
16. SVENDSEN P. - *Inhibition of cecal motility in sheep by volatile fatty acids. Nor
    Vet. Med., 1972, 24, 393-396.*
17. VAN GENDEREN H. - *Farmacologie van de pensmotiliteit. Tijdschr. Diergeneesk.,
    1972, 93, 1392-1401.*
18. VAN MIERT A.S.J.P.A.M. - *Inhibition of gastric motility by endotoxin (bacterial
    lipopolysaccharide) in conscious goats and modification of this response by
    splanchnectomy, adrenalectomy or adrenergic blocking agents. Arch. int. Pharmaco-
    dyn., 1971, 193, 405-414.*
19. VAN MIERT A.S.J.P.A.M., VAN VUGT F. - *The effect of dopamine on gastric adrener-
    gic receptors in the goat. Zbl. Vet. Med., 1974, 21, 96-104.*
20. WALKER D.M., GIBNEY M.J., KIRK R.D. - *Acidosis in preruminant lambs : Effect of
    sodium bicarbonate on nitrogen utilization and voluntary feed intake. Aust. J.
    agric. Res., 1978, 29, 123-132.*
21. WEEKES T.E.C., BUENO L., GARCIA-VILLAR R. - *Insulin release and inhibition of
    forestomach motility in sheep. Horm. metab. Res., 1976, 8, 238-239.*
22. WILSON R.C., GOETSCH D.D., HUBER T.L. - *Studies of mechanisms of action of secre
    tin and pancreozymin on rumen motility. Am. J. vet. Res., 1976, 37, 1131-1134.*

TACHYKININS AND FORESTOMACHS

R. FAUSTINI, P. ORMAS, A. GALBIATI and C. BERETTA
Institute of Veterinary Pharmacology and Toxicology University of Milan - Italy
Research carried out with a grant of C.N.R.

ABSTRACT

Eledoisin proved to be lacking of hypotensive effects in sheep but exerted remarkable stimulatory actions on the smooth musculature of the forestomachal apparatus of ruminants both when investigated *in vitro* (isolated preparations from cattle) and *in vivo* (anaesthetized or awake sheep). The peptide showed moreover a noticeable activity in increasing amplitude and rate of myoelectric potentials of the viscera of the digestive tract of ruminants. Following these findings tachykinins seem to be a good tool to study the physiological and pathological features of these viscera and to open a new field of investigation on the therapeutic equipment to treat their dysfunctions.

INTRODUCTION

The control of motility of ruminant forestomachs is a subject special to veterinary research. The most important findings in this field refer to the involvement of structures of CNS and ANS in controlling and coordinating the motor functions of these viscera. We have now good information on the role of some structures in the cerebral cortex as well as medulla oblongata, on the parasympathetic or sympathetic efferent pathways and moreover on the reflex phenomena which occur through their reciprocal interaction after mediating activities of afferent fibers (1-2-3). Bij contrast little attention has been paid to the possible roles of polypeptides in regulating motor and secretory functions of the various gastrointestinal organs of ruminants in spite of the powerful effects that many of these substances (e.g. gastrins, CCK-PZ, secretin etc.) exert both on visceral smooth muscles and on secretory glands of different animal species. Preliminary investigation performed by Ruckebusch (pentagastrin)(4) and by ourselves (caerulein) (5-6) revealed that this field of investigation might have a promising future in elucidating the physiological role of gastrointestinal hormones on the gastrointestinal apparatus of ruminants, thus preconizing the conclusions of a recent paper of Bell et al. (7): "Experimental investigation of the effects of gastrointestinal hormones on motor, secretory and other functions of the alimentary tract (of ruminants) may make important contributions to the understanding of the development of disease conditions in animals as they have already in man."

OUR OWN EXPERIENCE

Sheep systemic blood pressure

During experiments carried out with caerulein in our laboratory, a peculiar finding resulted at first about the effects of this peptide on sheep blood pressure: moderate hypertension instead of the marked hypotension observed in dogs and rabbits (8). Through a specific experiment (9) we also investigated the effects of another polypeptide, eledoisin, well known as a hypotensive drug more active than caerulein. This tachykinin, when administered intravenously to sheep at doses 1000 times higher than the threshold hypotensive ones in dogs, was ineffective or produced weak hypertensive effects. In animals pretreated with alpha-adrenolytic drugs, these doses of eledoisin exerted only feeble and short lasting depressor effects. This finding revealed that the hypertension observed in intact animals was due to a catecholamine releasing activity of the peptide and moreover that sheep vascular bed was nearly insensitive to its vasodilating properties (fig. 1).

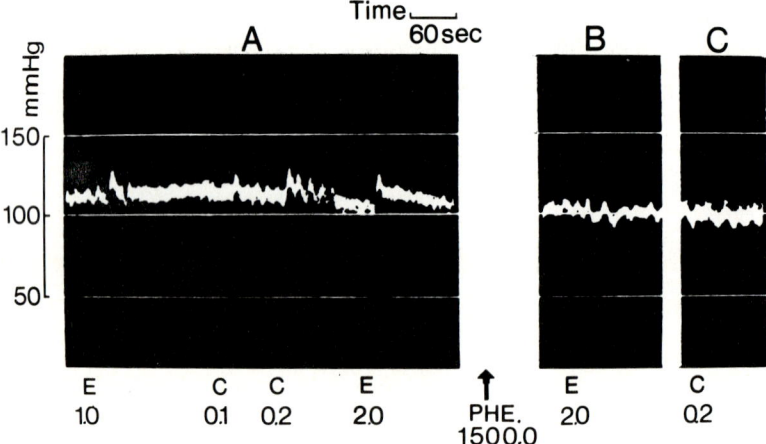

Fig. 1. Blood pressure of a sheep (kg 36) under pentobarbitone anaesthesia. Note the weak hypertensive effects of eledoisin and caerulein (µg/kg) and the lack of hypotensive effects after phentolamine.

The direct observation of movements of the abdominal wall and of evacuation of the bowel after eledoisin, supported in our mind the idea of potent excitatory effects of this drug on visceral smooth muscles of sheep and increased our interest towards tachykinins on ruminant's digestive tract. To study the properties of eledoisin (or physalemin as a second, powerful and representative member of the tachykinin family) some different pharmacological and electrophysiological assays were designe often by employing Substance P as a reference drug.

Spasmogenic effects on ruminant's gastrointestinal sections

The first investigation (10) was directed on isolated preparations *in vitro* of the reticulo-omasal sphincter of cattle which is a critical structure of the forestomachal apparatus of ruminants. The results were as follows: a) eledoisin elicited contraction of the sphincter starting from threshold doses as small as 15-20 ng/ml, while physalemin was inactive up to 500-1000 ng/ml; b) the effects of eledoisin showed a particular and complex pattern in which the presence of a tonic component lacking a good dose-response relationship and of a phasic "up and down" component, whose intensity and rate was proportional to the increasing doses administered in the organ bath was clear (Fig. 2); c) eledoisin was the most potent among different drugs tested for a comparison since bradykinin was 3-7 times less active, acetylcholine 50-100 times, epinephrine 10 times and histamine 60 times (Fig. 3);

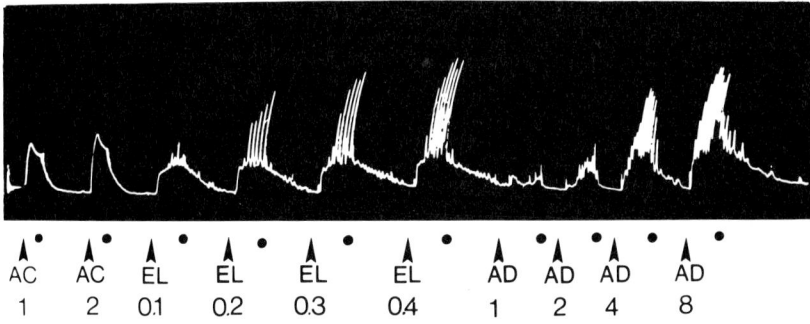

Fig. 2. Isolated reticulum-omasal sphincter. Tyrode at 38°C. Doses of acetylcholine (AC), eledoisin (EL) and epinephrine (AD) in μg/ml. Note the tonic and phasic components of the effects of eledoisin. ● = washing the organ bath.

d) the effects of eledoisin were partially inhibited by papaverine (20 μg/ml) but were resistant to pretreatments of the preparation with hexamethonium (100 μg/ml), cocaine (10 μg/ml), morphine (200 μg/ml), BOL (10 μg/ml), mepyramine (1 μg/ml), atropine (1 μg/ml) and tetradotoxin (2 μg/ml).

DRUGS	ELEDOISIN	BRADYKININ	ACETYLCHOLINE	EPINEPHRINE	HISTAMINE
ACTIVITY RATIO	100	15 - 30	1 - 2	10	1 - 2

Fig. 3. Potency ratio (on the basis of dose response relationship) among different agonists tested on isolated reticulum-omasal sphincter.

A second set of *in vitro* experiments was done to study the responsiveness of the different sections of cattle forestomachs and abomasum to eledoisin (11-12). The results obtained revealed that eledoisin was always the most potent among the various agonists tested i.e. acetylcholine, histamine, 5-HT, epinephrine and Substance P. The potency ratio with Substance P varied from 5 to 20 in favour of eledoisin in the various sections examined.

The most responsive section proved to be abomasum (Fig. 4), since strips from this organ were stimulated by doses of the peptide as small as 2.5-10 ng/ml.

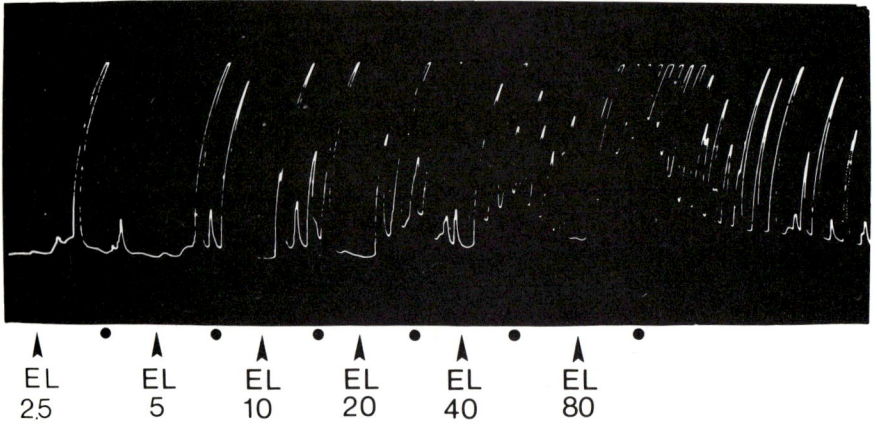

Fig. 4. Isolated strip of bovine abomasum. Tyrode at 38°C. The doses of eledoisin are in ng/ml. ● = washing the organ bath.

As a decreasing order of sensitivity we scored: reticulum and rumen (threshold doses of eledoisin = 20-30 ng/ml) and omasum (threshold doses of eledoisin = 100-150 ng/ml). Since the isolated preparations of the omasum were the most difficult to study (Fig. 5) owing to frequent lacks of spontaneous and acetylcholine-stimulated activity, we cannot really attest to the accuracy of this last determination.

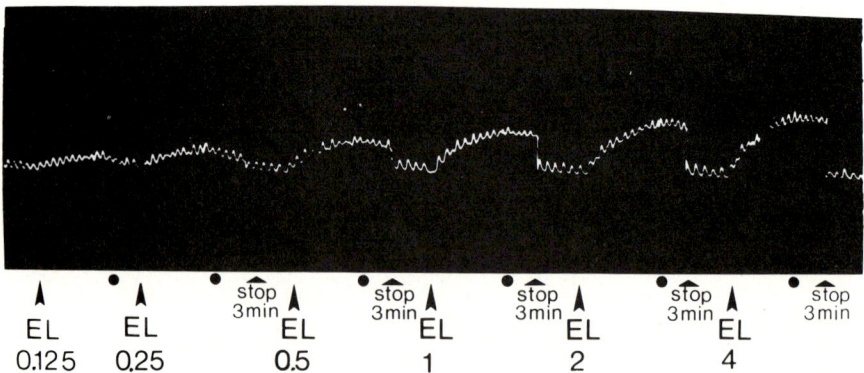

Fig. 5. Isolated strip of bovine omasum. Tyrode at 38°C. The doses of eledoisin are in µg/ml. ● = washing the organ bath.

The conclusions drawn from these experiments revealed that the smooth musculature of forestomachs and abomasum of cattle are responsive to eledoisin and encouraged us to pursue our experiments and to study it also *in vivo*.

For these purposes we decided to employ sheep as experimental animals. The animals were put under pentobarbitone anaesthesia and strain-gauges were surgically applied to the serosal surface of reticulum, omasum, rumen (dorsal sac) and abomasum. The experiments were performed by administering the drugs intravenously either to anaesthetized animals or to animals (24 hours after the surgical operation) awake and standing. The results (11-12-13-14) confirmed the previous findings of the *in vitro* experiments and may be summarized as follows:

a) eledoisin stimulated motility both of the anterior gastric section (rumen, reticulum, omasum) and of abomasum; b) omasum was the most sensitive section,

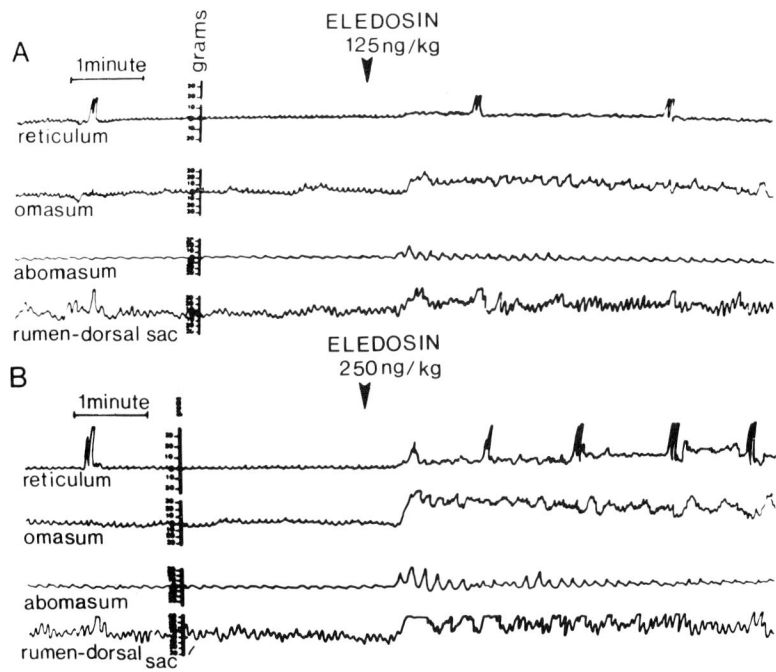

Fig. 6. Effects of 125 (a) and 250 (b) ng/kg of eledoisin administered intravenously on the mechanical activities of reticulum, omasum, abomasum and rumen (dorsal sac).

the threshold doses of eledoisin being 25-50 ng/kg; c) the other stomachs were
sensitive to eledoisin starting from 50-100 ng/kg; d) reticulum activity could be
restored by eledoisin also when it was silent following a previous administration
of caerulein which had been proved to block its rythmical motility when intravenously
infused at a rate of 0.1 ng/kg/min (6); e) the effects of eledoisin were always
proportional to the doses administered both for intensity and duration. Reticulum
showed an exceptional behaviour with doses of eledoisin higher than 0.5 μg/kg
because at these dose levels the peptide evoked immediately a burst of rapid and
superficial waves of contraction (as observed through the recording system employed)
which only later on, were followed by enlarged and frequent contractions of the
organ; f) parasympatholytic, ganglionic blocking, antihistaminic, alpha and beta
adrenolytic and anti-5-HT drugs always failed to affect the stimulating properties
of eledoisin; g) synthetic Substance P up to 1.0 - 1.5 μg/kg i.v. was completely
inactive in provoking any stimulation of motor functions of all the sections
examined; h) the effects of eledoisin on gastric musculature were nowhere accompanied
by any modification of artial blood pressure (monitored) or of heart performances
(at least at a clinical evaluation) (Fig. 6a and b). On account of this set of
assays we might state that the effects of eledoisin were due to a direct stimulation
of the ruminant visceral smooth musculature, that sheep offered a good experimental
model to study these properties of eledoisin without any cardiovascular interference
and that eledoisin might be a possible therapeutic tool for treatment of the
frequent event of forestomach atonia in ruminants.

Spasmogenic effects on extra-gastrointestinal structures

In the meantime, both for a further study of the extravascular effects of
eledoisin and for a comparison of them with analogous anatomical structures from
different animal species, new experiments were performed $in\ vitro$ on isolated
preparations of urinary bladder of swine, cattle and horses (15) on the basis
that this test was useful (16-17-18) for qualitative discrimination of tachykinins
and caerulein-like peptides and for their quantitative assays.

Through this assay eledoisin also revealed good dose-related effects on cattle
urinary bladder, although the preparations obtained from swines were 2-10 times
more sensitive to the polypeptide spasmogenic properties.

Myoelectrical recordings

The last approach we made in studying eledoisin effects was performed by means
of drawings of the electromyograms from the wall of the different sections of the
gastric apparatus of sheep (Fig. 7).

The muscular potentials were recorded through extracellular bipolar electrodes
prepared with silver wire (Ø = 0.4 mm) and surgically implanted in the muscular
layers (serosal sides) of rumen (posterior part of the dorsal sac), reticulum

(apical part of the ventral area), omasum (great curvature), abomasum (pyloric region) and duodenum (10 - 15 cm caudal to the pylorus). The electrode connections passed across the abdominal wall through a teflon plug sutured on it and were connected to a paper photokymographic system. The animals were tested only on the 10th - 12th day after the surgical operation in order to avoid the recording of non specific events following the acute inflammation of the handled tissues. The experiments were always performed on awake and standing animals which had fasted 24 - 36 hours, since the intense myoelectrical activity recorded during feeding was found to disguise the stimulant effects of the drugs injected intravenously.

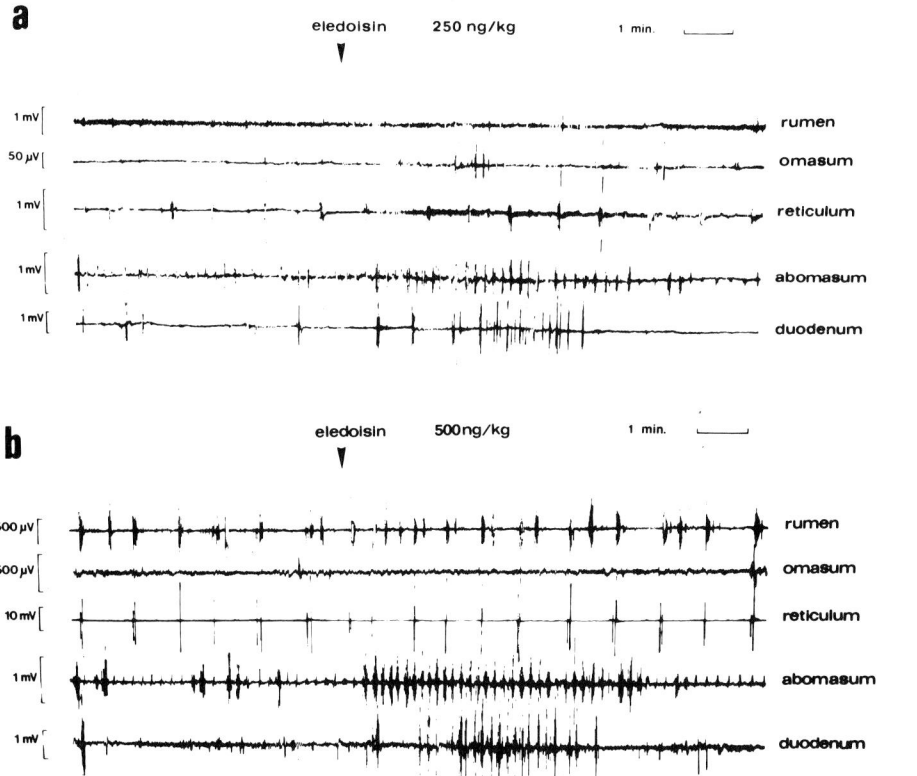

Fig. 7. Myoelectric potentials of rumen, omasum, reticulum, abomasum and duodenum. Effects of 250 (a) and 500 (b) ng/kg i.v. of eledoisin.

The results recently obtained may be summarized as follows: 1) starting from 50 - 100 ng/kg i.v. eledoisin increased both amplitude and rate of abomasal and duodenal spike potentials; 2) increasing doses of the peptide evoked increasing effects, provided a 60 min interval period elapsed between two succesive administrations: otherwise tachyphylaxis often occurred; 3) increases of amplitude and rate of spike potentials of rumen and reticulum were excited by eledoisin only at doses as high as 250 - 500 ng/kg i.v.; 4) the basal muscular potentials of omasum were too inconstant and the effects of eledoisin too incoherent to allow definitive conclusions; 5) the slow wave potentials, which were detected only as a basal electric rythm (BER) of abomasal activity during periods of silence of spike potentials, were not affected by eledoisin; 6) some of the antagonists employed in order to investigate the mechanism of action of eledoisin sometimes exerted effects by themselves: for instance Methysergide (250 μg/kg i.v.) strongly excited electric activity of rumen-reticulum, abomasum and duodenum, while hexamethonium (8 mg/kg i.v.) inhibited ruminal spikes and abolished those of the other sections. Obviously these findings tangled up the effects of the peptide which often could not be correctly discriminated; 7) physalemin behaved exactly like eldoisin having only a weaker activity (80 - 90%).

By summing up these still incomplete results we may however confirm that eledoisin stimulates the myoelectric activity of visceral musculature of the whole gastric apparatus of ruminants.

Concluding remarks

The introduction of a new family of compounds such as polypeptides of the tachykinin type as drugs affecting forestomach and abomasal motor functions seems to be a good approach to the study of the physiological and pathological features of these viscera and to open a new field of investigation on the therapeutic equipment required to treat their dysfunctions.

By employing eledoisin as a characteristic member of this class of substances we always observed (isolated preparations *in vitro*, contractions *in vivo*, myoelectric potentials *in vivo*) stimulations of the motor activities of these gastric sections. Some discrepancies were recorded as regards the effective doses of eledoisin on the different sections examined, according to the different methods of investigations used. These discrepancies are difficult to interpret to date since they may be due to possible interactions of neural and humoral mechanisms involved in the control of these motor functions

These mechanisms require further investigation.

REFERENCES

1. Titchen, D.A.: "Nervous control of motility of the forestomach of ruminants" in Handbook of Physiology - Section 6 - "Alimentary Canal". Ed. by C.F. Code & W. Heidel - American Physiological Society Washington D.C. 1968.
2. Ruckebusch, Y.: Physiologie, pharmacologie, therapeutique animales? Maloine, S. Editeur - Paris 1979.
3. Leek, B.F. & Harding, R.H.: "Sensory nervous receptors in the ruminant stomach and the reflex control of reticulo-ruminal motility" p. 60-76 in "Digestion and metabolism in the ruminant." Ed. I.N. McDonald and A.C.I. Warner - IV Int. Symp. - Sydney - Australia - Univ. of New Publishing Unit (1975).

4. Ruckebusch, Y. - Experientia 27 (1971), 1185-1186
5. Beretta, C., Calvari, A.R., Leonardi, L. & Faustini, R. - Pharmac. Res. Comm. 5 (1973), 11-15
6. Faustini, R., Beretta, C., Cheli, R. & DeGresti, A. - Pharmac. Res. Comm. 5 (1973), 383-387
7. Bell, F.R., Titchen, D.A. & Watson, D.J. - Res. Vet. Sci. 23 (1977), 165-170
8. Bertaccini, G., DeCaro, G., Endean, R., Erspamer, V. & Impicciatore, M. - Brit. J. Pharmacol. 33 (1968), 59-71
9. Ormas, P., Pompa, G., Beretta, C. & Faustini, R. - Folia Vet. Latina 5 (1975) 45-54
10. Ormas, P., Beretta, C., Pompa, G., Andreini, G.C. & Villalobos, S.J. - Atti S.I.S. Vet. 28 (1974), 408-411
11. Ormas, P., Beretta, C., Villalobos, S.J., Pompa, G., Andreini, G.C., Beretta, C.M. & Faustini, R.: Pharmac. Res. Comm. 7 (1975), 527-534
12. Ormas, P., Beretta, C., Villalobos, S.J., Andreini, G.C., Beretta, C.M., Pompa, G. & Faustini, R.: 20th World Vet. Congress. - Salonicco - July 1975 - p. 344-346
13. Beretta, C., Faustini, R., Ormas, P. & Pompa, G.: Brit. J. Pharmacol. 52 (1974),, 468P
14. Faustini, R.: Deutsch. Tierärztl. Wochenschr. 83 (1976), 169-172
15. Ormas, P., Villalobos, S.J., Beretta, C.M. & Pompa, G.: Atti S.I.S. Vet. 30 (1976), 305-308
16. Falconieri Erspamer, G., Negri, L. & Piccinelli, D.: Naunyn Schmied. Arch. Pharm. 279 (1973), 61-74
17. Angelucci, L., Falconieri Erspamer, G. & Negri, L.: J. Pharm. Pharmac. 26 (1974), 193-196
18. Erspamer, V.: Ann. Rev. Pharmac. 11 (1971), 327-350

FEVER AND RETICULO-RUMINAL DYSFUNCTION

A.S.J.P.A.M. VAN MIERT

Department of Veterinary Pharmacology and Toxicology, Utrecht University, Utrecht
(The Netherlands)

ABSTRACT

   Injection of exogenous pyrogens cause fever and stasis of forestomach contraction
sequences in ruminants. The reactions of conscious goats and anesthetized sheep
to *E.coli* endotoxin administration were studied in more detail. Latency time, the
time during which shivering could be observed, the shape of the temperature curves
and the magnitude of the inhibition of the rumen contractions were all dose-dependent.
The stasis of forestomach contractions is 1. not secondary to the effects of
endotoxin on thermoregulation, 2. not mediated by endogenous pyrogen, 3. not
mediated by adrenaline or an increase in sympathetic activity, 4. not mediated
by histamine, serotonin or bradykinin. There is, however, a lot of evidence which
indicates that the stasis is the result of, initially, a reduced afferent drive
to the gastric centres and, later, a central nervous depression involving the
gastric centres. Antipyretic agents, which inhibit the synthesis of prostaglandins,
abolished fever and partly blocked the inhibition of reticulo-rumen motility due
to exogenous pyrogens. Therefore, it appears that prostaglandins are not predominant
involved in pyrogen-induced reticulo-ruminal stasis.

INTRODUCTION

   In 1762 Van Cour (33) accurately described the inhibition of forestomach
motility in febrile ruminants. This illustrates that for centuries fever and
associated clinical symptoms were recognized signs of disease. However, only during
the past six decades have the mechanisms by which gastric dysfunction develops
during fever begun to be clarified.

   The first contributions in this field appear to be those of Meyer and Carlson
(23,24). They observed that dogs with distemper or pneumonia refused food, and
showed complete atony of the stomach with absence of hunger contractions especially
during the fever episodes. In addition, they did some experiments in which fever
was evoked by pyrogens such as sodium nucleinate and a killed culture of *Serratia
marcessens*. Their conclusions were: first, that gastric secretion and the hunger

contractions were absent in marked fever and that these effects were associated with anorexia as long as fever was present; secondly, that these effects were present even after transection of the splanchnic nerves; and thirdly, that these effects were dependent on mechanisms which used parasympathetic pathways. Furthermore, the pyrogens used did not show any direct effect on gastric smooth muscles. Since then, other investigators confirmed the inhibition of gastric secretion by pyrogens, although less effort was expended to elucidate the mechanisms underlying this inhibitory effect (6,7,8,9,28,56). Moreover, little attention has been devoted to the effect of pyrogens on gastric emptying rate (27).

This report reviews our experimental work as a contribution towards the knowledge of fever and reticulo-ruminal dysfunction.

METHODS

Goats were trained to stand quietly during actual recording sessions by repeatedly placing them in the experimental cage, for several hours at a time, after passing nasal catheters to the rumen. Recordings of the intragastric pressure changes were made by means of an open-ended water-filled polyethylene tube passed into the rumen, while the other end was connected to a pressure transducer. The frequency (RF) and the amplitude (RA) of the rumen contractions were measured every 15 min and expressed in percentages of the initial value. These values were plotted on graph paper, with 1 h equal to 2 cm and 10% equal to 1 cm. Rectal temperatures were measured with an electrothermometer. The fever curves were plotted on graph paper with 1 h equal to 2 cm and $1^{\circ}C$ equal to 5 cm. Next a fever-index was calculated, this being the area in square cm under the fever curves. A frequency and amplitude index for rumen contractions was calculated in the same way.

EXOGENOUS PYROGENS

Intravenous injection of exogenous pyrogens induced fever, changes in heart rate (46,47) and inhibition of the reticulo-rumen contractions (Figures 1 and 2; Table 1). From these experiments we concluded that in conditions associated with fever, there is an inhibition of the forestomach contractions. This is in agreement with the observations made in patients during febrile episodes (10,12,13).

HYPERTHERMIA AND ENDOGENOUS PYROGEN

It is known that a physically induced rise of body temperature affects gastric secretion (6,9) and motility (23,25) in monogastric species. Therefore it seemed of interest to investigate the effect of hyperthermia on rumen contractions. The result of this experiment confirmed that body temperature elevation itself is a factor in the depression of gastric motility (5,36). The presence of endogenous pyrogens in the blood of goats during endotoxin-induced fever has been

Table 1.   FEVER AND INHIBITION OF RUMEN MOTILITY BY EXOGENOUS PYROGENS

Pyrogen	Dose per kg i.v.	Fever Index[1] $\pm$ SEM	Rumen contractions Amplitude Index[1]	Frequency Index[1]	N
Saline	1 ml	-1.5 $\pm$ 1.6	9.7 $\pm$ 1.6	6.5 $\pm$ 1.6	9
Poly 1:Poly C	30 µg	30.4 $\pm$ 7.8	40.0 $\pm$ 0.8	29.2 $\pm$ 0.5	4
Johnin[o]	5 µg	48.8 $\pm$ 5.5	33.9 $\pm$ 6.4	30.7 $\pm$ 6.8	8
NCD virus[*]	0.7 ml	54.1 $\pm$ 6.3	39.3 $\pm$ 5.9	27.1 $\pm$ 5.2	7
Nucleinate	10 mg	41.6 $\pm$ 4.0	60.4 $\pm$ 6.8	46.6 $\pm$ 7.2	7
E.coli LPS					
batch 481424	0.01 µg	23 $\pm$ 4.1	13 $\pm$ 4.2	7 $\pm$ 2.6	5
	0.025 µg	36 $\pm$ 5.9	27 $\pm$ 7.6	15 $\pm$ 5.4	5
	0.05 µg	49 $\pm$ 6.1	60 $\pm$ 3.6	43 $\pm$ 5.6	5
	0.1 µg	65 $\pm$ 6.7	64 $\pm$ 6.2	44 $\pm$ 7.6	5
	1 µg	47 $\pm$ 6.8	73 $\pm$ 3.9	53 $\pm$ 5.9	5
	10 µg	29 $\pm$ 6.6	81 $\pm$ 4.7	65 $\pm$ 5.3	5
batch 487989	0.1 µg	48.8 $\pm$ 4.8	68.1 $\pm$ 4.5	55.5 $\pm$ 5.1	8
batch 614378	0.1 µg	45.6 $\pm$ 4.3	67.4 $\pm$ 3.8	60.7 $\pm$ 4.4	14
S. typhimurium					
batch 514553	0.1 µg	49.6 $\pm$ 4.0	58.1 $\pm$ 5.1	50.5 $\pm$ 3.1	9
batch 488866	0.3 µg	55.1 $\pm$ 7.5	63.1 $\pm$ 3.4	46.9 $\pm$ 4.6	7
E.coli LPS					
batch 487989	0.01 µg[3]	10.6 $\pm$ 2.4[2]	9.6 $\pm$ 3.2[2]	6.1 $\pm$ 2.9[2]	4
	0.01 µg[4]	27.8 $\pm$ 4.5[2]	33.9 $\pm$ 8.7[2]	23.5 $\pm$ 7.3[2]	

N = number of goats per group

1) = index $\pm$ standard error of the mean calculated for 5 hours

2) = index $\pm$ standard error of the mean calculated for 4 hours

3) = total dose i.v.;   4) = total dose injected into the third ventricle
                            of the brain

o) = in previously vaccinated animals

* = La Sota strain, haemagglutination titre 1:240

demonstrated (40,41,46). Endogenous pyrogen evoked typical short lasting febrile
responses, while a marked inhibitory effect upon the rumen contractions could not
be observed (46). Moreover, an inhibition of rumen motility could not be recorded
during fever induced by intramammary administered endotoxin (54). In vitro
experiments showed that neither endogenous pyrogen nor endotoxins had any effect
on ruminal smooth muscles (37).

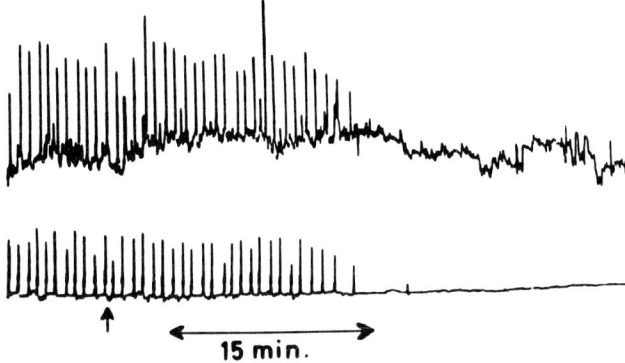

Fig. 1. Simultaneous inhibition of the extrinsic reticular and ruminal contractions
after i.v. injection (= ↑) of LPS E.coli 0.2 µg per kg body weight. Upper
tracing: contractions of dorsal rumen-sack; lower tracing: reticulum
contractions.(After Van Miert (1971), Arch. Int. Pharmacodyn., 193: 405-414)

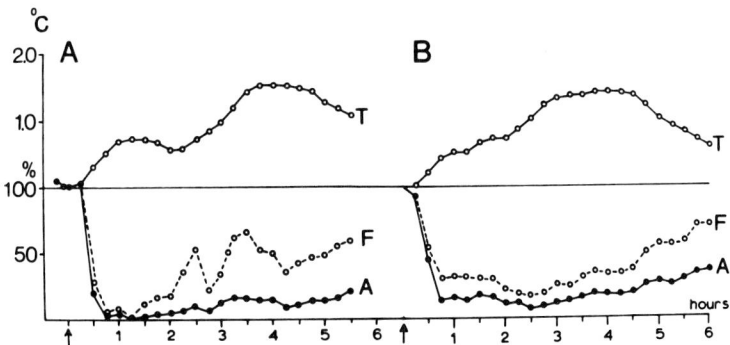

Fig. 2. The effect of LPS E.coli (↑ = 0.2 µg per kg body weight i.v.) on the extrinsic
reticular (A, left side) and ruminal (B, right side) contractions in groups
of 4 conscious goats. T = rise in body temperature; F = frequency of
contractions per 15 min expressed in % of the initial value; A = summation
derived from 15 min intervals of amplitude expressed in % of the initial
value. Mean values are given.

ENDOTOXINS

The reactions of adult goats to the intravenous administration of $E.coli$ endotoxin
were studied in more detail (39,50). Latency time, the time during which shivering
could be observed, the area under the temperature curves and the magnitude of the
inhibition of the rumen contractions were all dose-dependent (Table 1). With higher
doses of endotoxin the inhibition of rumen contractions was more pronounced while
the rise in body temperature was less prominent. The conclussion based on these
observations was that endotoxin-induced ruminal stasis in not secondary to the

effects of this pyrogen on thermoregulation (38,39). This is in agreement with
the observations made in rats after endotoxin administration. *E.coli* endotoxin
did not induce fever in this species (43). Nevertheless, an inhibition of gastric
secretion (22) and gastric emptying rate (42) could be observed. In other words,
the effects of endotoxin on thermoregulation and on the stomach seem to be due
to different mechanisms.

HUMORAL INTERMEDIATES

From the literature it is known that during hyperthermia (4,31) but also during
endotoxin-induced fever (29,32), a marked release of catecholamines occurs. Within
the intact animal both, α- and β- adrenergic drugs interfere with the reticular
and rumen contractions (35), probably by reflex inhibition. An intravenous infusion
with α- and β-adrenergic receptor blocking agents did not oppose the action of
endotoxin upon heart rate and rumen motility. Moreover, adrenalectomy or transection
of the splanchnic nerves did not antagonize the inhibition of reticular and rumen
contractions to endotoxin either (38).

A large number of vasoactive and spasmogenic agents are released during endotoxin-
induced shock (3,18,19,30,55). These include histamine, serotonin, bradykinin and
prostaglandins. Furthermore, these tissue hormones seem to be liberated during
immediate hypersensitivity (1,2,14). Clinical symptoms observed during endotoxin
shock or during experimentally induced, acute, systemic anaphylaxis in ruminants
include inhibition of rumen contractions, ruminal tympany and hypothermia occasional
followed by an increase in body temperature (1,2,11,17,26). However, little is
known about the influence of low pyrogenic doses of endotoxin upon the synthesis
and/or release of these substances. The question as to which humoral substances
is primarily responsible for mediating the forestomach responses induced with
pyrogenic doses of endotoxin cannot be answered conclusively from our experiments.
Certain conclusions can, however, be drawn. Neither histamine, serotonin nor
bradykinin are important humoral intermediates in the pyrogen-induced reticulo-
ruminal stasis (49,51,52). This conclusion is partly based on the finding that
endotoxin-induced ruminal stasis cannot be modified by pretreatment with specific
inhibitors of these agents, including H_1- and H_2 receptor blocking agents and
serotonin antagonists. Moreover, no significant changes in plasma serotonin (52)
and prostaglandin concentrations (53) could be found during endotoxin-induced
fever and only a small increase of the whole blood bradykinin-like activity could
be detected (52). On the other hand, nonsteroidal anti-inflammatory agents, which
inhibit the synthesis of prostaglandins (16,34), abolished fever and had a
significant partial antagonistic influence upon endotoxin-induced ruminal stasis
(45,47,53). It is well known that circulating prostaglandins are rapidly inactivated
by enzyme systems especially within the lung (15). Therefore, we cannot exclude

the possibility that pyrogenic doses of endotoxin increase prostaglandin production by ruminal tissue.

RESULTS OF ELECTROPHYSIOLOGICAL STUDIES

General anesthesia depresses thermoregulation. Nevertheless, the reticulo-ruminal responses of conscious sheep and goats to endotoxin were obtained similarly in halothane-anesthetized sheep (20), which therefore allowed a more profound analysis of the mode of action of this pyrogen. Dr. B.F. Leek and I did a number of experiments in which single-fibre techniques were used for recording both afferent vagal activity from nerves fibres innervating tension perceptors in the reticulo-rumen and efferent vagal activity in preganglionic fibres from the gastric centres to the reticulo-ruminal smooth muscles (20,21). After intravenous endotoxin administration four phases could be recognized, namely a latent period of 10 to 20 min, the onset of the stasis (approximately 8 min) and a prolonged depression of the extrinsic contractions followed by an episode during which the contractions reappeared and gradually returned to normal. During the latent period no changes were observed in the characteristics of the spike discharges from both afferent and efferent fibres. At the onset of the stasis there was little or no afferent activity (Figure 4) and no efferent activity.During this period it was possible to restore the extrinsic contractions by stimulating vagal afferent fibres electrically, by increasing tension perceptors activity passively by distending the reticulum (Figure 3) or by increasing tension perceptors activity actively by increasing

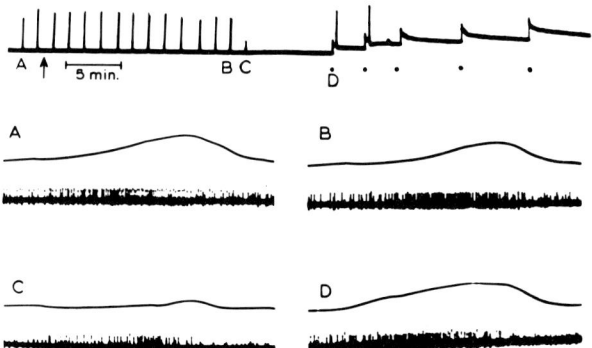

Fig. 3. The effect of LPS E.coli (↑ = 0.2 µg per kg body weight i.v.) on the extrinsic reticular contractions in a halothane-anesthetized sheep (upper tracing). A-D: Records showing the discharge patterns in an efferent gastric vagal unit. A: control; B: 17 min after LPS injection (normal discharge pattern); C: last spontaneous contraction (smaller size with a reduced number of spikes); D: reticulum contraction induced by distending the reticulum At . the volume of air in the reticular balloon was increased by 100 ml (After Van Miert et al. (1976) with permission of the editors Dtsch. Tierärzt. Wschr., 83: 188-192).

190

smooth muscle tonus with spasmogenic agents such as phenylephrine (21,44). During
the third phase, afferent activity became normal or supranormal but efferent activity
and extrinsic contractions remained absent (Figure 4). Electrical stimulation of the
afferent vagal fibres was ineffective in restoring extrinsic contractions. However,
electrical stimulation of the efferent fibres evoked contractions similar to those
obtained before endotoxin administration (Figure 5). Therefore, it was obvious that

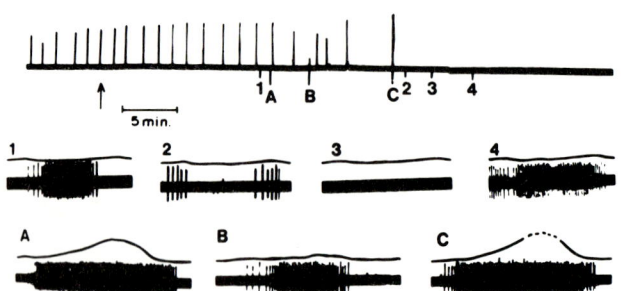

Fig. 4. The effect of LPS E.coli (↑ = 0.2 µg per kg body weight i.v.) on the extrins
(upper tracing) and intrinsic reticular contractions in a halothane-anesthetized sheep. 1-4: Records showing the discharge patterns in an afferent
unit innervating reticular tension perceptors, when extrinsic contractions
were absent. 1: normal activity, 2: reduced activity, 3: no activity,
4: supranormal activity. A-C: afferent discharge patterns, when the
reticulum contracted. (After Van Miert et al. (1976) with permission of
the editors Dtsch. Tierärztl. Wschr., 83: 188-192).

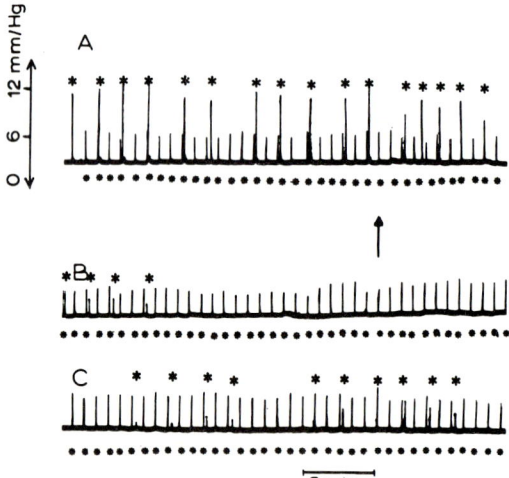

Fig. 5. The effect of LPS E.coli (↑ = 0.2 µg per kg body weight i.v.) on the extrins
reticular contractions in a halothane-anesthetized sheep. The spontaneous
contractions (*) stopped 16 min (B) after LPS administration, while there
was no influence upon the contractions evoked by stimulating motor fibres
in a branch of the thoracal vagus nerve. The spontaneous contractions
reappeared gradually after 57 min (C). At *, trains of stimuli (12 V) at
a frequency of 30 per sec were given at intervals of 1 min for durations
of 2 sec.

the pyrogen had an inhibitory action upon the central nervous system. This central effect was unaffected by complete transection of the brain stem at levels 10 mm rostal or 5 mm caudal to the obex, thereby leaving the gastric centres and their vagal connections intact (20). In other words, during the third phase, the pyrogen induced a prolonged depression of the gastric centres in the medulla oblongata. The results obtained from experiments in which endotoxin was given by intracerebral injections were in agreement with these observations.

EFFECTS OF INTRACEREBRAL INJECTION

The changes in arterial blood pressure and reticulum motility that resulted from endotoxin injection near the left and right dorsal vagal nucleus were similar to those produced by intravenous injection of this pyrogen (48). However, on intravenous injection about a 100 times larger dose of endotoxin was required than on injection into the medulla oblongata, which demonstrated that these effects were not due to a leakage of the pyrogen into the systemic circulation. The administration of a small dose of endotoxin (0.01 µg LPS *E.coli*, Table 1) into the third ventricle of conscious goats induced shivering, a biphasic rise in body temperature and inhibition of the extrinsic rumen contractions (48). A similar dose of this pyrogen given intravenously was much less effective. These findings prove that these effects can be reproduced by an action of endotoxin within the central nervous system. However, the symptoms were preceded by a certain time lag, which suggests that the action of endotoxin within the CNS is an indirect one. What is still required is a detailed study of these processes within the CNS.

REFERENCES

1. Aitken, M.M., Deline. T.R. and Eyre, P. (1975), J. Comp. Path., 85: 351-360
2. Aitken, M.M., Sanford, J., and Evans, D.P. (1975), Res. Vet. Sci., 18: 41-48
3. Al-Kaisi, N., Parratt, J.R., Siddiqui, H.H., and Zeitlin, I.J. (1975), J. Physiol., 256: 24P-25P
4. Andersson, B., Gale, C.C., Hökfelt, B., and Ohga, A. (1963), Acta Physiol. Scand., 61: 182-191
5. Atteberg, J.T., and Johnson, H.D. (1969), J. Animal Sci., 29: 734-737
6. Bandes, J., Hollander, F., and Bierman, W. (1948), Gastroenterol., 10: 697-707
7. Baume, P.E., Nicholls, A., and Baxter, C.H. (1967), Nature, 215: 59-60
8. Blickenstaff, D., and Grossman, M.I. (1950), Am. J. Physiol., 160: 567-571
9. Brodie, D.A., and Kundrats, S.K. (1964), Gastroenterol., 47: 171-178
10. Brunaud, M. (1954), Rev. Méd. Vét., 105: 535-580
11. Campbell, S.G. (1970), Cornell Vet., 60: 240-253
12. Clark, R. (1956), J.S.Afr. Vet. Med. Ass., 27:75-104
13. Diernhofer, K. (1959), Dtsch. tierärztl. Wschr. 66: 141-149
14. Eyre, P., and Burka, J.F. (1978), J. Vet. Pharmacol. Therap., 1: 97-109
15. Ferreira, S.H., and Vane, J.R. (1967), Nature, 216: 868-873
16. Flower, R.J., and Vane, J.R. (1972), Nature, 240: 410-411
17. Griel, L.C., Zarkowa, A., and Eberhart, R.J. (1975), Can. J. Comp. Med., 39: 1-6
18. Hall, R.C., and Hodge, R.L. (1971), J. Physiol., 213: 69-84
19. Hinshaw, L.B. (1964) in: Bacterial Endotoxins. ed. M. Landy and W. Braun Rutgers The State University, 118-125

20. Leek, B.F., and Van Miert, A.S.J.P.A.M. (1971), J. Physiol., 215: 28P-29P
21. Leek, B.F., and Van Miert, A.S.J.P.A.M. (1971), Rendic. R. Gastroenterol.,
    3: 163-167
22. Leenen, F.H.H. and Van Miert, A.S.J.P.A.M. (1969), Eur. J. Pharmacol.,
    8: 228-231
23. Meyer, J., and Carlson, A.J. (1917), Am. J. Physiol., 44: 222-233
24. Meyer, J., Cohen, S.J., and Carlson, A.J. (1918), Arch. Int. Med., 21: 354-365
25. Misiewicz, J.J., Waller, S.L., Fox, R.H., Goldsmith, R., and Hunt, T.J. (1968),
    Clin. Sci., 34: 149-159
26. Mullenax, C.H., Keller, R.F., and Allison, M.J. (1966), Am. J. Vet. Res.,
    27: 857-868
27. Necheles, H., Dommers, P., Weiner, M., Olson, W.H., and Rychel, W. (1942),
    Am. J. Physiol., 137: 22-29
28. Olson, W.H., Walker, L., and Necheles, H. (1954), Am. J. Physiol., 176: 393-395
29. Ouellette, H.H., Chosy, J.J., and Reed, C.H. (1967), J. Allergy, 39: 234-237
30. Parratt, J.R., and Sturgess, R.M. (1977), Br. J. Pharmac., 60: 209-219
31. Robertshaw, D., and Whittow, G.C. (1966), J. Physiol., 187: 351-360
32. Serafimov, N. (1962), Acta Physiol. Scand., 54: 354-358
33. Van Cour, P.A. (1762), Verhandelingen van allerlei ziektes van het rundvee,
    schapen, varkens, etc. ed. Ottho van Thol, 's-Gravenhage
34. Vane, J.R. (1971), Nature New Biol., 231: 232-235
35. Van Miert, A.S.J.P.A.M. (1969), J. Pharm. Pharmac. 21: 697-699
36. Van Miert, A.S.J.P.A.M. (1969), Acta Physiol. Pharmacol. Neerl., 15: 57-58
37. Van Miert, A.S.J.P.A.M. (1970), Ph. D. Thesis, University of Utrecht
38. Van Miert, A.S.J.P.A.M. (1971), Arch. Int. Pharmacodyn., 193: 404-415
39. Van Miert, A.S.J.P.A.M. (1973), Zbl. Vet. Med. Reihe A, 20: 614-623
40. Van Miert, A.S.J.P.A.M., and Atmakusuma, A. (1970), Zbl. Vet. Med. Reihe A,
    17: 174-184
41. Van MIert, A.S.J.P.A.M., and Atmakusuma, A. (1971), J. Comp. Path., 81: 119-127
42. Van Miert, A.S.J.P.A.M., and de la Parra, D.A. (1970), Arch. Int. Pharmacodyn.,
    184: 27-33
43. Van Miert, A.S.J.P.A.M., and Frens, J. (1968), Zbl. Vet. Med., Reihe A,
    15: 532-543
44. Van Miert, A.S.J.P.A.M., and Huisman, E.A. (1968), J. Pharm. Pharmac., 20:
    495-496
45. Van Miert, A.S.J.P.A.M., Van der Wal-Komproe, L.E., and Van Duin, C.Th.M.
    (1977), Arch. Int. Pharmacodyn., 225: 39-50
46. Van Miert, A.S.J.P.A.M., and Van Duin, C.Th.M. (1974), Zbl. Vet. Med. Reihe A,
    21: 692-702
47. Van Miert, A.S.J.P.A.M., and Van Duin, C.Th.M. (1979), J. Vet. Pharmacol. Thera
    2: 69-79
48. Van Miert, A.S.J.P.A.M., Van Duin, C.Th.M., and Leek, B.F. (1978), Zbl. Vet. Me
    Reihe A, 25: 718-726
49. Van Miert, A.S.J.P.A.M., Van Duin, C.Th.M., and Veenendaal, G.H. (1976), Zbl.
    Vet. Med. Reihe A, 23: 819-826
50. Van Miert, A.S.J.P.A.M., Veenendaal, G.H., and Van Genderen, H. (1976), Dtsch.
    Tierärztl. Wschr., 83: 188-192
51. Veenendaal, G.H. (1979), Ph.D. Thesis, University of Utrecht
52. Veenendaal, G.H., Van Miert, A.S.J.P.A.M., Van de Ingh, T.S.G.A.M., Schotman,
    A.J.H., and Zwart, D. (1976), Res. Vet. Sci., 21: 271-279
53. Veenendaal, G.H., Woutersen-Van Nijnanten, F.M.A., Van Duin, C.Th.M., and Van
    Miert, A.S.J.P.A.M. (1980), Res. Vet. Sci. in press
54. Verheijden, J.H.M. (1979), Ph.D. Thesis, University of Utrecht
55. Vick, J.A., Mehlman, B., and Heiffer, M.H. (1971), Proc. Soc. Exptl. Biol. Med.
    137: 902-906
56. Wyllie, J.H., Limbosch, J.M., and Nijhuis, L.M. (1967), Nature, 215: 879

TISSUE HORMONES AND RUMEN MOTILITY

G.H. VEENENDAAL

Institute of Veterinary Pharmacology and Toxicology, Faculty of Veterinary

Medicine, The State University, Biltstraat 172, 3572 BP Utrecht (The Netherlands)

ABSTRACT

   Concentration-response curves obtained for contraction of goat rumen strips

showed that PGE_1, $PGF_{2\alpha}$, bradykinin and serotonin are very potent agents. On a

molar basis the following rank order of potency can be given PGE_1 >BK >5-HT

>$PGF_{2\alpha}$. Histamine was rather inactive on this preparation. Polyphloretinphosphate

antagonized the smooth muscle stimulating action of both PGE_1 and $PGF_{2\alpha}$. The

shift to the right, apparently in parallel of the concentration-response curve

for $PGF_{2\alpha}$ suggests that the antagonism is competitive in nature. Sodiummeclo-

fenamate antagonized the smooth muscle stimulating action of bradykinin; the

5-HT blocking agents xylamidine and methysergide diminished the contractile

effects of serotonin. The results suggest a non competitive antagonism. In situ

prostaglandin E_1 and $F_{2\alpha}$ as well as histamine, bradykinin and 5-HT caused a

dose dependent inhibition of rumen contraction sequences. On a molar basis the

rank order of potency for inhibition of rumen motility was: BK >PGE_1> $PGF_{2\alpha}$

>5-HT > H. This inhibition is probably due to an increase in ruminal smooth

muscle tone, resulting in reflex inhibition of the normal cyclical

contraction sequences. In conscious goats bradykinin, histamine and PGE_1 caused

tachycardia, while 5-HT produced only minor changes in heart rate and $PGF_{2\alpha}$

caused bradycardia. The BK induced inhibition of rumen motility could be

prevented by sodiummeclofenamate or phenylbutazone. Pretreatment with the 5-HT

blocking agents only partly reduced serotonin induced effects. Pretreatment

with the H_1 antagonist clemastine completely reduced the histamine induced

inhibition of rumen contraction sequences while the H_2 antagonist cimetidine

had only a partial blocking effect.

INTRODUCTION

   In a number of species a large number of vasoactive and spasmogenic agents

are released during endotoxin shock. These include histamine (H), serotonin

(5-HT), bradykinin (BK) and prostaglandin (PG). Furthermore these tissue hormones

seem to be liberated during immediate hypersensitivity. Clinical symptoms observed
during endotoxin shock or during experimentally induced acute systemic anaphylaxis
in ruminants include dyspnoe, salivation, lacrimation, coughing, erection of
hair, muscle trembling, hypothermia occasionally followed by an increase in
body temperature, bradycardia followed by tachycardia, anorexia, inhibition of
rumen motility and ruminal tympany (14). Despite attempts to correlate clinical
symptoms with the release of these agents the relevance of the release of these
highly active substances under these pathological conditions is still unclear.
This presentation concerns the mechanism of action of these agents on rumen
motility. Therefore experiments were done (first) to determine in vitro the log
concentration-effect relationships of histamine, serotonin, bradykinin and
prostaglandins and (second) to learn if small doses given intravenously (i.v.)
would alter rumen motility. In these experiments we have investigated further
the blocking activity of the histamine antagonists clemastine (H_1) and cimetidine
(H_2) and of the serotonin antagonists xylamidine and methysergide. Furthermore
we have investigated the blocking activity of the prostaglandin antagonist
polyphloretinphosphate (PPP) and the bradykinin blocking activity of sodiummeclofenamate, which drug provides protection against anaphylaxis and endotoxin
shock.

MATERIALS AND METHODS

Methods for recording contractions of goat ruminal smooth muscle in vitro have
been described previously by Veenendaal et al. (14,16). The methods for recording
extrinsic ruminal contractions, heart rate and body temperature were described
previously (12, 16). The animals used were crossbred goats, females and castrated
males, varying in weight from 25 to 51 kg. The following drugs were used: histamine
dihydrochloride, clemastine, cimetidine, serotonin creatinin sulphate, methysergide
bimaleate, xylamidinetosylate, synthetic bradykinin, sodiummeclofenamate, phenylbutazone, prostaglandins E_1 and $F_{2\alpha}$ and polyphloretinphosphate.

RESULTS

In vitro experiments

The smooth muscle preparations were exposed to cumulative concentrations of
histamine, bradykinin, prostaglandin E_1 or prostaglandin $F_{2\alpha}$. The ruminal strip
preparation proved to be very insensitive to histamine, the threshold concentration
being about 12.8 µg per ml. Half maximal contraction was achieved by about 2 mg
per ml of histamine (14). The concentration-response curves obtained for 5-HT,
BK, PGE_1 and $PGF_{2\alpha}$ are shown in fig. 1. The threshold concentrations were 0.2 ng
for BK and PGE_1 and 3.2 ng for 5-HT and $PGF_{2\alpha}$. The mean concentrations ($\pm$ sem)
required for half maximal contraction were respectively 0.14 ± 0.02 µg (5-HT),
0.23 ± 0.04 µg (BK), 9.8 ± 2.8 ng (PGE_1) and 4.1 ± 1.0 µg per ml for $PGF_{2\alpha}$.

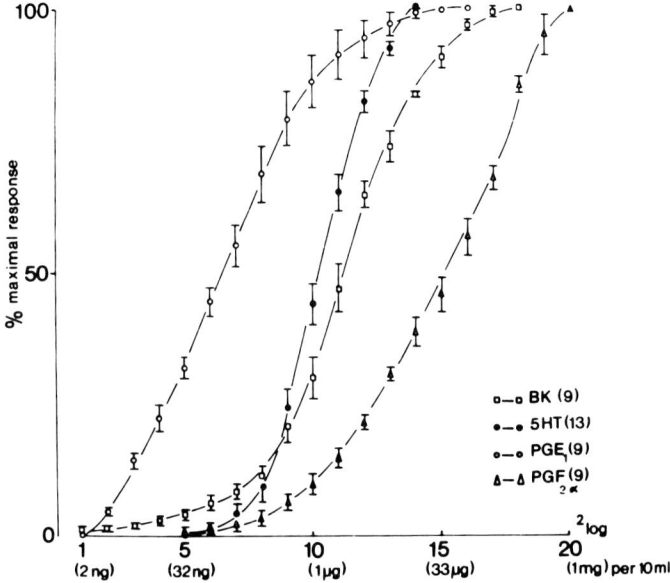

Fig. 1. Log dose-response curves for contraction of goat ruminal smooth muscle strips by bradykinin (BK), serotonin (5-HT), prostaglandin E_1 and $-F_{2\alpha}$ (PGE_1 and $PGF_{2\alpha}$). Each point represents the mean $\pm$ standard error. Number of experiments in parenthesis.

Next in a number of experiments the influence of xylamidine (5 ng per ml; n = 13) and methysergide (0.4 ng per ml; n = 5) was studied on the effect of 5-HT. Both drugs antagonized the 5-HT induced contractions of the ruminal strip and caused a non parallel shift to the right of the concentration-response curve for 5-HT (14, 18).

In 3 experiments sodiummeclofenamate (10 µg per ml) was added to the organ bath. This resulted in a diminished sensitivity to the contractile effects of BK. The change in concentration-response curve for BK on the ruminal strip in the presence of sodiummeclofenamate suggested a non competitive antagonism (14, 18).

In 7 experiments the prostaglandin antagonist PPP (100 µg per ml) was added to the bath, resulting in a diminished sensitivity to the contractile effects of PGE_1. The antagonism of the $PGF_{2\alpha}$ induced contractions of ruminal strips by PPP was manifested by a parallel shift of the concentration-response relationship (14, 17).

In vivo experiments

Intravenous injection or infusion of histamine caused a sudden increase of the heart rate and induced a short lasting inhibition of rumen contractions (Fig. 2, left side). The influence on the extrinsic ruminal contractions following histamine infusion was completely prevented by treatment

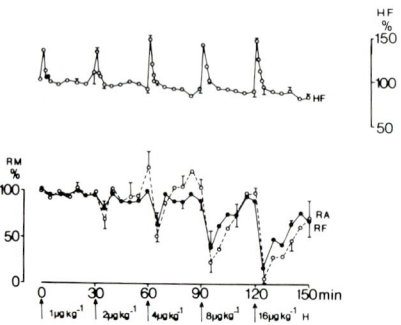 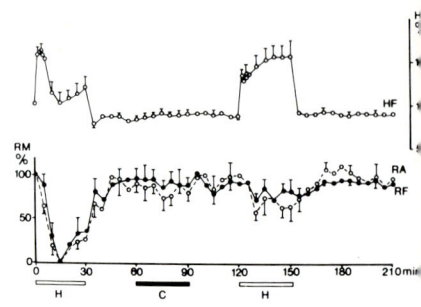

Fig. 2. Left side: changes in rumen motility (RF and RA) and heart rate (HF) after
i.v. injection of histamine (H). RF = frequency of rumen contractions per 5 min
expressed as percentages of the initial value. RA = summation derived from 5 min
intervals of amplitude expressed as percentages of the initial value. Mean values
± sem are given for a group of 4 goats. Right side: changes in rumen motility
(RF and RA) and heart frequency (HF) during i.v. infusion of histamine (2 μg/kg/min,
H) before and after an i.v. infusion of cimetidine (0.5 μg/kg/min, C). Mean values
± sem are given for a group of 5 goats.

with clemastine (50 mg per kg, i.v.) (13,14). Infusion of cimetidine partially

blocked the inhibition of ruminal contractions following histamine infusion

(fig. 2, right side). Intravenous injections of BK induced a sudden tachycardia

and a dose dependent inhibition of rumen contraction sequences (14,18). Repeated

i.v. injections with a short interval did not induce tachyphylaxis. The influence

of BK on rumen motility was prevented by phenylbutazone or sodiummeclofenamate

(14,18). In contrast 5-HT evoked only minor changes in heart rate, although a dose

dependent inhibition of rumen contraction sequences could be observed (14,18).

No signs of tachyphylaxis were seen after repeated i.v. injections (4x30 μg per kg)

with intervals of 30 minutes. The effects of a single i.v. injection of 5-HT on

rumen motility were partly prevented by xylamidine pretreatment or methysergide

pretreatment (14,18). An i.v. injection or infusion of PGE_1 induced a sudden

increase in heart rate and a dose dependent inhibition of the extrinsic rumen

contraction sequences (fig. 3, left side; ref. 14,15,17).

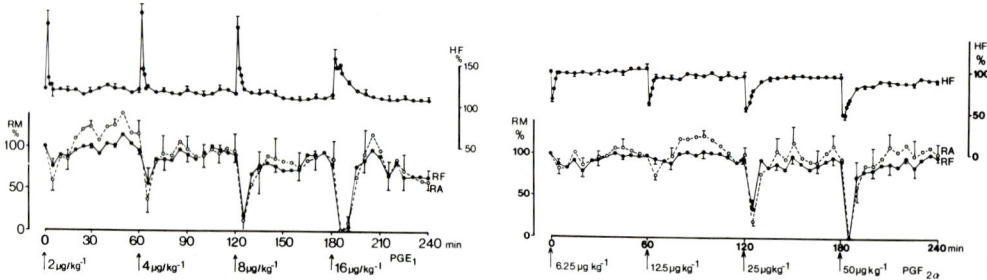

Fig. 3. The effect of PGE_1 (left side) and $PGF_{2\alpha}$ (right side) on goat rumen motility
(RM) and heart rate after i.v. injection (↑) into the jugular vein (RF, RA and HF
as in fig. 2). Mean values are given (n=5).

In contrast substantially higher doses of $PGF_{2\alpha}$ were required to depress the ruminal contractions. Moreover $PGF_{2\alpha}$ evoked bradycardia (14,17). Similar effects on heart rate and rumen motility were induced by i.v. $PGF_{2\alpha}$ infusions (fig. 3, right side, ref. 14,17).

DISCUSSION

The present study was designed to investigate the effects of BK, H, 5-HT and $PGE_1/PGF_{2\alpha}$ on ruminal motility, particularly the direct myogenic action of these tissue hormones. The isolated goat rumen strip proved to be a simple and reproducible in vitro preparation for studying the direct effect of 5-HT, BK, PGE_1 and $PGF_{2\alpha}$ on the smooth muscle of this organ. Comparison of the log concentration-response curves (fig. 1) shows that on a molar basis the following rank order can be given $PGE_1 > BK > 5\text{-}HT > PGF_{2\alpha}$. Histamine was rather inactive on this preparation (14).

The present results demonstrate clearly that sodiummeclofenamate antagonizes the rumen smooth muscle stimulating actions of BK. Other investigators found that this drug inhibited bronchoconstriction by BK (2,4). The mechanism of this antagonism is not clear. However, the shape of the concentration-response curve in the presence of sodiummeclofenamate suggests an antagonism being non competitive in nature. Moreover it has been demonstrated that sodiummeclofenamate is an antagonist of $PGF_{2\alpha}$ on human isolated bronchial smooth muscle (5). The non parallel shift to the right of the concentration-response curves for 5-HT in presence of xylamidine or methysergide suggests that the antagonism is non competitive in nature. On the other hand 5-HT stimulates the isolated guinea pig ileum partly by acting directly upon it (D-receptors) and partly by exciting intramural ganglion cells (M-receptors); only the direct action is blocked by various 5-HT blocking agents (6). Therefore a more detailed analysis would be necessary to confirm the existence of D- and M receptors in the ruminal smooth muscle layers.

The dose-response relationships obtained for inhibition of rumen motility in situ show that BK is more potent than 5-HT (14,18). The short duration of these effects is probably due to rapid inactivation by enzyme systems such as mono-amino oxidase (MAO) and carboxypeptidases (kininases). A short lasting inhibition · of the rumen contraction sequences can also be induced by prostaglandins; PGE_1 being more potent than $PGF_{2\alpha}$ (fig. 3). This type of inhibition is probably due to an increase in ruminal smooth muscle tone, resulting in reflex inhibition of the normal cyclical contraction sequences. Using a "single fibre" technique for recording afferent vagal activity from nerve fibres connected with tension perceptors in the reticulo-rumen, spasmogenic substances like carbachol and phenylephrine induced an exaggerated tension perceptor activity (i.e. a supranormal excitatory input to the gastric centres) accompanied by a short lasting inhibition of the rumen contraction sequences (8,9,11).

On the other hand, histamine, vasopressin and octapressin are potent inhibitors

of rumen motility in situ (fig. 4; ref. 10,14), although these substances are
rather inactive on isolated ruminal smooth muscle (10,14). Therefore other mechanisms
like local changes in gastric blood flow may be involved. A more detailed
investigation concerning the influence of changes in local blood flow on
rumen motility has to be done. The inhibitory effect on ruminal contractions
following i.v. histamine administration could be completely blocked by the H_1
antagonist clemastine (13,14) and partially blocked by the H_2 antagonist cimetidine
(14).

Comparison of the dose-response relationships obtained in situ learn that on a
molar basis these tissue hormones have the following rank order of potency for
inhibition of rumen motility: BK > PGE_1 > $PGF_{2\alpha}$ > 5-HT > H. The changes in heart
rate induced by PGE_1, $PGF_{2\alpha}$, BK, H, octapressin and vasopressin may be reflex in
origin, due to systemic arterial pressure responses. This is however only one
possibility.

The inhibitory effect of BK upon rumen motility was prevented by sodiummeclofenamate or phenylbutazone pretreatment. These drugs did not however antagonize
BK induced tachycardia. These results agree with data reported for other species
(1,3,7). Pretreatment with xylamidine or methysergide only partly reduced 5-HT
induced effects, probably by D-receptor blockade. A more detailed analysis of the
D- and M-receptors in the ruminal wall would be necessary to confirm this suggestion

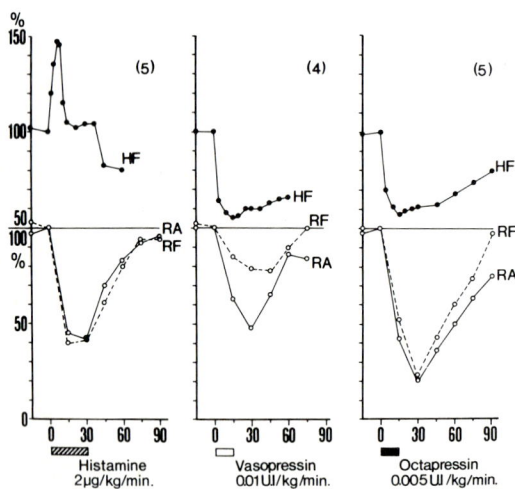

Fig. 4. Changes in rumen motility (RF and RA) and heart rate (HF) during intravenous
infusion of histamine, vasopressin and octapressin into the jugular vein. RA and
RF as in fig. 2 (per 15 min). Each point represents a mean value. Number of
goats in parenthesis (Courtesy Dr. A.S.J.P.A.M. van Miert).

REFERENCES

1. Aarsen, P.N.: Br. J. Pharmacol., 27 (1966), 196
2. Berry, P.A. and Collier, H.O.J.: Br. J. Pharmacol., 23 (1964), 210
3. Collier, H.O.J. in: Hypotensive peptides. Ed. E.G. Erdös, H. Back and F. Sicuteri Springer Verlag, New York (1966), p. 305
4. Collier, H.O.J. and Shorley, P.G.: Br. J. Pharmacol., 20 (1963), 345
5. Collier, H.O.J. and Sweatman, W.J.F.: Nature, 219 (1968), 864
6. Goodman, L.S. and Gilman, A., The pharmacological basis of therapeutics, fifth edition, MacMillan Publ. Co. Inc. New York (1975)
7. Lecomte, J.: Arch. Int. Pharmacodyn. Ther., 161 (1966), 463
8. Leek, B.F.: Ph.D. Thesis, Edinburgh (1967)
9. Leek, B.F. and Van Miert, A.S.J.P.A.M.: Rendic. R. Gastroenterol., 3 (1971), 163
10. Miert, A.S.J.P.A.M. van: Tijdschr. Diergeneesk., 93 (1968), 1402
11. Miert, A.S.J.P.A.M. van: Ph. D. Thesis, Utrecht (1970)
12. Miert, A.S.J.P.A.M. van and Van Duin, C.Th.M.: Eur. J. Pharmacol., 44 (1977), 197
13. Miert, A.S.J.P.A.M. van, Van Duin, C.Th.M. and Veenendaal, G.H.: Zentralbl. Veterinaermed. Reihe A, 23 (1976), 819
14. Veenendaal, G.H.: Ph.D. Thesis, Utrecht (1979)
15. Veenendaal, G.H. and Van Miert, A.S.J.P.A.M.: Ann. Rech. Vét. 10 (1979), 202
16. Veenendaal, G.H., Van Miert, A.S.J.P.A.M., Van den Ingh, T.S.G.A.M., Schotman, A.J.H. and Zwart, D.: Res. Vet. Sci., 21 (1976), 271
17. Veenendaal, G.H., Woutersen-van Nijnanten, F.M.A., Van Duin, C.Th.M. and Van Miert, A.S.J.P.A.M.: Res. Vet. Sci., (1979), in the press
18. Veenendaal, G.H., Woutersen-van Nijnanten, F.M.A. and Van Miert, A.S.J.P.A.M.: Am. J. Vet. Res., (1979), in the press.

COMPARATIVE ASPECTS OF CORPUS LUTEUM FUNCTION IN DOMESTIC ANIMALS

A.P.F. FLINT, F.A. HARRISON, R.B. HEAP, F.M. MAULE WALKER and L.D. STAPLES

A.R.C. Institute of Animal Physiology, Babraham, Cambridge CB2 4AT, U.K.

INTRODUCTION

The corpus luteum and luteal progesterone synthesis have been exploited during the evolution of viviparity as a preferred mode of reproduction in eutherian and marsupial mammals. Although luteal structures are found in the ovaries of non-mammalian vertebrates, where they develop the capacity to synthesize and secrete progesterone, it is principally among mammals that progesterone is indispensible for the establishment and maintenance of gestation. For this reason the mechanisms by which the life-span of the corpus luteum is extended in gestation, or curtailed after an infertile mating, are of particular interest. Among eutherian mammals the corpus luteum of pregnancy differs between species. It may grow larger, live longer and become more active (e.g. the rat), or simply live longer (e.g. sheep, and cow); it may also be similar during pregnancy or pseudo-pregnancy (e.g. ferret, dog) displaying an inherent life-span unaffected by pregnancy. An inherent life-span is also indicated in animals in which hysterecto prolongs luteal function for a period approximately equivalent to pregnancy. The control of luteal function is important not only in the context of the maintenance of pregnancy and the return to oestrus after an infertile mating, but also in event leading to parturition among animals dependent on ovarian progesterone throughout gestation. In this review we shall consider some of the recent advances in our understanding of these processes.

MECHANISMS OF LUTEAL REGRESSION

The removal of a uterine luteolysin (uterine luteolytic factor, ULF), released towards the end of each oestrous cycle, has been postulated to explain the prolongation of luteal function caused by hysterectomy. Since prostaglandin $F_{2\alpha}$ ($PGF_{2\alpha}$) is luteolytic on administration, and appears in the uterine venous blood at the expected time, it has been proposed that this compound is the ULF; the evidence for this, which is circumstantial, is best in the sheep and guinea-pig (ref. 1,2) but controversial in the cow (ref. 3). One property of $PGF_{2\alpha}$ which makes it a good candidate for the role of ULF is its rapid metabolism in the pulmonary circulation, in most species investigated. This is consistent with the unilateral, rather than systemic actions of ULF in the sheep and guinea-pig, in which hemihysterectomy causes ipsilateral luteal maintenance. Early work in the pig showed that in this species also, the uterus exerts a local action on the corpus luteum (ref. 4); however the pig differs from the guinea-pig and the sheep in that cyclic ovarian function continues after hemihysterectomy or after separation of the uterus and ovary by autotransplantation (ref. 5,6,7,8). This is probably due to relatively slow pulmonary clearance of circulating $PGF_{2\alpha}$ (Harrison & Maule Walker, unpublished observations). However, evidence for an additional endometrial ULF in the pig has been presented (ref. 9), and it appears, therefore, that $PGF_{2\alpha}$ may not be the only ULF in every species.

Mechanisms controlling uterine $PGF_{2\alpha}$ production. Although there is a considerable amount of evidence suggesting $PGF_{2\alpha}$ is a ULF, it is not certain how its uterine production is controlled. Recently it has been suggested that oxytocin may be involved, and that rising levels of oestrogen (produced by the ovarian follicles) facilitate the $PGF_{2\alpha}$-releasing effect of oxytocin by stimulating synthesis of the endometrial oxytocin receptor (ref. 10). Evidence in support of this has been obtained in sheep immunized against oxytocin (ref. 11). Active immunization against oxytocin during the reproductive season prolongs the oestrous cycle (Fig. 1); the effect is related to the circulating antibody titre and appears to result from lengthening of the secretory life of the corpus luteum. This finding does not contradict the proposed role for oestrogen in the control of uterine $PGF_{2\alpha}$ production, but clarifies the mechanism by which it may act.

CORPUS LUTEUM FUNCTION IN EARLY PREGNANCY

The maintenance of corpus luteum function is essential during early pregnancy in the domestic animals considered here, and is one of the earliest effects which the developing conceptus exerts on the mother. Mechanisms by which this is brought about are thought to differ between species.

Establishment of pregnancy in the ewe. The corpus luteum is rescued from cyclic regression by the presence of a conceptus in the ipsilateral uterine horn before Day 12 after mating (ref. 12). It can be mimicked by intrauterine infusion of homogenized conceptuses (ref. 13); the active component (trophoblastin) appears to be a high molecular weight, heat-labile, soluble protein, which disappears from the conceptus by Day 25 (ref. 13,14,15).

The mechanism of action of the antiluteolytic factor may involve either suppression of $PGF_{2\alpha}$ release, or its re-direction away from the venous blood towards the uterine lumen, as postulated by Bazer and his colleagues from studies in the pig (ref. 16). If a substance produced by the conceptus acts by redistributing uterine $PGF_{2\alpha}$ away from the uterine vasculature, levels of $PGF_{2\alpha}$ in uterine venous

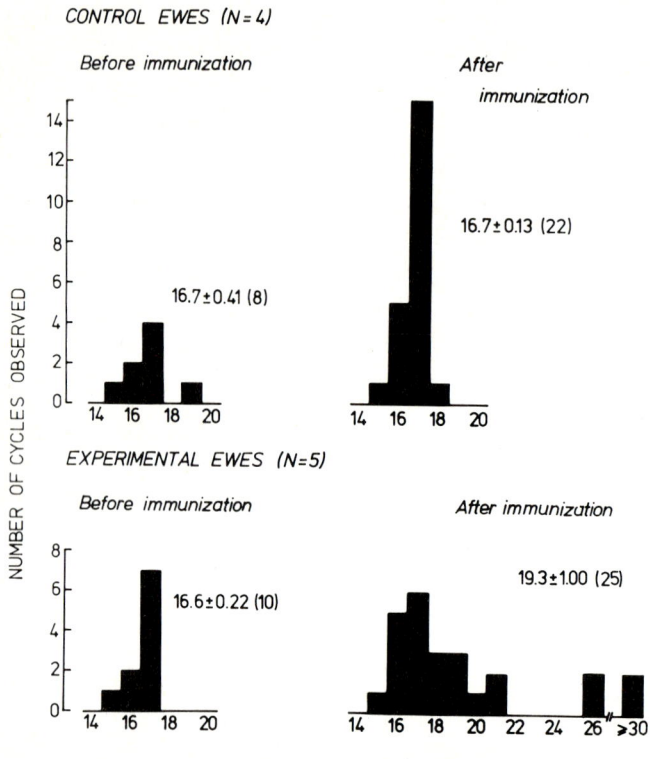

Fig. 1. Distribution of cycle lengths before and after starting immunization. Means ± S.E.M. are given for numbers of cycles in parentheses. Control ewes were immunized against bovine serum albumin; experimental ewes against oxytocin-BSA conjugate. Post-immunization cycles include those in which immune response was low or absent; after immunization cycle length (y) was related to oxytocin antibody titre (x) as follows: y = 0.09x + 16.55, r = 0.6034, P <0.001 (n = 25).

blood should be reduced in early pregnancy. However, different studies have produced conflicting results (ref. 17,18,19,20,21,22,23). The majority of these reports demonstrate that although there may be some decrease in utero-ovarian venous concentrations of $PGF_{2\alpha}$, the endometrium retains an extensive capacity to produce $PGF_{2\alpha}$ in early pregnancy, and therefore the redirection of $PGF_{2\alpha}$ secretion must be considered as a possible means of luteal protection at this time.

Recent experiments have shown that injection of a large dose of $PGF_{2\alpha}$ into an ovarian follicle ipsilateral to the corpus luteum caused luteolysis (ref. 24). When the experiment was performed with pregnant ewes the luteolytic effect was reduced (ref. 25,26,27) suggesting that the products of conception protected the corpus luteum. Additional evidence for the local release of an active agent

from the gravid uterus comes from the surgical procedures of Mapletoft and his
colleagues (ref. 28,29).   Uterine venous effluent from a pregnant uterine horn
neutralised the luteolytic influence of venous blood from a contralateral non-
gravid horn, implying the production of a luteotrophic substance.   Other studies
show luteal maintenance may result from competitive interaction of PGE_2 and $PGF_{2\alpha}$
for prostaglandin receptors (ref. 30).   However, the relative role of luteotrophic
and anti-luteolytic factors in early gestation remains unresolved.

Establishment of pregnancy in the pig.   The rescue of the corpus luteum in the
pig occurs between Days 11 and 12 p.c., at which time the conceptus becomes capable
of synthesizing oestrogens.   Since administration of oestrogen prolongs the
oestrous cycle, the possibility has been considered that the embryonic antiluteolysin
is an oestrogen (see ref. 31).   No alternative antiluteolysin has been proposed;
embryonic homogenates are antiluteolytic (ref. 32), possibly because they contain
oestrogens.

The time at which oestrogen synthesis begins is critical, and is difficult to
determine accurately because of methodological limitations.   It can be shown in
some circumstances to precede the phase of rapid elongation of the blastocyst on
Days 12-14 (ref. 31), and therefore to precede the time of rescue of corpora lutea.
This is consistent with the suggestion of Bazer & Thatcher (ref. 16) that oestrogen
may act directly on the endometrium to re-direct endometrial $PGF_{2\alpha}$ secretion away
from the stroma and towards the lumen of the uterus.   This proposal is supported
by the high levels of $PGF_{2\alpha}$ that appear in luminal flushings (ref. 16) and the
reduction in utero-ovarian venous levels both after administration of oestradiol
(ref. 33) and in early pregnancy (ref. 34).

MAINTENANCE OF LUTEAL FUNCTION IN MID-GESTATION

In the sheep, the antiluteolytic component of conceptus homogenates disappears
by Day 25 p.c. (ref. 13), although the placenta does not produce sufficient
progesterone to maintain pregnancy until about Day 50.   In the goat and pig, luteal
function is required throughout gestation.   Whether an antiluteolytic or luteotrophic agent is required between Days 25 and 50 is not certain, but the
disappearance of antiluteolytic activity from embryo homogenates suggests that
other factors may be involved.   These may be of either pituitary or embryonic
origin; since hypophysectomy causes luteal regression in sheep, goats and pig,
some contribution (either luteinizing hormone or prolactin or both) from the
pituitary is evidently required.   The interactions between pituitary and embryonic
luteotrophins are likely to be complex (see ref. 35).

Recent work has contributed particularly to our knowledge of the embryonic
factors involved.   Of the ruminant embryonic luteotrophins ovine and caprine
placental lactogens (oPL and cPL) are the most thoroughly studied.   oPL is present

as early as Day 16 p.c., but is not secreted in large quantities until about Day 50, when placental progesterone and oestrogen production also rise (see ref. 36). Maintenance of luteal function in the goat requires a luteotrophic complex of both luteinizing hormone and a lactogen; both prolactin and cPL are effective, and hypophysectomy experiments show that cPL levels are sufficiently high after Day 90 (ref. 37). Hysterectomy near term results in a drop in circulating progesterone levels of about 50% (ref. 38), suggesting that fetal luteotrophins account for that proportion of the total luteotrophic effect. Bovine PL also appears in the conceptus before attachment (ref. 39). No PL has been identified in the pig, rabbit or dog.

REGRESSION OF THE CORPUS LUTEUM AT PARTURITION

In sheep, progesterone production in late gestation is largely placental. After Day 50, the time at which the corpora lutea regress is of no significance to the course of pregnancy. In the goat and the pig ovariectomy at any stage of pregnancy results in abortion, and this can be blocked by giving progesterone; in these animals, therefore, it appears the regression of the corpus luteum is a necessary prelude to parturition (see ref. 40).

The mechanisms of luteal regression have been examined in detail in the goat (Fig. 2). The rise in fetal cortisol, which precedes the onset of labour and

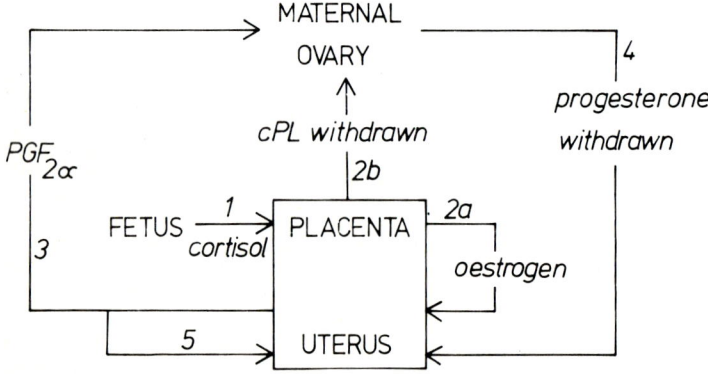

Fig. 2. Control of luteal function in the goat at parturition. Events thought to be involved are: [1] fetal cortisol rises; [2a] this causes increased placental oestrogen synthesis, which [3] increases uterine $PGF_{2\alpha}$ production; [4] luteal regression results, and the withdrawal of progesterone results in further $PGF_{2\alpha}$ synthesis [5], leading to uterine contractions. High fetal cortisol levels are also associated with reduced secretion of cPL [2b] (ref. 41).

causes maturation of many fetal systems (most notably pulmonary surfactant production) appears to cause increased placental production of oestrogens, through an effect on placental enzyme activities (ref. 41). Oestrogens are luteolytic

during pregnancy in the goat, presumably through stimulation of uterine prostaglandin secretion (ref. 42) so that luteal regression results. At the same time
there is a decline in cPL production (ref. 43).

Although similar endocrine changes precede parturition in the pig, the mechanism
by which luteal regression is triggered is not certain. Prostaglandin $F_{2\alpha}$ is
luteolytic near term (ref. 44); but whether increased uterine $PGF_{2\alpha}$ release precedes
progesterone withdrawal, and what stimulates its production, is not known.
Oestrogens are not luteolytic at term, and no alternative factors capable of
transmitting the luteolytic signal from the placenta to the ovary have been
identified (see ref. 40, 45).

Relaxin. The recent discovery that relaxin inhibits uterine contractility in a
number of laboratory and domestic animals has emphasized the possible importance
of this protein hormone in the maintenance of pregnancy (ref. 46). Although
alternative sources have been suggested, the corpora lutea are considered the
most important source of relaxin, and are used as a starting point in its
purification. In addition to controlling uterine contractions, relaxin induces
dilatation of the symphysis pubis, and it is in this role that it is most likely
to act late in pregnancy; its release at luteal regression in the pig, for instance
(ref. 47) seems likely to be important in this respect. Relaxin has recently
been shown to have structural similarities to insulin (ref. 48).

CONCLUSIONS

This review has concentrated on some of the recent advances in our understanding
of the control of luteal function in the oestrous cycle, in pregnancy and at
parturition. These have emphasized the role of the trophoblast and placenta and
the production by them of antiluteolysins and luteotrophins; however the importance
of pituitary luteotrophins should not be underestimated (see ref. 49). Recent
work on the corpus luteum in the rat has suggested that prolactin or placental
lactogen, together with oestrogen, may influence luteal function through LH
receptor concentrations (ref. 50), thereby drawing attention to the importance of
circulating LH in this connection.

REFERENCES

1. Flint, A.P.F. and Hillier, K., 1975. Prostaglandins and reproductive
      processes in female sheep and goats. In: S.M.M. Karim (Editor), Prostaglandins
      and Reproduction. MTP Press Ltd., Lancaster, pp. 271-308.
2. Horton, E.W. and Poyser, N.L., 1976. Uterine luteolytic hormones: a physio-
      logical role for $PGF_{2\alpha}$. Physiol. Rev., 56:595-651.
3. Hansel, W. and Fortune, J., 1978. The applications of ovulation control.
      In: D.B. Crighton, N.B. Haynes, G.R. Foxcroft and G.E. Lamming (Editors).
      Control of Ovulation. Butterworth & Co., London. pp. 237-263.
4. Anderson, L.L., 1966. Pituitary-Ovarian-Uterine relationships in pigs.
      J. Reprod. Fertil., Suppl., 1:21-32.

5. Du Mesnil du Buisson, F., 1961. Regression unilatérale des corps jaunes après hysterectomie partielle chez la truie. Ann. Biol. anim. Bioch. Biophys. 1:105-112.

6. Martin, P.A., Bevier, G.W. and Dziuk, P.J., 1978. The effect of disconnecting the uterus and ovary on the length of gestation in the pig. Biol. Reprod., 18:428-433.

7. Binns, R.M., Harrison, F.A. and Heap, R.B., 1967. Transplantation of the ovary in the pig and in the pregnant sheep. Acta endocr. (Kbh). Suppl. 119:193.

8. Harrison, F.A., 1979. Luteolysin in the pig. J. Physiol. (Lond.), 290:36P.

9. Maule Walker, F.M. and Watson, J., 1977. Effect of prostaglandin $F_{2\alpha}$ on non-pregnant and early pregnant porcine luteal steroid secretion. J. Endocrinol., 73:26-27P.

10. Roberts, J.S., McCracken, J.A., Gavagan, J.E. and Soloff, M.S., 1976. Oxytocin-stimulated release of prostaglandin $F_{2\alpha}$ from ovine endometrium in vitro: correlation with estrous cycle and oxytocin-receptor binding. Endocrinology, 99:1107-1114.

11. Sheldrick, E.L., Mitchell, M.D. and Flint, A.P.F., 1980. Delayed luteal regression in ewes immunized against oxytocin. J. Reprod. Fertil. (in press)

12. Moor, R.M., 1968. The corpus luteum of the sheep: functional relationship between the embryo and corpus luteum. J. Anim. Sci., 27, Suppl., 1:97-118.

13. Rowson, L.E.A. and Moor, R.M., 1967. The influence of embryonic tissue homogenate infused into the uterus on the life-span of the corpus luteum in the sheep. J. Reprod. Fertil., 13:511-516.

14. Staples, L.D., Lawson, R.A.S. and Findlay, J.K., 1978. Maintenance of the corpus luteum in the ewe by intrauterine infusion of a soluble extract of ovine conceptus. Proc. VIth Asia and Oceania Congress of Endocrinology, Singapore p.195 Abs.

15. Martal, J., Lacroix, M.-C., Loudes, C., Saunier, M. and Winterberger-Torres, S. 1979. Trophoblastin, an antiluteolytic protein present in early pregnancy in sheep. J. Reprod. Fertil., 56:63-73.

16. Bazer, F.W. and Thatcher, W.W., 1977. Theory of maternal recognition of pregnancy in swine based on estrogen controlled endocrine versus exocrine secretion of prostaglandin $F_{2\alpha}$ by the uterine endometrium. Prostaglandins, 14:397-401.

17. Thorburn, G.D., Cox, R.I., Currie, W.B., Restall, B.J. and Schneider, W., 1973. PGF and progesterone concentrations in the utero-ovarian venous plasma of the ewe during the oestrous cycle and early pregnancy. J. Reprod. Fertil., Suppl., 18:151-158.

18. Barcikowski, B., Carlson, J.C., Wilson, L. and McCracken, J.A., 1974. The effect of endogenous and exogenous estradiol-17β on the release of prostaglandin $F_{2\alpha}$ from the ovine uterus. Endocrinology, 95:1340-1349.

19. Peterson, A.J., Tervit, H.R., Fairclough, R.J., Hawick, P.G. and Smith, J.F., 1976. Jugular levels of 13,14-dihydro-15-keto-prostaglandin F and progesterone around luteolysis and early pregnancy in the ewe. Prostaglandins, 12:551-558.

20. Nett, T.M., Staigmiller, R.B., Akbar, A.M., Diekman, M.A., Ellinwood, W.E. and Niswender, G.D., 1976. Secretion of $PGF_{2\alpha}$ in cycling and pregnant ewes. J. Anim. Sci., 42:876-880.

21. Pexton, J.E., Weems, C.W. and Inskeep, E.K., 1975. Prostaglandin F in uterine venous plasma, ovarian arterial and venous plasma and in ovarian luteal tissue of pregnant and non-pregnant ewes. J. Anim. Sci., 491:154-159.

22. Lewis, G.D., Wilson, L., Jr., Wilks, J.W., Pexton, J.E., Fogwell, R.L., Ford, S.P., Butcher, R.L., Thayne, W.V. and Inskeep, E.K., 1977. $PGF_{2\alpha}$ and its metabolites in uterine and jugular venous plasma and endometrium of ewes during early pregnancy. J. Anim. Sci., 45:320-327.

23. Wilson, L., Jr., Butcher, R.L. and Inskeep, E.K. 1972. Prostaglandin $F_{2\alpha}$ in the uterus of ewes during early pregnancy. Prostaglandins, 1:479-482.

24. Fogwell, R.L., Lewis, G.D., Butcher, R.L. and Inskeep, E.K., 1977. Effects of ovarian bisection on response to intrafollicular injection of $PGF_{2\alpha}$ and on follicular development in ewes. J. Anim. Sci., 45:328-335.

25. Inskeep, E.K. and Pexton, J.E., 1974. Effect of pregnancy on response of ewes to PGF$_{2\alpha}$. J. Anim. Sci., 39:212 Abs.
26. Inskeep, E.K., Smutney, W.J., Butcher, R.L. and Pexton, J.E., 1975. Effects of intrafollicular injections of prostaglandins in non-pregnant and pregnant ewes. J. Anim. Sci., 41:1098-1104.
27. Pratt, B.R., Butcher, R.L. and Inskeep, E.K., 1975. Intrafollicular PGF$_{2\alpha}$ on Day 13 in bred and non-bred ewes. J. Anim. Sci., 41:374 Abs.
28. Mapletoft, R.J., Del Campo, M.R. and Ginther,O.J., 1975. Unilateral luteotrophic effect of uterine venous effluent of a gravid uterine horn in sheep. Proc. Soc. Exp. Biol. Med., 150:129-133.
29. Mapletoft, R.J., Lapin, D.R. and Ginther, O.J., 1976. The ovarian artery as the final component of the local luteotropic pathway between a gravid uterine horn and ovary in ewes. Biol. Reprod., 15:414-421.
30. Henderson, K.M., Scaramuzzi, R.J. and Baird, D.T., 1977. Simultaneous infusion of prostaglandin E$_2$ antagonizes the luteolytic action of prostaglandin F$_{2\alpha}$ _in vivo_. J. Endocrinol., 72:379-383.
31. Flint, A.P.F., Burton, R.D., Gadsby, J.E., Saunders, P.T.K. and Heap, R.B., 1979. Blastocyst oestrogen synthesis and the maternal recognition of pregnancy. In: J. Whelan (Editor), Maternal Recognition of Pregnancy. Ciba Foundation Symposium 64, Excerpta Medica, Amsterdam, pp. 209-228.
32. Longenecker, D.E. and Day, B.N., 1972. Maintenance of corpora lutea and pregnancy in unilaterally pregnant gilts by intrauterine infusion of embryonic tissue. J. Reprod. Fertil., 31:171-177.
33. Frank, M., Bazer, F.W., Thatcher, W.W. and Wilcox, C.J., 1977. A study of prostaglandin F$_{2\alpha}$ as the luteolysin in swine. III. Effects of estradiol valerate on prostaglandin F, progestins, estrone and estradiol concentrations in the utero-ovarian vein of non-pregnant gilts. Prostaglandins, 14:1183-1196.
34. Moeljono, M.P.E., Thatcher, W.W., Bazer, F.W., Frank, M., Owens, L.J. and Wilcox, C.J., 1977. A study of prostaglandin F$_{2\alpha}$ as the luteolysin in swine. II. Characterization and comparison of prostaglandin F, estrogens and progestin concentrations in utero-ovarian vein plasma of non-pregnant and pregnant gilts. Prostaglandins, 14:543-555.
35. Thorburn, G.D., 1979. Physiology and control of parturition:reflections on the past and ideas for the future. Anim. Reprod. Sci., 2:1-27.
36. Flint, A.P.F., Ricketts, A.P. and Craig, V.A., 1980. Control of endocrine function of the trophoblast and placenta in domestic animals. J. Reprod. Fertil., Suppl. (in press).
37. Buttle, H.L., 1978. The maintenance of pregnancy in hypophysectomized goats. J. Reprod. Fertil., 52:255-260.
38. Currie, W.B. and Thorburn, G.D., 1974. Luteal function in hysterectomized goats. J. Reprod. Fertil., 41:501-504.
39. Flint, A.P.F., Henville, A. and Christie, W.B., 1979. Presence of placental lactogen in bovine conceptuses before attachment. J. Reprod. Fertil., 56:305-308.
40. Flint, A.P.F., Ricketts, A.P. and Craig, V.A., 1979. The control of placental steroid synthesis at parturition in domestic animals. Anim. Reprod. Sci., 2:239-251.
41. Flint, A.P.F., Kingston, E.J., Robinson, J.S. and Thorburn, G.D., 1978. Initiation of parturition in the goat: evidence for control by foetal glucocorticoid through activation of placental C$_{21}$-steroid 17α-hydroxylase. J. Endocrinol., 78:367-378.
42. Currie, W.B. and Thorburn, G.D., 1976. Release of prostaglandin F, regression of corpora lutea and induction of premature parturition in goats treated with estradiol-17β. Prostaglandins, 12:1093-1103.
43. Currie, W.B., Kelly, P.A., Friesen, H.G. and Thorburn, G.D., 1977. Caprine placental lactogen: levels of prolactin-like and growth hormone-like activities in the circulation of pregnant goats determined by radioreceptor assays. J. Endocrinol., 73:215-226.

208

44. Ash, R.W. and Heap, R.B., 1973. The induction and synchronization of parturition in sows treated with I.C.I. 79,939, an analogue of prostaglandin $F_{2\alpha}$. J. agric. Sci., 81:365-368.

45. First, N.L. and Bosc, M.J., 1979. Proposed mechanisms controlling parturition and the induction of parturition in swine. J. Anim. Sci., 48:1407-1421.

46. Porter, D.G., 1979. The myometrium and the relaxin enigma. Anim. Reprod. Sci., 2:77-96.

47. Sherwood, O.D., Nara, B.S., Cruekovic, V.E. and First, N.L., 1978. Relaxin concentrations in pig plasma after the administration of indomethacin and prostaglandin $F_{2\alpha}$ during late pregnancy. Endocrinol., 104:1716-1721.

48. Bedarker, S., Turnell, W.G., Blundell, T.L. and Schwabe, C., 1977. Relaxin has conformational homology with insulin. Nature (Lond.), 270:449-451.

49. Denamur, R., 1974. Luteotrophic factors in the sheep. J. Reprod. Fertil., 38:251-259.

50. Gibori, G. and Richards, J.S., 1978. Dissociation of two distinct luteotropic effects of prolactin: regulation of luteinizing hormone-receptor content and progesterone secretion during pregnancy. Endocrinol., 102:767-774.

THE MECHANISM OF LUTEAL REGRESSION

K.M. HENDERSON

Department of Biochemistry, University of Edinburgh Medical School, Teviot Place, Edinburgh EH8 9AG, Scotland.

INTRODUCTION

Following ovulation, the collapsed follicle differentiates into the corpus luteum (CL), the function of which is to provide the progesterone essential for the maintenance of pregnancy should the ovum be successfully fertilized. In the event that the ovum is not fertilized, there must be a return to estrous so that a fresh attempt to achieve pregnancy can be made. This requires the regression of the CL since its presence prevents any return to estrous. In many species including the sheep, cow, pig and horse, the natural luteolysin is uterine in origin while in others such as the dog, cat, monkey and perhaps most notably the human, the uterus plays no role (1). Most research has been concerned with understanding luteal regression in those species in which the uterus participates, and so will be the subject of this paper. It should, however, be borne in mind that our understanding of the mechanism of luteal regression in those species in which the uterus does not participate is still largely obscure.

Prostaglandin $F_{2\alpha}$ - the uterine luteolysin

There is now a substantial body of evidence to indicate that prostaglandin $F_{2\alpha}$ ($PGF_{2\alpha}$) is the natural uterine luteolysin in several species including the ewe, cow, pig, horse, guinea-pig, rabbit and rat (see ref. 2 for review). Studies in the ewe (3) indicate that $PGF_{2\alpha}$ reaches the CL from the uterus by a so-called "counter current" mechanism of transfer whereby on being released into the uterine vein $PGF_{2\alpha}$ passes through it into the ovarian artery which is tightly adherent to the uterine vein and coiled on it. The anatomical structure of the utero-ovarian vasculature is such that similar transfer mechanisms may also exist in the cow, sow, rat, hamster and possibly the guinea-pig (4).

$PGF_{2\alpha}$ is synthesized and released from the uterus in a pulsatile fashion, as indicated by studies in the ewe (5). While both progesterone and estradiol are almost certainly involved in regulating this (6), the pulsatile nature of the release makes it difficult to explain by steroid action alone. Recent evidence suggests that oxytocin released by the posterior pituitary may also be involved. The luteolytic action of oxytocin has long been known (7) and recent studies indicate that oxytocin can stimulate the release of $PGF_{2\alpha}$ from the uterus, a process which is enhanced by estradiol, both in vivo (8) and in vitro (9). Moreover, towards the end of the luteal phase there is an increase in uterine oxytocin receptors, the formation of which is most likely regulated by estradiol (10). Since appreciable amounts of both estradiol and oxytocin are present in blood throughout the luteal phase, it has been suggested that estradiol, through interaction with its uterine receptors, induces the formation of uterine oxytocin receptors thereby sensitizing the uterus to synthesize $PGF_{2\alpha}$ in response to the endogenous levels of oxytocin (11). Although progesterone priming of the uterus is required for maximum production of $PGF_{2\alpha}$, continued high levels reduce the amount of $PGF_{2\alpha}$ released through inhibiting the formation of uterine estradiol receptors (12), inhibiting oxytocin release from the pituitary (13) and stimulating prostaglandin dehydrogenase activity (14). These actions of progesterone may explain why maximum amounts of $PGF_{2\alpha}$ are not released from the uterus until the very late luteal phase when luteal regression has already commenced and serum progesterone levels have declined substantially.

Mechanism of action of $PGF_{2\alpha}$

$PGF_{2\alpha}$ is a potent venoconstrictor and it was originally proposed that $PGF_{2\alpha}$ might cause luteal regression through reducing blood flow to the ovary (15); luteolysis resulting from anoxia. However, there is little evidence for anoxic damage during the early stages of luteal regression (16) and studies in the rabbit (17), ewe (18) and rat (19) indicate that during $PGF_{2\alpha}$ induced luteolysis serum levels of progesterone start to decline prior to any reductions in blood flow to the ovary or CL. Luteolysis may arise from a biochemical action of $PGF_{2\alpha}$ on the CL since $PGF_{2\alpha}$ can inhibit progesterone production by luteal tissue in vitro (20-23). This is illustrated in Figure 1 where it can be seen that $PGF_{2\alpha}$ abolishes the stimulatory action of human chorionic gonadotrophin (hCG) on progesterone production by rat luteal cells during 4 hour incubation periods in vitro. A clue to the site of action of $PGF_{2\alpha}$ is provided by the finding that $PGF_{2\alpha}$ fails to inhibit the stimulatory action of dibutyryl cyclic AMP (DBC) on progesterone production. This suggests that $PGF_{2\alpha}$ may be acting by inhibiting the activation of adenylate cyclase by hCG, and recent studies have demonstrated directly that $PGF_{2\alpha}$ does indeed inhibit luteal adenylate cyclase activity, thereby indirectly suppressing progesterone synthesis (21,24). Interestingly, $PGF_{2\alpha}$ also fails to inhibit PGE_2 stimulated progesterone production (Fig. 1) which like that of hCG is mediated through cAMP. Thus $PGF_{2\alpha}$ may act to inhibit specifically hCG and LH (luteinizing hormone) activated adenylate cyclase. While inhibition of adenylate cyclase activity is thought to be the initial event in $PGF_{2\alpha}$ inhibition of luteal

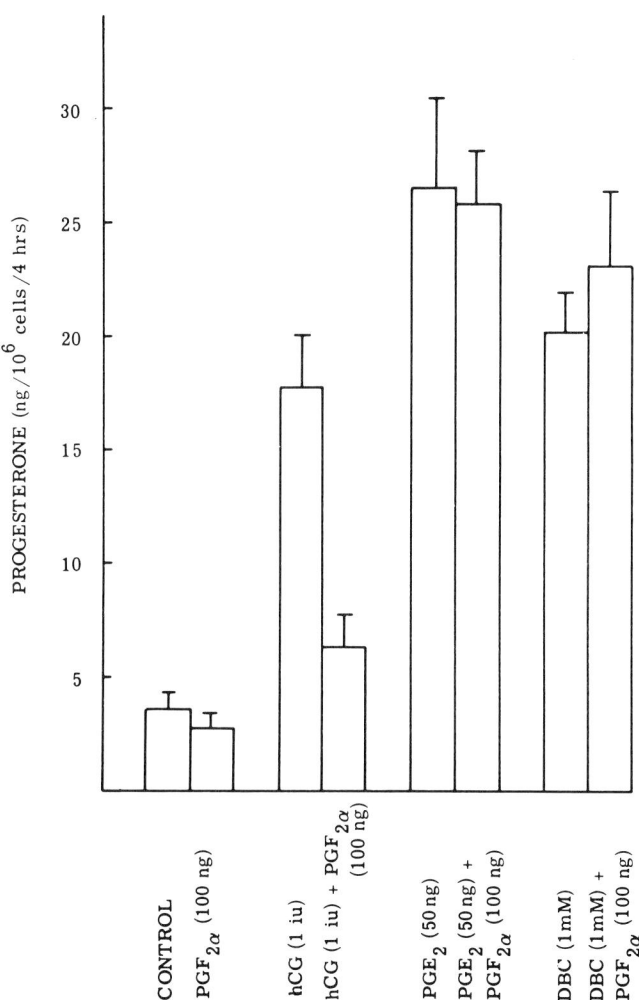

Fig. 1.   Effect of hCG, PGF$_{2\alpha}$, PGE$_2$ and DBC on progesterone production by rat luteal cells _in vitro_.   Each point is the mean + S.D. of 5 replicates.

progesterone production (21), PGF$_{2\alpha}$ also has a secondary later effect of causing a loss of receptors for LH in the luteal cell (25,26).   Together, these two actions of PGF$_{2\alpha}$ can bring about a rapid and sustained inhibition of luteal progesterone production.   The possibility that PGF$_{2\alpha}$ initiates luteal regression _in vivo_ by similar actions is strengthened by the fact that during natural and PGF$_{2\alpha}$ induced luteolysis in the sow there is a reduction in luteal adenylate cyclase activity (27) and cAMP content (28), while in the ewe there is a marked reduction in luteal LH receptors (29,30).   In addition, PGE$_2$ can antagonize the luteolytic action of PGF$_{2\alpha}$ _in vivo_ (31) which is also consistent with the _in vitro_ findings.

Morphological deterioration of the corpus luteum in response to PGF$_{2\alpha}$ only becomes apparent several hours after serum progesterone levels have started to

decline (16). While $PGF_{2\alpha}$ may initiate luteal regression, as indicated by a decline
in progesterone secretion, through its biochemical actions as discussed above, whether
these actions also trigger morphological deterioration is uncertain. Labilization
of lysosomal membranes with the consequent release of stored hydrolases is associated
with morphological regression of the CL (32,33), and indeed $PGF_{2\alpha}$ has been
reported to induce some release of lysosomal hydrolase from luteal tissue in vitro
(34). Morphological regression however is also associated with a reduction in blood
flow to the CL (35) and while this may be a consequence of morphological regression
rather than its cause, the possibility that a venoconstrictor action of $PGF_{2\alpha}$ may be
involved in causing the final irreversible morphological deterioration of the CL
cannot be excluded. Interestingly, this final morphological deterioration of the CL
in the ewe is coincident with the release of large amounts of $PGF_{2\alpha}$ from the uterus,
compared to the levels of $PGF_{2\alpha}$ associated with the initiation of luteolysis (36,37)
Thus, while the release of relatively small amounts of $PGF_{2\alpha}$ from the uterus on days
12-14 of the cycle may be sufficient to initiate functional regression of the CL of
the ewe i.e. to trigger the decline in progesterone production, they may be inadequate
to cause complete morphological regression. The final irreversible structural demise
of the CL may require the much larger amounts of $PGF_{2\alpha}$ released from the uterus in the
very late luteal phase on days 15 and 16.

The refractory CL

While the lytic action of $PGF_{2\alpha}$ is well established, the newly formed CL shows
considerable resistance to $PGF_{2\alpha}$. In the horse (38), sheep (39) and cow (40) the CL
is refractory to $PGF_{2\alpha}$ for the first 4 days after its formation, and in the pig this
refractory period is about 12 days (41). In studies in which follicular granulosa
cells (the precursor cells of the CL) were induced to luteinize in tissue culture,
and so provide an in vitro model of the newly formed CL, it was found that while PGF
could inhibit progesterone production prior to cellular luteinization when progesterone production was low, $PGF_{2\alpha}$ had little effect on progesterone production when the
cells were fully luteinized and producing maximum amounts of **progesterone** (42,43).
This loss of response to $PGF_{2\alpha}$ was accompanied by a decrease in the capacity of the
luteinized cells to bind $PGF_{2\alpha}$ (43). Since progesterone production by granulosa-
luteal cells in vitro may be related to the cellular response to LH, it was
suggested (42,43) that increasing amounts of LH interacted with the cells during
luteinization and in so doing 'masked' plasma membrane receptors for $PGF_{2\alpha}$ (44).
A similar situation may exist in vivo in that following the ovulatory LH 'surge'
saturation of luteal plasma membrane LH receptors may mask those for $PGF_{2\alpha}$, thereby
rendering the CL refractory to $PGF_{2\alpha}$. This view is consistent with in vivo findings
that LH or hCG antagonizes the luteolytic action of $PGF_{2\alpha}$ in the rat (45,46) and
guinea-pig (47) while in the sheep (48) and cow (49), both species in which $PGF_{2\alpha}$ is
thought to be the natural luteolysin, exogenous LH or hCG prolongs the life-span

of the CL. The variation in refractory periods between different species may be due to differences in the rate of unmasking of receptors for $PGF_{2\alpha}$ as luteal bound LH is gradually depleted through either internalization and degradation by lysosomes or by gradual dissociation from its receptor sites.

The CL of pregnancy

Progesterone secreted by the CL is essential for the maintenance of early pregnancy, thus during a fertile estrous cycle the CL must be maintained. Studies in the guinea-pig (50) and pig (51) indicate that the levels of $PGF_{2\alpha}$ found in uterine venous blood during a fertile cycle at the time luteolysis would normally have occurred are very much lower than the levels occurring during a non-fertile cycle. In the guinea-pig this is likely due to an inhibition of uterine prostaglandin synthesis (52), but in the pig uterine prostaglandin synthesis may not be inhibited but rather the $PGF_{2\alpha}$ is released into the uterine lumen instead of the uterine vein (53). While uterine venous blood levels of $PGF_{2\alpha}$ in the pregnant ewe have also been reported to be reduced compared to the non-pregnant state (5) this has been disputed (54). However, uterine venous (55) and ovarian arterial (56) blood on the side of a gravid uterus in the ewe have luteotrophic properties indicating that the CL may be maintained by an anti-luteolytic action at the ovary. Interestingly, it has been suggested that these anti-luteolytic factors may include PGE_2 (57, 58) which as discussed above has the capacity to override the luteolytic action of $PGF_{2\alpha}$.

Concluding remarks

While most research, as reviewed above, has focussed attention on the role of $PGF_{2\alpha}$ in regulating luteal regression, recent findings raise the possibility that $PGF_{2\alpha}$ may not, after all, be the actual natural luteolysin, but a side-product, with some luteolytic activity, of the principle luteolysin. Studies in the rat (59) and sheep (60) indicate that the major PG produced by the uterus is not $PGF_{2\alpha}$ but $6\text{-keto-}PGF_{1\alpha}$ the stable metabolite of PGI_2 (prostacyclin); both these PG's like $PGF_{2\alpha}$ being breakdown products of the prostaglandin endoperoxides. While PGI_2 is thought to play a key role in haemostasis (61) its luteolytic activity has not yet been determined. However, its metabolite $6\text{-keto-}PGF_{1\alpha}$ has been found to inhibit luteal progesterone production in pregnant hamsters through interacting with what was thought to be the luteal receptor for $PGF_{2\alpha}$ (44).

REFERENCES

1. Anderson, L.L. (1973) Handbook of Physiology, Section 7: Endocrinology, vol. 2, pp. 69-86.
2. Horton, E.W. and Poyser, N.L. (1976) Physiological Reviews 56, 595-651.

214

3. McCracken, J.A., Carlson, J.C., Glew, M.E., Goding, J.R., Baird, D.T., Green, K. and Samuelsson, B. (1972) Nature (New Biology) 238, 129-134.

4. Ginther, O.J. (1974) J. Anim. Sci. 39, 550-564.

5. Thorburn, G.D., Cox, R.I., Currie, W.B., Restall, B.J. and Schneider, W. (1973) J. Reprod. Fert. Suppl. 18, 151-158.

6. Scaramuzzi, R.J., Baird, D.T., Boyle, H.P., Land, R.B. and Wheeler, A.G. (1977) J. Reprod. Fert. 49, 157-160.

7. Armstrong, D.T. and Hansel, W. (1959) J. Dairy Sci. 42, 533-542.

8. Roberts, J.S. and McCracken, J.A. (1976) Biol. Reprod. 15, 457-463.

9. Small, M.G., Gavagan, J.E. and Roberts, J.S. (1978) Prostaglandins 15, 103-112.

10. Roberts, J.S., McCracken, J.A., Gavagan, J.E. and Soloff, M.S. (1976) Endocrinology 99, 1107-1114.

11. McCracken, J.A., Gammal, L.M., Glew, M.E. and Underwood, L.F. (1978) 60th Annual Meeting of the Endocrine Society, Miami, U.S.A., abstract no. 440.

12. Koligian, K.B. and Stormshak, F. (1977) Biol. Reprod. 17, 412-416.

13. Roberts, J.S. and Share, L. (1970) Endocrinology 84, 1076-1081.

14. Alan, N.A., Russel, P.T., Tabor, N.W. and Moulton, B.C. (1976) Endocrinology 98, 859-863.

15. Pharriss, B.B. (1970) Perspect. Biol. Med. 13, 434-444.

16. Stacy, B.D., Gemmell, R.T. and Thorburn, G.D. (1976) Biol. Reprod. 14, 280-291.

17. Bruce, N.W. and Hillier, K. (1974) Nature (New Biology) 249, 176-177.

18. Einer-Jensen, N. and McCracken, J.A. (1976) Recent Advances in Prostaglandin and Thromboxane Research. Eds. R. Paoletti and B. Samuelsson. New York, Raven, vol. 2, pp.201-207.

19. Pang, C.Y. and Behrman, H.R. (1978) 11th Annual Meeting of the Society for the Study of Reproduction, Southern Illinois University. Abstract no. 136.

20. O'Grady, J.P., Kahorn, E.I., Glass, R.A., Caldwell, B.V., Brock, W.A. and Speroff, L. (1972) J. Reprod. Fert. 30, 153-156.

21. Thomas, J.-P., Dorflinger, L.J. and Behrman, H.R. (1978) Proc. Natl. Acad. Sci. 75, 1344-1348.

22. Evrard, M., Leboulleux, P. and Hermier, C. (1978) Prostaglandins 16, 491-500.

23. Hall, A.K. and Robinson, J. (1979) J. Endocr. 81, 157-165.

24. Khan, M.I. and Rosberg, S. (1979) J. Cyclic Nucleotide Res. 5, 55-63.

25. Grinwich, D.L., Hichens, M. and Behrman, H.R. (1976) Biol. Reprod. 14, 212-218.

26. Torjesen, P.A., Dahlin, R., Haug, E. and Aakvaag, A. (1978) Acta Endocrinol. (Kbh) 87, 617-624.

27. Andersen, R.N., Schwartz,F.L. and Ulberg, L.C. (1974) Biol. Reprod. 10, 321-326

28. Krzymowski, T., Kotwica, J., Okrasa, S., Doboszynska, T. and Ziecik, A. (1978) J. Reprod. Fert. 54, 21-27.

29. Diekmann, M.A., O'Callaghan, P., Nett, T.M. and Niswender, G.D. (1978) Biol. Reprod. 19, 999-1009.

30. Diekmann, M.A., O'Callaghan, P., Nett, T.M. and Niswender, G.D. (1978) Biol. Reprod. 19, 1010-1013.

31. Henderson, K.M., Scaramuzzi, R.J. and Baird, D.T. (1977) J. Endocr. 72, 379-383

32. Dingle, J.T., Hay, M.E. and Moor, R.M. (1968) J. Endocr. 40, 325-326.

33. Lahav, M., Meidan, R., Amsterdam, A., Gebauer, H. and Lindner, H.R. (1977) J. Endocr. 75, 317-324.

34. Kaley, G. and Weiner, R. (1975) Prostaglandins 10, 685-688.

35. Nett, T.M., McClellan, M.C. and Niswender, G.D. (1976) Biol. Reprod. 15, 66-78.

36. Thorburn, G.D., Cox, R.I., Currie, W.B., Restall, B.J. and Schneider, W. (1972) J. Endocr. 53, 325-326.

37. Baird, D.T. and Scaramuzzi, R.J. (1975) Ann. Biol. Anim. Bioch. Biophys. 15, 161-174.

38. Allen, W.R. and Rowson, L.E.A. (1973) J. Reprod. Fert. 33, 539-543.

39. Hearnshaw, H., Restall, B.J. and Gleeson, A.R. (1973) J. Reprod. Fert. 32, 322-323.

40. Henricks, D.M., Long, J.T., Hill, J.R. and Dickey, J.F. (1974) J. Reprod. Fert. 41, 113-120.

41. Moeljono, M.P.E., Bazer, F.W. and Thatcher, W.W. (1976) Prostaglandins 11, 737-743.

42. Henderson, K.M. and McNatty, K.P. (1975) Prostaglandins 9, 779-798.

43. Henderson, K.M. and McNatty, K.P. (1977) J. Endocr. 73, 71-78.

44. Kimball, F.A. and Porteous, S.E. (1978) Prostaglandins 16, 427-432.

45. Fuchs, A.R., Mok, E. and Sundaram, K. (1974) Acta Endocrinol. (Kbh) 76, 583-596.

46. Chatterjee, A. (1976) Prostaglandins 12, 525-534.

47. Tso, E.C. and Tam, W.H. (1978) Can. J. Physiol. Pharmacol. 56, 828-833.

48. Karsch, F.J., Roche, J.R., Noveroske, J.W., Foster, D.L., Norton, H.W. and Nalbandov, A.V. (1971) Biol. Reprod. 4, 129-136.

49. Donaldson, L.E. and Hansel, W. (1965) J. Dairy Sci. 48, 903-904.

50. Blatchley, F.L., Maul Walker, F.M. and Poyser, N.L. (1975) J. Endocr. 67, 225-229.

51. Moeljono, M.P.E., Thatcher, W.W., Bazer, F.W., Frank, M., Owens, L.J. and Wilcox, C.J. (1977) Prostaglandins 14, 543-555.

52. Walker, F.M. and Poyser, N.L. (1978) Br. J. Pharmacol. 62, 177-183.

53. Frank, M., Bazer, F.W., Thatcher, W.W. and Wilcox, C.J. (1978) Prostaglandins 15, 151-160.

54. Lewis, G.S., Wilson, L. Jr., Wilks, J.W., Pexton, J.E., Fogwell, R.L., Ford, S.P., Butcher, R.L., Thayne, W.V. and Inskeep, E.K. (1977) J. Anim. Sci. 45, 320-327.

55. Mapletoft, R.J., Del Campo, M.R. and Ginther, O.J. (1975) Proc. Soc. Expt. Biol. Med. 150, 129-133.

56. Mapletoft, R.J., Lapin, D.R. and Ginther, O.J. (1976) Biol. Reprod. 15, 414-421.

57. Pratt, B.R., Butcher, R.L. and Inskeep, E.K. (1977) J. Anim. Sci. 46, 784-791.

58. Lewis, G.S., Jenkins, P.E., Fogwell, R.L. and Inskeep, E.K. (1978) J. Anim. Sci. 47, 1314-1323.

59. Fenwick, L., Jones, R.L., Naylor, B., Poyser, N.L. and Wilson, N.H. (1977) Br. J. Pharmacol. 59, 191-199.

60. Jones, R.L., Poyser, N.L. and Wilson, N.H. (1977) Br. J. Pharmacol. 59, 436P.

61. Moncada, S. and Vane, J.R. (1978) Br. Med. Bull. 34, 129-135.

A LABORATORY MODEL FOR THE STUDY OF FUNCTIONAL LUTEOLYSIS

J. ROBINSON, A.K. HALL[†] and B.J. MERRY

Department of Zoology, University of Hull, Hull, HU6 7RX (U.K.)

ABSTRACT

A procedure is described for the synchronous induction of pseudopregnancy by administration of exogenous gonadotropins to immature female rats. Premature luteolysis, as indicated by falls in plasma progestogen levels, was induced in these animals by injection of µg amounts of 16-aryloxy $PGF_2\alpha$. The sensitivity to $PGF_2\alpha$ increased with the duration of pseudopregnancy. Plasma levels of both progesterone and 20α dihydroprogesterone declined within minutes of $PGF_2\alpha$ administration. Luteal cells isolated from ovaries of pseudopregnant rats synthesized greatley reduced amo of progesterone, in the presence of $PGF_2\alpha$ or its synthetic analogue. Similarly, ovarian mitochondria, isolated from pseudopregnant rats previously injected with $PGF_2\alpha$, showed diminished steroidogenic competence. Preliminary studies indicated that in vitro, the antigonadotropic effects of $PGF_2\alpha$ were Ca^{2+}-sensitive.

INTRODUCTION

The induction of pseudopregnancy by means of exogenous gonadotropin administrati in laboratory rats, can provide a suitable and practicable model for investigation corpus luteum function. In this way corpora lutea of synchronous age can be obtain in amounts adequate to sustain biochemical and sub-cellular investigations (1,2). present work describes the use of this animal preparation for investigation of the initial stages of the luteolytic process.

METHODS

Animal treatment

Immature (24-day old) female rats (Sprague-Dawley, CFY strain) received 50 i.u. pregnant mare serum gonadotropin (Gestyl; Organon Laboratories Ltd, Surrey, U.K.) s in 0.2ml 0.9% saline, followed 72h later by 25 i.u. human chorionic gonadotropin (hCG; Pregnyl; Organon Laboratories Ltd.), s.c. in 0.2ml 0.9% saline. The day of t hCG injection was designated day 0 of pseudopregnancy. Various characteristics of this animal preparation have been described previously (1,2).

[†] Dept. of Obstetrics & Gynecology, School of Medicine, University of Yale, U.S.A.

Preparation of ovarian cell suspensions

Suspensions of isolated luteal cells were routinely obtained from 2g (wet wt) rat ovaries, by a procedure involving collagenase digestion, described elsewhere (3).

Steroid radioimmunoassays

The extraction and estimation of progesterone and 20α dihydroprogesterone in blood and ovarian tissue samples was carried out according to previously validated methods (2,3).

RESULTS

Pseudopregnancy initiated by gonadotropin pretreatment (as above) was found to resemble that resulting from an infertile mating, in terms of duration, and profile of steroid secretion (4); the major difference was that ovarian size (although not individual corpus luteum size) was much greater in hormonally induced pseudopregnancy and this was reflected in the much higher plasma levels of progestational steroid (2).

In pseudopregnant rats the administration of prostaglandin (PG)F$_2$α can induce premature luteolysis. Its onset can be determined by measuring the decline in plasma progesterone levels. For _in vivo_ use, several synthetic analogues of PGF$_2$α are available which show greatly enhanced luteolytic potency. We routinely use a 16-aryloxy derivative of PGF$_2$α, ICI 80996 ('Estrumate"; ICI Ltd, Pharmaceuticals Division, Cheshire, U.K.); quantities (per rat) of 1μg or greater caused a maximal depression of plasma progesterone, measured 1h following subcutaneous injection.

The sensitivity of the animal preparation to luteolytic challenge was shown to be a function of the age of the corpora lutea (see Fig. 1). Groups of animals (n=4) were injected (s.c.) with either 2.5μg 16-aryloxy PGF$_2$α or control vehicle, and trunk blood collected after sacrifice at 1h. This procedure was repeated at different stages of pseudopregnancy. The newly formed corpus luteum (day 2) was relatively refractory to luteolytic induction, whilst in later pseudopregnancy the same dose of PG elicited dramatic declines in plasma progesterone levels. Similar resistance to PGF$_2$α in the early luteal phase has been reported in the cow (5), sheep (6) and pig (7,8).

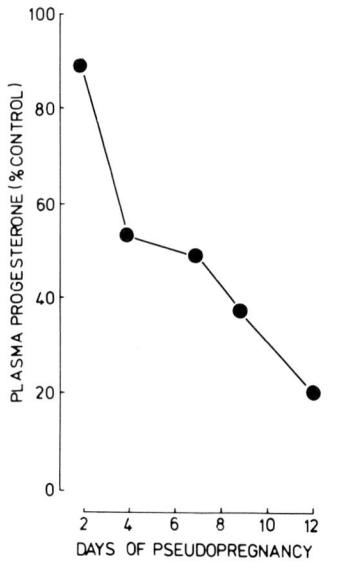

Fig. 1. Increasing luteal sensitivity to PGF$_2$α as pseudopregnancy progresses. Values are means of plasma progesterone measured 1h after s.c. injection of 2.5μg ICI 80996, expressed as % pre-injection levels.

218

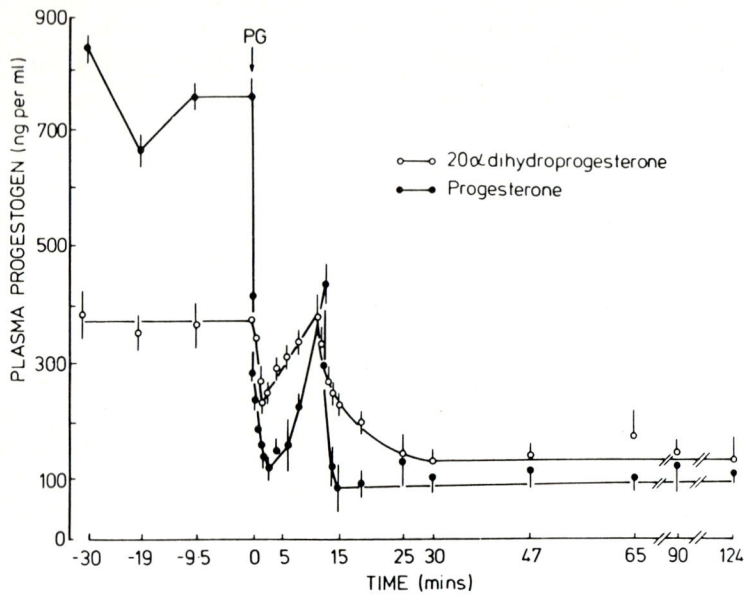

Fig. 2. Rapid onset of functional luteolysis induced by PGF$_2\alpha$ (2.5µg ICI 80996) <u>in vivo</u>: changes in plasma levels of progesterone and 20α dihydroprogesterone. Values are means ± SD.

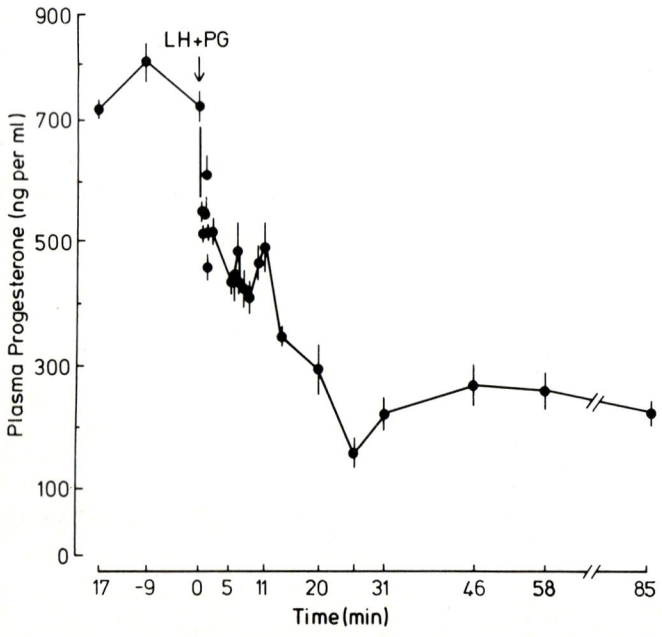

Fig. 3. Antigonadotropic effects of PGF$_2\alpha$: plasma progesterone levels after injec of 10µg LH (NIH–LH–B9) and PGF$_2\alpha$ (2.5µg ICI 80996). Values are means ± S.D.

The time course of the onset of luteolysis was determined in concious rats bearing indwelling carotid cannulae (9). Basal blood samples (5μl) were taken, and then 2.5μg 16-aryloxy PGF₂α injected via the cannula. Rapid samples of blood were obtained during the following 2h period. The levels of progesterone and 20α dihydroprogesterone in plasma both fell rapidly following PG administration (see Fig. 2); the levels of these steroids were minimal after 15 and 30 min respectively. In the intervening period however, transient rises following the initial precipitous falls were evident. The precise cause of these is unknown, but might represent an haemodynamic or injection artefact; we have more recently found them reduced if PGs are administered via the jugular vein, and blood samples taken via the carotid artery. The onset of PG-induced functional luteolysis in this rat model is apparently characterized by a rapid fall in total progestogenic secretion; this confirms similar findings (10), and emphasizes

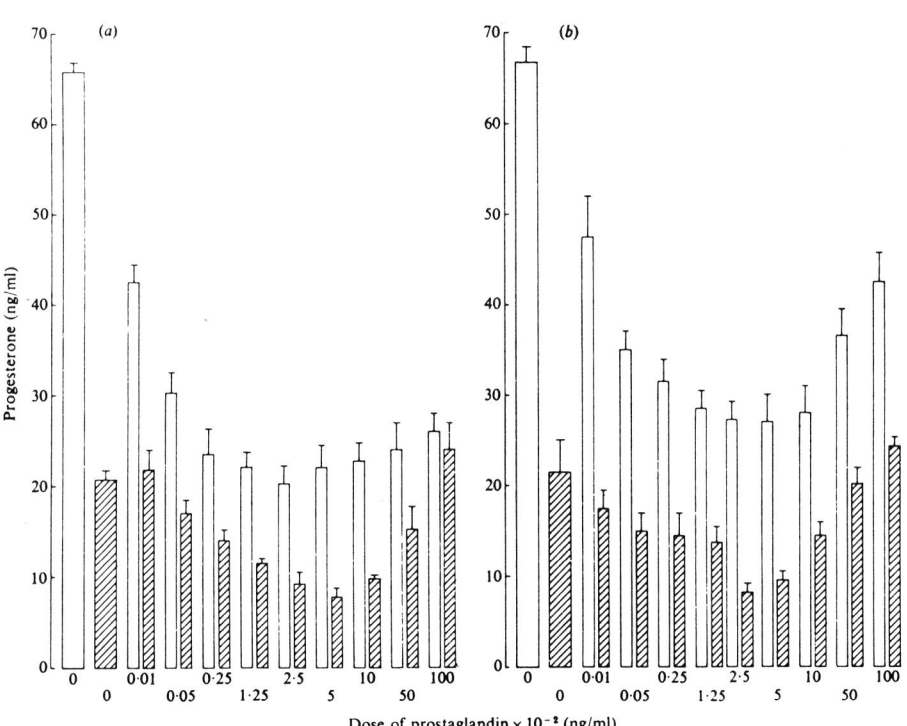

Fig. 4. Effect of (a) prostaglandin F₂α and (b) 16-aryloxy prostaglandin F₂α (ICI 80996) on progesterone biosynthesis by luteal cell suspensions in vitro. Hatched bars show the control value when ethanol vehicle alone was added, open bars show the effect of the presence of 1μg LH/ml. The values indicated by the histograms are those for progesterone synthesized during 60 min incubations of luteal cells, corrected by subtraction of the content of progesterone at zero time (means ± S.D.) (3).

that rises in 20α dihydroprogesterone – previously held to be an index of luteolysis in this species (11) – are associated with later events in the luteolytic process.

In similar acute experiments the effect of simultaneous administration of LH (10μg NIH-LH-B9) and 16-aryloxy-PGF$_2$α (2.5μg) was investigated (see Fig. 3). Plasma progesterone levels again rapidly fell: the usual stimulatory effect of LH in this system (1) was completely abolished.

Attempts to demonstrate inhibitory effects of PGF$_2$α on luteal progesterone biosynthesis in vitro have in the past produced inconsistent results: paradoxically, steroidogenesis was often shown to be stimulated in such experiments (12). More recently McNatty, Henderson and co-workers have shown that PGF$_2$α could diminish progesterone secretion in long-term cultures of granulosa cells (13,14). Ovaries taken from pseudopregnant rats can provide a convenient source of tissue to prepare suspensions of isolated luteal cells for in vitro investigations. In a recent study we were able to demonstrate that such isolated luteal cells could respond rapidly and sensitively to luteolytic prostaglandins in vitro (3) (see Fig. 4). Both natural PGF$_2$α, and its synthetic 16-aryloxy analogue were unambiguously luteolytic in this system in terms of inhibition of progesterone secretion. The equipotency of these two PGs in vitro is in marked contrast to their relative potencies in vivo.

The luteotrophic effects of LH are thought to reside ultimately in the ability of this gonadotropin to control the rate of cholesterol side chain cleavage occuring in luteal mitochondria (15). Since many of the effects of PGF$_2$α appear to be anti-gonadotrophic it was of interest to investigate the possibility that the luteolytic effect of PGF$_2$α might be mediated via an inhibitory action at the mitochondrial level (see Fig. 5). Four groups

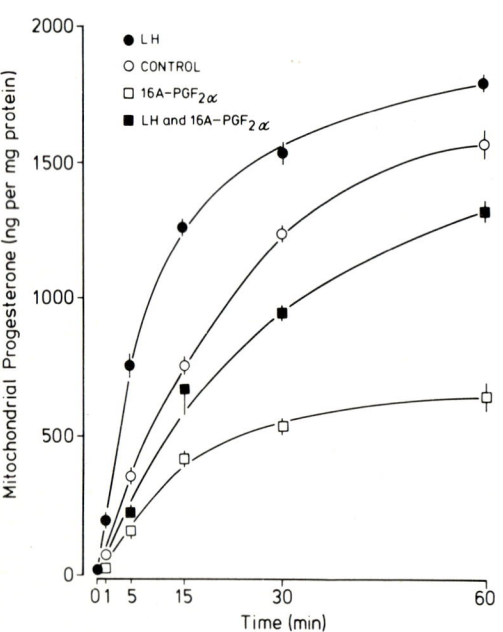

Fig. 5. Effects of prior administration in vivo of 10μg LH (10μg) and 2.5μg PGF$_2$α (ICI 80996) on ovarian mitochondrial progesterone biosynthesis.

rats (n=15) on day 7 of pseudopregnancy received (s.c.) either 10μg LH (NIH-LH-B9), 2.5μg ICI 80996, 10μg LH plus 2.5μg ICI 80996, or control vehicle. Rats were killed 30 min later, and ovarian mitochondria prepared (1). Mitochondrial preparations corresponding to the treatment groups were incubated under conditions as described elsewhere (1), in the presence of 10mM D,L-isocitrate (respiratory substrate). The data clearly show that prior exposure to PGF$_2\alpha$ results in greatly impaired mito-chondrial steroidogenic capability (Fig. 5).

Ca^{2+} is an important intracellular regulator in many physiological systems, in-cluding some involving cyclic 3'5' AMP. Our recent preliminary studies indicate that PGF$_2\alpha$-induced luteolysis shows Ca^{2+} sensitivity (see Fig. 6). Isolated luteal cells were prepared as previously described (3) and incubated for 1h in the presence or absence of LH (1μg/ml), PGF$_2\alpha$ (500ng/ml), and a range of incubation media containing varying $[Ca^{2+}]$. The amounts of progesterone synthesized under these different treat-ments are shown in Fig. 6. The maximal antigonadotropic effect of PGF$_2\alpha$ occured in Ca^{2+}-free medium.

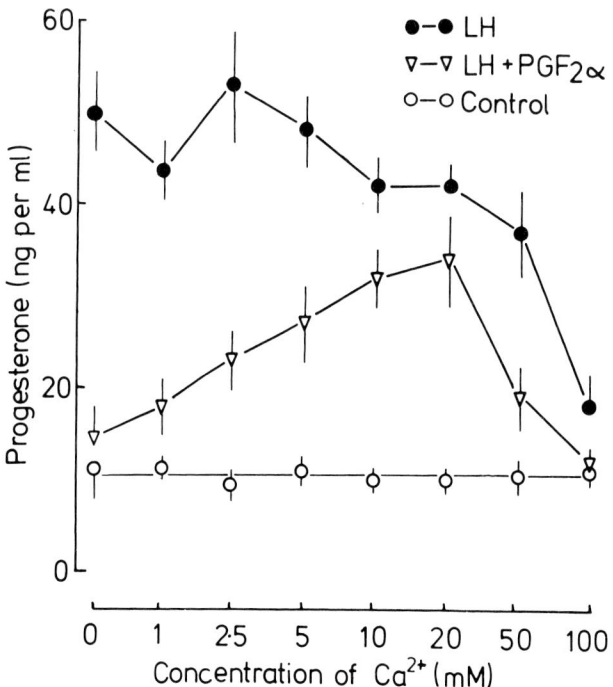

Fig. 6. Effects of $\left[Ca^{2+}\right]$ upon PGF$_2\alpha$ and LH modulation of progesterone biosynthesis in luteal cells. Values are means ± S.D.

DISCUSSION

A great deal of evidence has accumulated to support the contention that $PGF_2\alpha$ is t physiological luteolysin in the rat and many other non-primate mammalian species (review, 16). Our present data demonstrates that hormonal induction of pseudopregnan in rats offers a suitable and practicable animal model for investigations on the luteolytic mechanism. $PGF_2\alpha$ was shown to be luteolytic both in vivo (Figs. 1-3,5) and in vitro (Figs. 4,6). It was apparent that $PGF_2\alpha$-induced luteal regression was of rapid onset in both situations (see also (3)), and characterized by reduced luteal secretion of both progesterone and 20α dihydroprogesterone. Luteal regression is kn to be associated with loss of LH-receptor (17,18,19) and induction of 20α hydroxy-steroid dehydrogenase (11,20); however these phenomena have a latency that effectiv excludes their involvement in the onset of the luteolytic process. It also appears unlikely that the binding affinity of LH for its luteal receptors is changed by PGF_2 (21). The antigonadotropic effect of $PGF_2\alpha$ may well initially involve disruption of the interaction between occupied LH receptors and the adenylate cyclase system (21,2 23) of luteal cells. How this might be achieved remains unknown. The experiments described in Fig. 6 indicate that Ca^{2+} may have a role in this, as in many other cel regulatory phenomena.

ACKNOWLEDGEMENTS

This work was supported by grants from the Wellcome Trust (J.R.), the Science Research Council (A.K.H.) and the Nuffield Foundation (B.J.M.).

REFERENCES

1. Tan, C.H. and Robinson, J. (1977) Endocrinology 101, 396.

2. Hall, A.K. and Robinson, J. (1978) Prostaglandins 15, 1013.

3. Hall, A.K. and Robinson, J. (1979) J. Endocr. 81, 157.

4. DeGreef, W.J., Dullart, J. and Zeilmaker, G.H. (1976) Endocrinology 98, 1228.

5. Rowson, L.E.A., Tervit, R. and Brand, A. (1972) J. Reprod. Fertil. 29, 145.

6. Hearnshaw, H., Restall, B.J. and Gleeson, A.R. (1973) J. Reprod. Fertil. 32, 32

7. Diehl, J.R. and Day, B.N. (1973) J. Anim. Sci. 37, 307.

8. Polge, C. (1975) Ann. Biol. Anim. Bioch. Biophys. 15, 663.

9. Popovic, V. and Popovic, P. (1960) J. Appl. Physiol. 15, 727.

10. Torjesen, P.A., Dahlin, R., Haug, E. and Aakvaag, A. (1978) Acta Endocr. 87, 6

11. Weist, G.W., Kidwell, W.R. and Balogh, K. (1968) Endocrinology 82, 844.

12. Pharriss, B.B., Wyngarden, L.J. and Gutknecht, G.D. (1968) In: "Gonadotrophin (ed. E. Rosemberg) pp 121-129. Palo Alto, California: Geron-X, Inc.

13. McNatty, K.P., Henderson, K.M. and Sawers, R.S. (1975) J. Endocr. 67, 231.

14. Henderson, K.M. and McNatty, K.P. (1977) J. Endocr. 73, 71.

15. Hall, P.F. and Koritz, S.B. (1965) Biochemistry 4, 1037.

16. Horton, E.W. and Poyser, N.L. (1976) Physiol. Rev. 56, 595.

17. Grinwich, D.L., Hichens, M. and Behrman, H.R. (1976) Biol. Reprod. 14, 212.

18. Grinwich, D.L., Hichens, M. and Behrman, H.R. (1976) Endocrinology 98, 146.

19. Torjesen, P.A. and Aakvaag, A. (1977) Acta Endocr. 86, 162.

20. Lamprecht, S.A., Herlitz, H.V. and Ahren, K.E.B. (1975) Molec. Cell Endocr. 3, 273.

21. Behrman, H.R., Grinwich, D.L. and Hichens, M. (1976) In: "Advances in prostaglandin and thromboxane research", Vol. 2 (Eds. B. Samuelsson and R. Paoletti) pp 655-666. New York: Raven Press.

22. Lahav, M., Freud, A. and Lindner, H.R. (1976) Biochem. Biophys. Res. Commun. 68, 1294.

23. Thomas, J.P., Dorflinger, J. and Behrman, H.R. (1978) Proc. Nat. Acad. Sci. U.S.A. 75, 1344.

PHARMACOLOGICAL INDUCTION OF LUTEOLYSIS

A.J. Mul

Research Laboratories, Intervet International B.V., P.O. Box 31, 5830 AA Boxmeer, The Netherlands.

In order to regulate reproduction or to treat some types of reproductive disorders, elimination of an existing corpus luteum may be desirable.

In the early days of veterinary intervention in reproduction, the only reliable and clearly understandable technique of eliminating a corpus luteum, was the manual enucleation. The disadvantages of this technique are well known. Not only is this technique not applicable in smaller species, there is also a real risk of bleeding, cystic degeneration and periovarian adhesions.

The need for a more elegant and safer technique is illustrated by the following sentence in a booklet by Austin & Short (ref. 3) :
"So far, most attemps to induce luteal regression by injection of hormones have been ineffective and much progress is unlikely to be made on this approach, until a substance has been found that will act directly on the ovary, in order to block luteal function".

From the foregoing papers in this session, it is clear that much more is known to day about this "luteolytic substance".

Much of the new data and their practical implications have been reviewed by different authors (ref. 16, ref. 19 and ref. 30).

This paper will only review the recent progress in understanding the mode of action of apparently total different treatments that shorten the functional life of the corpus luteum.

To understand the role of the corpus luteum in the oestrus cycle of various species, the following table may be helpfull (After Jöchle, W.).

Table I   Types of ovarian cycle

Type	Ovulation	Formation of CL	Species
I	induced	spontaneous	rabbit, cat
II	spontaneous	induced	rat, mouse, hamster
III	spontaneous	spontaneous	cow, sheep, goat, horse, pig, dog, guinea pig, primates

From this table it is clear that many economically important domestic animals have "true cycles" or "complete biphasic cycle", including a spontaneous CL-fase of predictable length after every ovulation.

Species also show variations in their utero-ovarian relationship. In the cow, sheep, pig, guinea pig, rabbit, hamster, mouse, rat, hysterectomy extends CL life. In the dog, monkey and man, hysterectomy does not influence the length of CL fase. Even within these groups differences exist. The uterine-ovarian relationship is much closer in sheep than in pigs. (ref. 25)

A number of treatments are known to shorten the active progesterone secreting lifetime of the CL. Some of these treatments were already in use long before anything was known about their mode of action. The expected difference between systemic and local treatments will turn out to be less striking. The various treatments will be discussed now.

Prostaglandins

Discovery of the physiological role of these tissue hormones has been the basis for an explosion in interest and research in luteolysis. The mechanism of action of prostaglandins of the F2α-type has been dealt with in the preceeding papers. More details of clinical use and species differences will be discussed in the last paper of this session. In this place, the large differences in sensitivity and tolerance should be mentioned.

In all species studied, PGF2α and analogues do not cause luteal regression in the freshly formed corpus luteum (3 - 5 days), but sensitivity increases as the CL matures and progesterone synthesis increases. At the onset of spontaneous luteolysis, the effect of a pharmacological application of PGF2α can not be detected any more. The period between this point is the period in which exogenous PGF2α can be used with a high success rate. The short period of sensitivity in the pig (day 12 - 14) has been a major disadvantage for the routine use in this species. (ref. 14 and ref. 22)

If synchronisation is wanted, this may be obtained by extending the CL life with oestrogens, by induction of accessory CL with PMSG-HCG or by using lysis of early corpora lutea of pregnancy from day 23 of pregnancy onwards.

Relative sensitivity is high in the mare, sheep, cow but low in the bitch and very low in primates and man. Sensitivity seems to be related to luteotrophic and luteolytic mechanisms in the various species.

Sensitivity for PGF2α induced luteolysis also seems to be dependent on the availability of oestrogens. (ref. 18)

It might be interesting to know whether the few % non responders at PGF2α treatment are those at the lowest oestrogen levels in the so-called follicular minicycle.

Sensitivity for luteolysis by exogenous PGF2α can be enhanced by synchronous application of one of the common non-steroidal anti-inflammatory drugs that act on the PG-synthetase and dehydrogenase systems (indomethacin, asperin etc.). In a patent application, it is claimed also that the responsive period in the pig can be extended by this method.

Tolerance for the natural PGF2α differs substantially between species. The dog is extremely intolerant, the ruminants are tolerant, whilst the horse and pig are intermediate. There is evidence that this tolerance difference correlates with differences in first-pass age degradation. Clinical use in the dog has been almost impossible up till now because of the combination of low sensitivity and low tolerance. (ref. 19, ref. 29 and ref. 9)

There is sufficient evidence now to assume that the site of action of PGF2α is a specific receptor on the CL cell surface.

Since the first synthesis of PGF2α, about 10 years ago, many analogues have been developed and tested for luteolytic action (ref. 15). A number of analogues are available now. Main advantage of these compounds seems to be a longer circulation half-life. Differences in receptor affinity and efficacy may cause some dissociation between luteolytic and smooth muscle activity. As a result of this structure modification, a better tolerance and/or a lower dose can be obtained. The overall pharmacological pattern is still very close to PGF2α however. The endocrine and physiological events following a pharmacologically induced luteolysis are fully comparable to those in spontaneous physiological luteolysis (Karg et al : 1978 (unpublished).

Oestrogens

Oestrogens, applied in physiological and pharmacological doses can cause luteolysis in cow and sheep. Oestrogens may cause the release of prostaglandins from the

endometrium, especially when this has been primed with progesterone. PGF2α
release from uteri has been detected about 60 - 90 min. after oestradiol 17 β -
infusions, corresponding with E2 levels of 10 pg/ml and above. (ref. 5)

A parallel to the natural mechanism is evident. The sequence of high progesterone and rising oestrogen is supposed to cause the secretion of the endogenous
luteolysin, which seems to be synonymous to PGF2α. The initial PGF2α release
is supported by a quick action on PG-synthetase and a secundary action to increase
the synthesis capacity. So, after the initial trigger, a self stimulating mechanism
seems to occur. This mechanism has been confirmed in the rat, guinea pig and cow
(ref. 19)

Some conflicting data have been published about luteotrophic action of oestrogens
when applied to sheep, guinea pigs and pigs in the late luteal phase. Some other
factors may interfere.

It must be noted that a completely different situation exists in the pig and
rabbit, since oestrogens are clearly luteotrophic in this species.

The mechanism of action of oestrogens in causing luteal regression in hyster-
ectomized animals and primates, cases in which no influence of the uterus on the
ovaries exists, has been discussed by many authors (ref. 19, ref. 17 and ref. 4)
Sufficient evidence exists that luteolysis is caused in these cases by a local
luteolysin, synthesised in the ovary. Indomethacin blocked the luteolytic effect
in various trials (ref. 2 and ref. 26).

The sensitivity pattern for this effect of oestrogens fits that for the action
of exogenous PGF2α. However, there may be some additional mechanisms involved
(ref. 31 and ref. 8). A direct effect on the corpus luteum cell, influenceing
the c-AMP system or the 20α-OHSD directly can not be excluded. Inhibition of
luteotrophins secretion may occur, but seems to be not mechanism of action
(ref. 19)

Progestagens

Some studies report a shortening of the luteal phase after application of proges-
tagens direct after ovulation (ref. 16). In general however, low and moderate
doses of progesterone are clearly luteotrophic in all species (ref. 11). Especially
in the pregnant pig, high levels of progesterone block the normal gonadotrophin
and oestrogen support of the corpus luteum (ref. 21, ref. 19 and ref. 27).
Not all data are consistent. Woody (ref. 16) failed to show shortening of cycle
in pigs after 10 daily injections of 200 mg progesterone, while comparable treatments did cause shortening of CL phase in cattle, sheep and guinea pig. (ref. 1).
Baird (ref. 5) suggested that early application of progesterone may act as an
"early priming" of the PGF2α synthesising tissues (minimal period about 10 days).
As a conclusion I would say that progesterone acts as a suppressor of CL activity

and does not act as a real luteolytic agent. This view is in accordance with the fact that progesterone application in a later stage of CL function, e.g. as a intra vaginal device, does not influence CL lifetime.

Gonadotrophins

There is a remarkable similarity between dose-effect relations of gonadotrophins and PGF2α. Both are luteotrophic in low doses and luteolytic in high doses (ref. 1). High doses of LH and/or FSH (HCG, PMSG) are reported to be luteolytic in cattle, sheep, horse, guinea-pig, rat and primates (ref. 6).

Excessive doses of LH cause an increase in the synthesis of PGF2α, which can be suppressed by indomethacin. These findings suggest that LH and HCG act on ovarian progesterone synthesis by a mechanism that is mediated by prostaglandins. PMSG is luteolytic in the pregnant rat by causing polyfolliculogenesis and subsequent abortion (ref. 13). Indomethacin and corticosteroids can block this effect. The same occurs in hamsters.

As clomiphene proved to block PMSG-induced abortion in rats very effectively, it is reasonable to explain the effect as an oestrogen-PGF2α mediated effect, again, mimicking exactly the normal luteolytic events (ref. 8). Specific effects on pathways of steroid genesis, favouring the synthesis of the less active 20α-dihydroxy progesterone may play a role, as well as induction of refractoriness by overstimulation of receptors.

Oxytocin

Oxytocin can cause luteolysis in the cow, sheep and pig, when applied daily in high doses. In the cow, 150 - 200 IU/day during days 0-5 of cycle are required to cause luteolysis and oestrus at day 8-12. The uterus is required for the effect (ref. 16 and ref. 12).

The mechanism of action may be a cascade effect of PGF2α and oxytocin, acting as a mutually positive feedback. Oestrogens may play a role in this cascade-effect as well, in sensitizing receptors and stimulating PG-synthesis. The fact that LH can overcome the action of oxytocin support the evidence of PGF2α mediation (ref. 16).

Chan (ref. 7) reported prostaglandin release by oxytocin stimulation in the late pregnant rat uterus. Contractile effects of oxytocin and PG releasing effect seem to be separated actions. There seems to be no evidence for a direct action of oxytocin on luteal cells, causing luteal regression.

Local stimuli

To this group of treatments, one may reckon I.U.D.'s, uterine irrigations with irritating substances, slight uterine infections and electrical or mechanical stimulations. Because of the present insight in luteolytic processes in normal cycle, this group of treatments can be taken as one entity.

Uterine distensions and I.U.D's are promoting the endometrial PGF2α release in at least cow, sheep, guinea pig, primates. It is also well known that absence of glandular epithelium in the uterus causes persisting CL, e.g. in the case of pyometra and severe endometritis.

Irrigation of the uterine cavity with anti-bacterial fluids like iodine and anti-biotics in irrirating solvents is well known to change the length of the ovarian cyle (ref. 16 and ref. 19). In the case of electrical or mechanical stimulation, both release of prostaglandins and triggering of oxytocin may occur. The mare seems to be very sensitive to uterine irritation. Flushing with normal saline already causes an immediate PGF2α release and a subsequent shortening of the oestrus cycle (ref. 23). In the cow, a more damaging irritation may cause a delayed PGF2α release after repair of the endometrium. Dependent on the moment of application, a shortened or extended cycle may occur. (ref. 24 and 28).

Specific drugs can alter the function of luteal cells. Possibilities are gonadotrophin blockers, colchicine and related alcaloids, most probably by causing PGF2α release, and specific blockers of steroid synthesis like aminoglutethimide. This groups of substances will not be discussed in detail in this paper.

Summarising the various treatments that cause luteal regression, it turns out that the luteolysin, which is most likely PGF2α plays a key role in all types of pharmacologically induced luteolysis. The most practicable treatments now are PGF2α and -analogues and oestradiol.

All modes of action fit quite well into the complex regulation scheme of oestrus cycle, as discussed recently by Lamming (ref. 20).

REFERENCES

1. Astwood, E.B. : Recent progress in hormone research. Proceedings of the 1971 Laurentian Hormone Conference. 28, 51-89 (1972).
2. Auletta, F.J., Caldwell, B.V. and Speroff, L. : Estrogen-induced luteolysis in the rhesus monkey / reversal with indomethacin. Prostaglandins 11 (4) 745-752 (1976).
3. Austin, C.R. and Short, R.V. : Reproduction in Mammals. 5. Artificial control of reproduction. p. 19 (1972).
4. Baird, D.T. : Content and secretion of steroids by the human ovary in vivo. James, V.H.T. Ed. Endocrinology - Ex. medica. 330-336 (1977).
5. Baird, D.T. : Local utero-ovarian relationships. In control of ovulation. Eds. D.B. Crighton, G.B. Foxcroft, N.B. Haynes & G.E. Lamming, Butterworths London 217-233 (1978).
6. Banik, U.K. : Pregnancy-terminating effect of human chorionic gonadotrophin in rats. J. Reprod. Fert. 42, 67-76 (1975).
7. Chan, W.Y. : Evidence for independent oxytocic and prostaglandin-releasing actions of oxytocin. Fed. Proc. 38 (3) 528-ev. (1979).
8. Chatterjee, A., Pal, A.K. and Gupta, T. : Pregnant Mare's Serum Gonado-trophin : II Reversal of the antifertility faculty of pregnant mare's serum gonadotrophin by using Clomiphene Citrate of reserpine in rats. Contraception 15 (5) 571-578 (1977).
9. Concannon, P.W. and Hansel, W. : Prostaglandin F2α induced luteolysis, hypothermia and abortions in beagle bitches. Prostaglandins 13 (3) 533-542 (1977).
10. Currie, W.B., Cox, R.I. and Thorburn G.D. : Release of Prostaglandin F, regression of corpora lutea and induction of premature parturition in goats treated with estradiol 17β. Prostaglandins 12 (6) 1093-1103 (1976).
11. Denamur, R. : Formation and maintenance of corpora lutea in domestic animals J. Anim. Sci., 27 (1) 163-180 (1968).
12. Ellendorff, F., Forsling, M., Parvizi, N., Williams, H., Taverne, M. and Smidt, D. : Plasma oxytocin and vasopressin concentrations in response to prostaglandin injection into the pig. J. Reprod. Fert. 56, 573-577 (1979).
13. Gupta, T. and Chatterjee, A. : Pregnant mare's serum gonandotrophin : V. indomethacin of cortisone and the reversal of antifertility efficacy of pregnant mare's serum gonadotrophin. Contraception (1978).
14. Guthrie, H.D. and Polge, C. : Luteal function and oestrus in gilts treated with a synthetic analogue of prostaglandin F2α (ICI 79,939) at various times during the oestrous cycle. J. Reprod. Fert. 48, 423-425 (1976).
15. Hammarström, S., Powell, W.S., Kyldén, U. and Samuelsson, B. : Some properties of a prostaglandin F2α receptor in corpora lutea. Prostaglandin and Thromboxane Research 1, 235-246 (1976).
16. Hansel, W., Concannon, P.W. and Lukaszewska, J.H. : Corpora lutea of the large domestic animals. Biology of Reproduction 8, 222-245 (1973).
17. Hawk, H.W. and Bolt, D.J. : Luteolytic effect of estradiol - 17β when administered after midcycle in the ewe. Biology of reproduction 2, 275-278 (1970).
18. Hixon, J.E., Gengenbach, D.R. and Hansel W. : Failure of prostaglandin F2α to cause luteal regression in ewes after destruction of ovarian follicles by X-irradiation. Biology of Reproduction 13, 126-135 (1975).
19. Horton, E.W. and Poyser, N.L. : Uterine luteolytic Hormone : A physiological role for prostaglandin F2α. Physiological Reviews 56 (4) 595-651 (1976).
20. Lamming, G.E. : Pharmacological control of reproduction cycles. Vet. Rec. 156-160 (1979).
21. Liptrap, R.M. : Oestrogen excretion by sows with induced cystic ovarian follicles. Res. Vet. Sci. 15, 215-219 (1973).
22. Moeljono, M.P.E., Bazer, F.W. and Thatcher, W.W. : A study of Prostaglandin F2α as the luteolysin in Swine. I. Effect of prostaglandin F2α in hyster-ectomized gilts. Prostaglandins 11 (4) 737-743 (1976).

23. Neely, D.P., Stabenfeldt, G.H. and Sauter, C.L. : The effect of exogenous oxytocin on luteal function in mares. J. Reprod. Fert. 55, 303-308 (1979).
24. Oxender, W.D. and Seguin, B.E. : Bovine intrauterine therapy. J.A.V.M.A. 168 (3) 217-219 (1976).
25. Patek, C.E., and Watson, J. : Prostaglandin production during the oestrous cycle by porcine and ovine corpus luteum tissue in vitro. J. Endocrinol. 71 (2) 47-48 (1976).
26. Poyser, N.L. : Involvement of prostaglandins in the female reproductive cycle. Biochemical society transactions 6, 718-721 (1978).
27. Rampacek, G.B. and Kraeling, R.R. : Effect of estrogen on luteal function in prepuberal gilts. J. Anim. Sci. 46 (2) 453-457 (1978).
28. Seguin, B.E. Morrow, D.A. and Oxender, W.D. : Intrauterine therapy in the cow. J.A.V.M.A. 164 (6) 609-612 (1974).
29. Sokolowski, J.H. : Effect of prostaglandin F2α .a-THAM in the bitch. J.A.V.M.A. 170 (5) 536-537 (1977).
30. Stabenfeldt, G.H., Edqvist, L.E., Kindahl, H., Gustafsson, B. and Bane, A. : Practical implications of recent physiologic findings for reproductive efficiency in cows, mares, sows and ewes. J.A.V.M.A. 172 (6) 667-675 (1978).
31. Williams, M.T., Roth, M.S., Marsh, J.M. and LeMaire, W.J. : Inhibition of human chorionic gonadotrophin-induced progesterone synthesis by estradiol in isolated human luteal cells. Journal of clinical endocrinology and metabolism 48 (3) 437-440 (1979).

CLINICAL CONSEQUENCES OF LUTEOLYSIS

A. de KRUIF and A. BRAND
Department of Herd Health and Ambulatory Clinic, Veterinary School, University of
Utrecht, Yalelaan 20, Utrecht, 3508 TD, The Netherlands

ABSTRACT

Because of their luteolytic effect prostaglandins can be used in the reproductive
field of farm animals. In this paper the possibilities of the use of prostaglandins
both for synchronization of oestrus and for various clinical indications in mares,
cows, sheep and pigs are discussed.

INTRODUCTION

The oestrous cycle of the mare, cow, ewe and goat can be manipulated by affecting
the life span of the corpus luteum with prostaglandins (PG). Administration of PGF
2 alpha or structurally-related compounds during the oestrous cycle induces a prema
ture regression of the corpus luteum and results in the onset of a fertile heat
two to five days later (12,16,17,33).

It has been shown that administration of prostaglandins mimic or closely approac
the natural oestrous cycle at the termination of the luteal phase (15). Prostaglandins are now used on a large scale as an aid to breeding management and as a
therapy for certain reproductive disorders. The application of prostaglandins in
these areas will be discussed.

Synchronization of oestrus

Prostaglandins are effective inducers of luteolysis only during a restricted
period of the oestrous cycle. In general, animals approaching oestrus or less
than 5 days after oestrus will not respond to PG. This means that in a group of
randomly cycling animals about 65 percent will react to a single treatment.
Theoretically this percentage can be increased to almost 100 by a double PG-treatment, 11 days apart. The first injection will result in luteolysis in those
animals that are between days 5 and 17 of a 20-day oestrous cycle while the
second injection will produce luteolysis in most of the remaining animals that
should be at day 7 to 10 of their cycle.

Synchronization of oestrus with PG means synchronization of luteolysis. This is normally achieved in 24 to 36 hours and generally provides good synchronization. The subsequent steps in the oestrous cycle, maturation of the follicle(s), onset of oestrus and ovulation, are not influenced by exogenous prostaglandins, but by endogenous hormone balances. In this respect it is better to speak of synchronization of luteolysis instead of synchronization of oestrus. This may also explain why the onset of oestrus varies from 2 to 5 days following a single PG injection.

Besides variation in the onset of oestrus, there is also a variation in the onset of ovulation in PG-treated animals. When insemination is not performed at oestrus, the spread of ovulation makes a double insemination schedule at predetermined times advisable. However the most important prerequisites for good synchronization and subsequent pregnancy results are that animals to be synchronized are cycling normally and have a normal reproductive tract.

Synchronization of oestrus in the cow

Prostaglandin treatment of a group of heifers or cows enables the farmer to:
- extend the genetic benefits of A.I. to maiden heifers which are naturally bred by a less valuable bull;
- batch cows and heifers for breeding and subsequent calving over the year, or just within a restricted period of a seasonally breeding programme;
- facilitate or restrict oestrus detection or even to eliminate oestrus detection.

For the synchronization of oestrus and the subsequent insemination the following procedures are used:
- single or double treatment and insemination at oestrus or at (a) set time(s).

Irrespective of the regime of the treatment chosen, it would be advisable whenever possible to conduct a rectal examination on every heifer or cow before treatment. This will exclude animals from treatment which are not cycling, show reproductive abnormalities, or are pregnant. This will reduce treatment costs for the farmer while ensuring that these animals are properly treated. The extra cost of drugs when a double-treatment schedule is used can be lowered by administering the first treatment to only those animals that have a functional corpus luteum. Animals that are thought to be in pro-oestrus or just past oestrus, or that did not respond to the first treatment can then be treated 11 days later. However, in some countries and under some conditions it may be more expensive to do rectal examinations, have two insemination periods and observe oestrus at two different times (34). In addition, silent heats may be missed when fixed time insemination(s) after the second treatment is not employed.

Fertility at the synchronized oestrus

The only valid assessment of the fertility of a PG-synchronized oestrus is by comparing the pregnancy rate of treated animals with that of untreated control animals from the same herd under the same conditions. The general conclusions that can be drawn from various well designed experiments are:

- pre-treatment identification of cycling animals by use of a bull or by rectal examination of the reproductive organs is a prerequisite for satisfactory pregnancy results in all categories of cattle (29, 34);
- high pregnancy rates can only be achieved if the oestrus synchronization rate is high, especially when fixed-time inseminations are used (10, 11, 32);
- the percentage of animals in oestrus within 4 days after a double PG treatment is higher in cycling heifers than in cycling cows (13, 24);
- the pregnancy rate in cycling heifers to a single A.I. at oestrus or a double A.I. at 72 hr and 96 hr after PG treatment is comparable to that of untreated control heifers (13);
- the pregnancy rate in cycling cows after set-time insemination(s) is lower than in untreated controls, possibly because of a delayed oestrous response (10, 29).

In adult dairy cows and suckler beef cows a significant increase in fertility is reported with a combined progestagen - prostaglandin treatment compared to treatment with a double PG injection (11, 32). This improved fertility with the combined progestagen - prostaglandin treatment may be due to a higher synchronization rate. In order to improve the synchronization rate and ovulation rate in both heifers and cows, additional hormones (GnRH, HCG, oestrogens) have been administrated in association with PG treatment (32). Although such treatments may hasten and synchronize the time of ovulation, they have not been shown to increase pregnancy rate (32).

Synchronization of oestrus in the horse

Prostaglandin F 2 alpha is a potent luteolysyn in mares (16) but it has some unwanted side effects such as sweating, diarrhea, increased heart and respiration rates and discomfort (30). These adverse side effects are eliminated with the use of a structurally related compound to PGF 2 Alpha, Equimate (ICI - 81008) in a dose of 250 ug (2). The average interval from treatment to onset of oestrus is 3 days but may show a wide variation from 2 to 6 days. This variation in onset of oestrus and subsequent ovulation is thought to be caused by endogenous factors which influence follicular growth and maturation of preovulatory follicles (31). This variation makes it difficult to use synchronization of oestrus as an aid in such stud management practices as, spacing heats to avoid stallion fatigue and facilitating service on nominated days. Experiments to increase the

synchronization of oestrus and ovulation in mares with PG in conjuction with other
hormones like GnRH or HCG, have not been consistently successful.

Synchronization of oestrus in the ewe

Administration of PG will induce luteolysis in ewes which are between days 4
and 14 of the oestrous cycle. Oestrus is shown 2 to 3 days after PG administration
(17). Due to its luteolytic action, prostaglandins can only be used during the
breeding season when the ovaries contain luteal tissue. It therefore does not
enhance the output potential of the ewe flock. During the breeding season synchronization of oestrus offers the sheep breeder the possibility to:
  - extend the genetic benefits of A.I. to many ewes;
  - restrict the breeding and the lambing period to about 10 days;
  - rear and sell fattened lambs in more uniform groups.
Prostaglandins are administered in either a single injection or double injection
regime, 9 - 14 days apart. Insemination is performed either naturally or artificially
at oestrus or at fixed times. However, variable fertility levels have been reported
following the use of PG. No significant difference in conception rate between treated
and control ewes could be found (4, 18, 20, 34). In contrast other workers (3, 5)
reported a lower conception rate following PG treatment. According to Boland et al.
(1978), PG treatment is not an acceptable alternative to orthodox progestagen treatment.

Synchronization of oestrus in the goat

Luteolysis can effectively be induced in goats between day 4 and 17 of the
oestrous cycle with PG (6, 21). Oestrus is induced 2 to 3 days after treatment.
To our knowledge no fertility results following prostaglandin treatment have been
published to date.

Synchronization of oestrus in the pig

In the sow synchronization of oestrus is limited due to the insensitivity of
corpora lutea to prostaglandin administered during the first 11 days of the
oestrous cycle. The limited period from day 12 to 16 in which luteolysis can be
induced with prostaglandins, makes synchronization impractical (34).

Clinical Indications
Cattle
Suboestrus

Suboestrous cows are those animals which by rectal examination have cyclic
ovarian activity and ovulate but fail to show overt oestrus. Suboestrus forms a
part of the syndrome of anoestrus. According to de Kruif (1977), 80% of cows in

which oestrus is not observed (apparent anoestrus) suffer from suboestrus.
The remaining 20% of cows classed as anoestus have inactive ovaries (genuine anoestrus), cystic luteinized follicles, pyometra or are pregnant. Treatment of suboestro
cows involves administration of PG at the time when an active corpus luteum is
present in one of the ovaries. It must be stressed that each anoestrous cow must be
clinically examined very carefully for pregnancy or other causes of anoestrus before
treatment. De Kruif and Brand (1976) examined 300 lactating suboestrous cows which
were divided in two groups; 150 cows with a palpable corpora lutea were treated
with PG and 150 herd mates served as controls. The expected date of oestrus was
predicted on the basis of ovarian examination. Sixty-four percent of treated cows
responded with oestrus within 5 days. The average interval between treatment and
insemination was 8,8 and 17,6 days in the treated and control group respectively.
The pregnancy rates were 56 and 58 per cent, respectively, for the two groups.

Pyometra

Pyometra is usually accompanied by a persistent corpus luteum and anoestrus.
The persistence of the corpus luteum is thought to be caused by an insufficient
release or synthesis of prostaglandins due to pathological changes in the endometriu
Administration of prostaglandins to pyometra cows will result in lutolysis of the
persistent corpus luteum and oestrus. This will be accompanied by relaxation of
the cervix and uterine contractions, followed by evacuation of the uterus (19,
23, 28). The fertility of the treated cows is reduced even if the uterus is completely evacuated. This may be due to permanent damage to the endometrium (28).

Cystic ovarian follicles

In dairy cows during the early post partum period cystic ovarian follicles
are often noticed but may regress spontaneously. Cystic follicles are characterized
clinically by short oestrus intervals or anoestrus and are thought to be caused
by a malfunction of the hypothalamus which results in an insufficient preovulatory
LH-release. In cases of anoestrus caused by luteinized follicles, PG treatment may
be effective. Prostaglandins will induce luteolysis of the luteinized tissue.
The subsequent oestrus may be accompanied by ovulation and a normal development
of the corpus luteum. An alternative treatment regime is administration of GnRH,
followed by PG treatment 9 days later (25). GnRH is given to induce luteinisation
of the wall of the cyst. This will enhance the progesterone production as well as
the chances of a fertile oestrus. The pregnancy rate at first insemination in
such treated cows is about 40%.

Non-pregnant inseminated cows

Prostaglandins are effective in cows that have been inseminated and have not
returned, but are not pregnant according to a rectal examination. Before treatment

with PG the ovaries should be examined rectally for the presence of a well developed
corpus luteum.

Superovulation and embryo transfer

The continued application of embryo transfer techniques in cattle necessitates
the recovery of large numbers of eggs from selected cows. This requires superovulation of donor cows. A standardised superovulation treatment is the intramusculair
injection of 2000 to 3000 i.u. PMSG between days 8 and 14 of the oestrous cycle,
followed by an injection of PG, 2 days later (9). Onset of oestrus can be expected
about 48 hours after prostaglandin treatment. Recipient cows can be synchronized
with the donor cows by PG treatment at the same time or half a day earlier than
the donor.

Termination of pregnancy

In the bovine the reasons for termination of pregnancy can be classified into
three categories:
- mismating and juvenile pregnancy;
- pathological gestation such as hydrops of foetal membranes, and mummification
  or maceration of the foetus;
- Induction of parturition in normal gestation.

Mismating and juvenile pregnancy

Treatment of mismating and juvenile pregnancy with PG is very effective after
the 7th day of mating. When the date of mating or insemination is not known, the
length of pregnancy has to be estimated by rectal examination. This is because
the success rate of treatment is decreased in cows pregnant for more than 5 months
(7) (Brand et al., 1975).

Hydrops of foetal membranes

Hydrops of the foetal membranes can be differentiated into hydrops allantois
and hydrops amnion. The former abnormality is more common and is normally recognized
in the 6th to 8th month of pregnancy. It is often complicated by dystocia, retained
foetal membranes, severe metritis and even shock at the time of either induced or
natural parturition. Administration of PG on two consecutive days will generally
induce parturition within 48 hours. In our opinion the use of PG may be preferred
over glucocorticosteroids because of the danger of the latter in the presence of
subclinical infections.

Mummified and macerated foetuses

Pathological gestations of mummified or macerated foetuses are generally
accompanied by a persistent corpus luteum which blocks expulsion of the foetus.

In these cases there is no functional foetal - placental unit and gestation is
maintained by progesterone from the corpus luteum. Administration of PG will induce
parturition after luteolysis of the corpus luteum. In most cases the mummified
foetus is lodged in the cervix after PG-treatment. This makes manual delivery
necessary.

Induction of parturition in normal gestation

The reasons for inducing premature parturition in cows include: synchronization
of calving and reduction of the incidence of dystocia; lengthening of the interval
from calving to the start of mating when a restricted breeding period is needed;
changes in farm policy which require an earlier mean calving date and occasionally th
treatment of stressed animals (14).

Administration of PG after 250 days of gestation will successfully induce parturition within 96 hours of treatment. The interval is shorter in cows which are
nearer to term. Induction of parturition with PG is of limited practical use due
to complications such as dystocia and more frequently retained placentae (22).
Cow and calf survival is generally normal. Reduction in the percentage of retained
after birth is possible with a combined treatment consisting of a depot corticostero
such as dexamethasone trimetyl—acetate followed 8 to 12 days later by PG (14).
On the other hand, using depot corticosteroids may increase calf mortality.

Horse
Anoestrus

Anoestrus in mares may be due to genuine anoestrus or to apparent anoestrus.
Genuine anoestrus is normally due to a persistent corpus luteum while apparent
anoestrus may be due to poor oestrus detection by the horse owner (1).

Unlike the cow, the corpus luteum of the mare is not palpable. Therefore, the
estimation of the stage of the oestrous cycle is not possible. Since administration
of PG is only effective from 5 days after ovulation, treatment may be ineffective
in some cycling mares. In such mares a second injection of PG, 7 days later, is
therefore advisable. Fertility rate following PG induced oestrus is normal (1).

Non-pregnant mated mares

Due to a seasonal breeding season, PG treatment for non-pregnant mated mares
is a valuable technique when a fertile oestrus is needed before the end of the
breeding season.

Induction of parturition

Induction of parturition in the mare is possible with oxytocin or with PG.
Use of PG is preferable due to a smoother induction of parturition. The mayority
of mares foal in the absence of attendents and this may increase the chances of

difficult parturitions. Since parturition occurs 2-5 hours after PG administration, the time of foaling is predictable and attendants can be present. This technique has few disadvangages if used after 330 days of gestation. In 100 induced foalings, 90% occurred within 6 hrs of PG administration. In the remainder a second injection was successful (Van Schie, personal communication).

Induction of parturition

In pigs PG will induce luteolysis of corpora lutea of pregnancy. This can be used to induce parturition at the end of pregnancy. The average interval between injection and parturition is approximately 28 hrs. Many authors conclude that induction of parturition from day 111 of gestation or later does not adversely affect litter lize, litter weight at three weeks and litter survival compared with supervised spontaneous parturition. Induction of parturition in piggeries may be used on a larger scale as soon as a good method of oestrus synchronization becomes available. Administration of PG at day 111 of gestations will then shorten the range of gestation length, which normally is about 10 days, to about 4 days This is especially valuable when the " all in-all out" system is used (35).

Unproductive pregnancies

Prostaglandins can be used in cases of mismating or when sows are suspected to carry nummified foetuses caused by a SMEDI virus infection. Treated sows will abort within 24-48 hours and may exhibit oestrus 4 to 5 days later. Fertility at the second oestrus after treatment seems to be unaffected (8).

Concluding remarks

As demonstrated PG can be used for a wide range of veterinary needs pertaining to large farm animals. During the last two years PG's have been increasingly used for cattle and horses. For sheep and pigs their use is more limited. The treatments described in this article are only related to the reproductive field, however it is to be expected that in the future PG will also be used in other areas.

REFERENCES

1. Allen, W.R., Stewart, F., Cooper, M.J., Crowhurst, R.C., Simpson, D.J., McEnery, R.J., Greenwood, R.E.S., Rossdale, P.D., and Ricketts, S.W. (1974). Equine. Vet. J., 6: 31 - 35.

2. Allen, W.R. and Cooper, M.J. (1975). Ann. Biol. Anim. Biochem. Biophys., 15: 461.

3. Allison, A.J. (1978). N.Z. Vet. J., 26: 34 - 35.

4. Bielanski, A.B. (1978). Theriogenology, 10: 241 - 245.

5. Boland, M.P., Lemainque, F. and Gordon, I. (1978). J. Agric. Sci. Camb., 91: 765 - 766.

6. Bosu, W.T.K., Serna, J., Barker, C.A.V. (1978). Theriogenology. 9: 371 - 390.

7. Brand, A., de Bois, C.H.W., Kommery, R. and de Jong, M.P. (1975). Tijdschr. Diergeneesk., 100: 432 - 435.

8. Brand, A., Trounson, A.O. and Straver, G.M. (1976). Diergeneesk. Memorandum. 23: 163 - 178.

9. Brand, A., Aarts, M.H., Zaaijer, D. and Oxender W.D. (1978). In: Control of Reproduction in the Cow. Ed. J.M. Sreenan. p. 281 - 292.

10. Chupin, D. and Pelot, J. (1978). Theriogenology, 10: 307 - 312.

11. Chupin, D., Pelot, J. and Mauleon, P. (1978). In: Control of Reproduction in the cow. Ed. J.M. Sreenan. p. 546 - 561.

12. Cooper, M.J. (1974). Vet. Rec., 95: 200 - 203.

13. Cooper, M.J. and Jackson, P.S. (1975). Proc. 20th World Vet. Congress. Thessaloniki, 1: 371 - 372.

14. Day, A.M. (1979). N.Z. Vet. J., 27: 22 - 29.

15. Dobson, H., Cooper, M.J. and Furr, B.J.A. (1975). J. Reprod. Fert., 42: 141 - 144.

16. Douglas, R.H. and Ginther, O.J. (1972). Prostaglandins 2: 265.

17. Douglas, R.H. and Ginther, O.J. (1973). J. Anim. Sci., 37: 990 - 993.

18. Fairnie, I.J., Martin, E.R. and Rogers, S.C. (1978). Proc. Aust. Soc. Anim. Prod. 12: 256.

19. Gustafsson, B., Bäckström, G. and Edqvist, L.E. (1976). Theriogenology, 6: 45 - 50.

20. Haresign, W. and Acritopoulou, S.A. (1978). Livest. Prod. Sci., 5: 313 - 319.

21. Hearnshaw, H., Restall, B.J., Nancarrow, C.D. and Mattner, P.E. (1974). Proc. Aust. Soc. Anim. Prod., (1) 242 - 245.

22. Henricks, D.M., Rawlings, N.C., Ellicott, A.R., Dickey, J.F. and Hill, J.R. (1977). J. Anim. Sci., 44: 438 - 441.

23. Jackson, P.S. (1977). Vet. Rec., 101: 441 - 443.

24. Kalis, C.H.J. and Dieleman S.J. (1978). In: Control of Reproduction in the cow. Ed. J.M. Sreenan. p. 596 - 605.

25. Kessler, D.J., Garverick, H.A., Caudle, A.B. Bierschwal, C.J., Elmore, R.G.
    and Youngquist R.S. (1978). J. Anim. Sci., 46: 719 - 725.

26. de Kruif, A. and Brand, A. (1976). Tijdschr. Diergeneesk. 101: 491 - 493.

27. de Kruif, A. (1977). Tijdschr. Diergeneesk. 102: 247 - 253.

28. de Kruif, A., van der Wielen, N.J.G.J., Brand, A. and Dieleman, S.J. (1977).
    Tijdschr. Diergeneesk. 102: 851 - 856.

29. Macmillan, K.L. (1978). N.Z. Vet. J., 26: 104 - 108.

30. Miller, P.A., Lauderdale, J.W. and Geng, S. (1976). J.Anim. Sci. 42: 901.

31. Nett, T.M., Pickett, B.W. and Squires, E.L. (1979). J. Anim. Sci., 48: 69 - 75.

32. Roche, J.F. (1977). Vet. Sci. Commum. 1: 121 - 129.

33. Rowson, L.E.A., Tervit, R. and Brand, A. (1972). J. Reprod. Fert., 29: 145.

34. Trounson, A.O., Brand, A. and Straver, G.M. (1976). Diergeneesk. Memorandum,
    23: 141 - 161.

35. Willemse, A.H., Taverne, M.A.M., Roppe, L.J.J.A. and Adams, W.M. (1979).
    The Vet. Quarterly, 1: 145 - 149.

242

MODE OF ACTION OF PYRETHROIDS

Joep VAN DEN BERCKEN

Department of Veterinary Pharmacology and Toxicology, Utrecht University, Utrecht
(The Netherlands)

ABSTRACT

   The principal action of pyrethroids in the vertebrate peripheral nervous system
is to induce repetitive activity, notably in sense organs and, for some pyrethroids,
also in sensory nerve fibres and in motor nerve endings. The repetitive activity is
entirely caused by a prolongation of the membrane sodium current, brought about by
a delay in the closing of sodium channels by these insecticides. It is concluded
that the sodium channel in the nerve membrane is one of the most important target
sites of pyrethroids.

INTRODUCTION

   In the past decade great progress has been made, notably by Elliott and co-
workers (6,7), in the development of highly active and stable synthetic pyrethroids,
based on the structure of the naturally occurring pyrethrins. These modern
pyrethroids combine excellent insecticidal activity with remarkably low oral
toxicity to mammals. Further, unlike the organochlorines, pyrethroids are rapidly
metabolized in mammals and, as far as we know, they leave no persistent residues in
the environment. Because of these favourable porperties, more widespread application
of pyrethroids in the near future, e.g. for vector control and against ectoparasites
can be expected.

   Like the other major classes of insecticides, pyrethroids act primarily on the
nervous system, both in insects and in higher animals, and symptoms of poisoning
usually include hyperexcitation, tremors and convulsions, eventually followed by
death. So far, however, inhibition of a specific enzyme system, - like cholinesteras
inhibition by organophosphates and carbamates -, or other biochemical mode of
action of pyrethroids has not been established. The available evidence indicates
that pyrethroids act directly on excitable membranes and interfere with the changes
in ionic permeability of the membrane that underly the generation and conduction
of the nervous impulse.

   This brief paper is restricted to the effects of pyrethroids on the vertebrate nervous system. For additional information the reader is referred to a recent review by Wouters and van den Bercken (16).

EFFECTS ON THE PERIPHERAL NERVOUS SYSTEM

Most experimental work on the effects of pyrethroids on the peripheral nervous system has been carried out on isolated preparations of the frog. Structural formulas of some pyrethroids presently under investigation in our laboratory are depicted in Fig. 1.

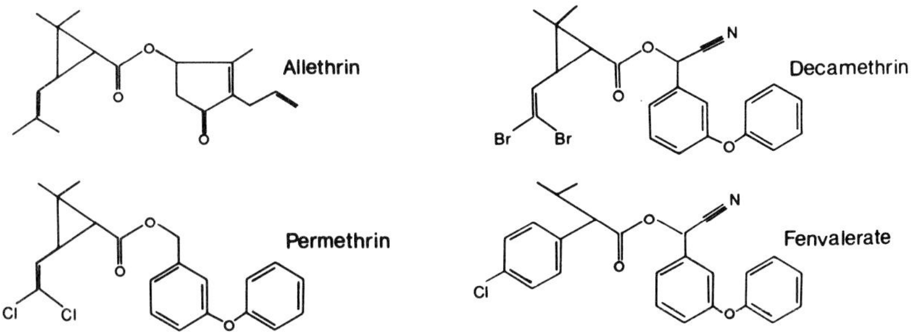

Fig. 1. Structural formulas of allethrin and of three recently synthetized pyrethroids

After exposure of excised frog nerves to allethrin, one of the early synthetic pyrethroids, the compound action potential of a sensory nerve branch was followed by pronounced repetitive activity (Fig. 2A), whereas motor nerve branches showed no or only slight repetitive activity, even after higher concentrations of allethrin (3). Permethrin, the first photostable pyrethroid, caused very similar repetitive activity in frog nerves, and as with allethrin this repetitive activity occurred in sensory fibres only (14). This difference in repetitive response between sensory and motor fibres on treatment with pyrethroids can be accounted for by differences in rate of recovery from sodium inactivation (4,16). On the other hand, decamethrin, the most active pyrethroid presently known, failed to induce repetitive activity in isolated frog nerve fibres (13). Preliminary experiments indicated that fenvalerate, a pyrethroid which lacks the classical cyclopropane ring (see Fig. 1), also failed to cause marked repetitive activity in frog nerves (14).

Sense organs appeared to be particularly sensitive to pyrethroids. Treatment with allethrin caused the cutaneous touch receptor of the frog to produce a train of impulses in response to a brief mechanical stimulus, instead of a single impulse, as illustrated in Fig. 2B (1). Allethrin also induced pronounced repetitive activity in the lateral-line organ of the clawed frog (3). The single impulses which occur spontaneously in this sense organ were all converted to trains of impulses (Fig. 2C).

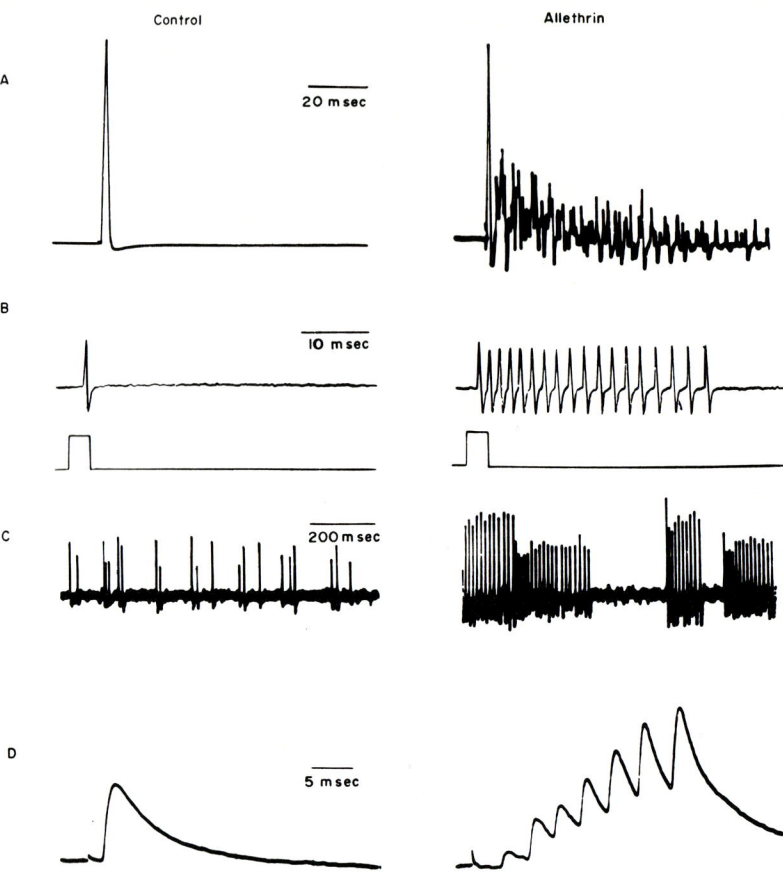

Control   Allethrin

A

20 m sec

B

10 m sec

C

200 m sec

D

5 m sec

Fig. 2. Repetitive activity induced by allethrin in various parts of the peripheral nervous system of the frog. Left hand traces; control. Right hand traces; after treatment with allethrin. (A) Compound action potential of a sensory nerve branch (ramus cutaneous cruris posterior) before and 40 min after exposure to 3.3×10^{-7}M allethrin. (B) Response of a cutaneous touch receptor to a brief mechanical stimulus (lower trace) before and 30 min after exposure to 1×10^{-5}M allethrin. (C) Spontaneous activity from a single lateral-line organ before and 60 min after exposure to 1×10^{-5}M allethrin. (D) Intracellularly recorded end-plate potentials of the sartorius muscle evoked by a single stimulus to the motor nerve before and 30 min after exposure to 1×10^{-6}M allethrin. (From Wouters & van den Bercken (16), with permission of Pergamon Press Ltd).

Further experimentation revealed that the allethrin-induced repetitive activity originated in the afferent nerve endings, possibly at the site of impulse generation. Very similar repetitive activity was observed after exposure of the lateral-line preparation to permethrin (14). Interestingly, decamethrin as well as fenvalerate, which both did not cause repetitive activity in nerve fibres, induced intense repetitive activity in the lateral-line organ (14). After treatment with these pyrethroids spontaneous trains of impulses which lasted for 10 sec or more were observed.

The effects of allethrin on synaptic transmission have been studied in the frog nerve-muscle preparation by means of intracellular micro-electrodes (17). Despite the absence of repetitive activity in allethrin-treated motor nerve fibres mentioned above, this pyrethroid caused marked repetitive firing of the presynaptic nerve endings resulting in trains of postsynaptic (end-plate) potentials in response to a single stimulus (Fig. 2D). By recording activity along the whole nerve innervating the muscle, it was demonstrated that the repetitive activity arose in the very fine intramuscular nerve branches. Apparently, motor nerve endings, like sensory nerve endings, are more susceptible to the induction of repetitive activity by pyrethroids than the more proximal parts of the nerve fibres. A significant effect of allethrin on transmitter release or on the postsynaptic membrane was not observed. Similar results have been obtained by Evans (8) in the frog nerve-muscle preparation treated with cismethrin.

Recently, Carlton (5) has reported that in the rabbit i.v. injection of cismethrin caused repetitive activity in skin sensory receptors as well as repetitive firing of the sural nerve. An increase in spontaneous afferent nerve activity was also observed.

These results show that the principal action of pyrethroids in the vertebrate peripheral nervous system is to induce repetitive activity, notably in sense organs and, for some pyrethroids, also in sensory nerve fibres and in motor nerve endings. This repetitive activity will no doubt play an important role in the development of symptoms of poisoning by pyrethroids.

EFFECTS ON THE CENTRAL NERVOUS SYSTEM

At the moment there is very little information on the effects of pyrethroids on the central nervous system. Since the mechanisms responsible for impulse generation and conduction are basically the same throughout the entire nervous system, it is conceivable that pyrethroids will cause similar repetitive activity in the central nervous system as was observed in the peripheral nervous system.

In the rabbit it was found that cismethrin caused an increase in spinal reflex activity which was mainly due to repetitive firing of afferent nerve fibres (5). An additional, direct effect of cismethrin on intraspinal structures could, however, not be excluded. Very recently, Ray and Cremer (12) have reported generalized spiking and evoked spike discharges in the EEG of decamethrin-poisoned rats. According to these authors the effects of this pyrethroid were suggestive of an action mediated via the basal ganglia. It seems likely, however, that the intense repetitive activity caused by decamethrin in the peripheral nervous system will contribute significantly to the effects observed in the brain of intact animals. The convulsions induced by cismethrin and decamethrin in the rat were found to be associated with a marked increase in c-GMP content of the brain, particularly in the cerebellum, without affecting c-AMP (2). Since the insecticide DDT as well as other convulsive poisons also produce an increase in the brain levels of c-GMP, this effect is probably a secondary one.

EFFECTS ON MEMBRANE IONIC CONDUCTANCES

Experiments with single myelinated frog nerve fibres showed that after treatment with allethrin the action potential was followed by a large depolarizing afterpotential upon which the repetitive action potentials were superimposed (H.P.M. Vijverberg, unpublished observations). Decamethrin caused a small but long-lasting depolarizing afterpotential, without repetitive activity (13).

A nerve action potential is brought about by a transient increase in sodium permeability, or conductance, of the membrane resulting in a brief inward flow of sodium ions, followed by an increase in potassium conductance leading to an outflow of potassium ions (see Fig. 3). These voltage dependent ionic currents through the nerve membrane, which are mediated by specialized molecular structures called sodium and potassium channels, can be studied in detail by a method known as the voltage clamp technique. Application of this technique to single myelinated frog nerve fibres revealed that allethrin as well as decamethrin caused a substantial prolongation of the sodium current associated with depolarization of the membrane (13, 15). After decamethrin, however, the sodium current was prolonged to a much greater extent than after allethrin, although its amplitude was significantly smaller. Further experimentation showed that the prolongation of the sodium current by allethrin may be explained by a delay in the closing of sodium channels on repolarization of the membrane (15).

The prolongation of the membrane sodium current by pyrethroids is directly responsible for the depolarizing afterpotential following the action potential and for the induction of repetitive activity in various parts of the peripheral nervous system described above (4,16). Fig. 3 shows the time courses of the action potential, the sodium conductance and the potassium conductance of the nerve membrane before and after application of pyrethroid. The amplitude of the prolonged sodium current after decamethrin is apparently too small to cause repetitive firing in nerve fibres, but sufficient to induce intense repetitive activity in the lateral-line sense organ.

Pyrethroids are known to induce pronounced repetitive activity in excitable membranes of insects and other invertebrates which is also primarily due to a prolongation of the membrane sodium current (see ref. 11,16). Thus it can be concluded that in the nervous system of vertebrates as well as invertebrates the sodium channel in the nerve membrane is one of the most important target sites of pyrethroids.

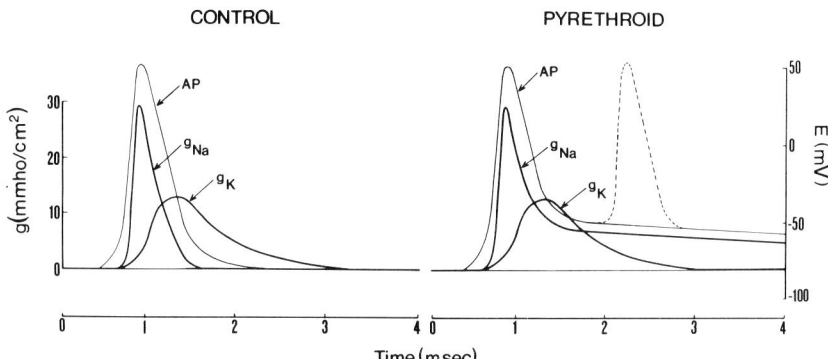

Fig. 3. Schematic drawing of the time courses of the nerve action potential (AP),
the membrane sodium conductance (g_{Na}), and the membrane potassium conductance (g_K) before and after application of pyrethroid. The occurrence of
a repetitive action potential superimposed on the large depolarizing
afterpotential is indicated. (After Hodgkin & Huxley (9) and Narahashi
(10)).

A last point worth mentioning is the striking similarity between the effects
of the insecticide DDT and those of pyrethroids (3,4,16). DDT also causes a
prolongation of membrane sodium current resulting in marked repetitive activity
in various parts of the vertebrate and invertebrate nervous system. On the basis
of a detailed analysis of sodium current kinetics in frog myelinated nerve fibres
it has been proposed that DDT, allethrin and probably other pyrethroids share a
common mechanism of action on the sodium channels in the nerve membrane (15).

REFERENCES

1. Akkermans, L.M.A., van den Bercken, J. and Versluijs-Helder, M.(1975),
   Pestic. Biochem. Physiol., 5: 451-457
2. Aldridge, W.N., Clothier, B., Forshaw, P., Johnson, M.K., Parker, V.H.,
   Price, R.J., Skilleter, D.N., Verschoyle, R.D. and Stevens, C. (1978),
   Biochem. Pharmacol., 27: 1703-1706
3. Bercken, J., van den, Akkermans, L.M.A. and van der Zalm, J.M. (1973),
   Eur. J. Pharmacol., 21: 95-106
4. Bercken, J., van den, Kroese, A.B.A. and Akkermans, L.M.A. (1979) in:
   Neurotoxicology of Insecticides and Pheromones, ed. T. Narahashi,
   Plenum Publishing Corporation, 183-210
5. Carlton, M. (1977), Pestic. Sci., 8: 700-712
6. Elliott, M. (1977), in: Synthetic Pyrethroids, ACS Symposium Series,
   ed. M. Elliott, ACS Washington, D.C., 42, 1-28
7. Elliott, M. and Janes, N.F. (1978), Chem. Soc. Rev., 7: 473-505
8. Evans, M.H. (1976), Pestic. Biochem. Physiol., 6: 547-550
9. Hodgkin, A.L. and Huxley, A.F. (1952), J. Physiol. 117: 500-544
10. Narahashi, T. (1971), Bull. Wld Hlth Org. 44: 337-345

11. Narahashi, T. (1976) in: Insecticide Biochemistry and Physiology, ed.
    C.F. Wilkinson, Plenum Press, New York, 327-352
12. Ray, D.E. and Cremer, J.E. (1979), Pestic. Biochem. Physiol., 10: 333-340
13. Vijverberg, H.P.M. and van den Bercken, J. (1979), Eur. J. Pharmacol., in
    the press
14. Vijverberg, H.P.M. and van den Bercken, J., in preparation
15. Vijverberg, H.P.M., van der Zalm, J.M. and van den Bercken, J., in preparation
16. Wouters, W. and van den Bercken, J. (1978), Gen. Pharmacol., 9: 387-398
17. Wouters, W., van den Bercken, J. and van Ginneken, A. (1977), Eur. J. Pharmacol.
    43: 163-171

THE TOXICITY OF SYNTHETIC PYRETHROIDS TO MAMMALS

J.A. JAMES BVetMed, MRCVS
Wellcome Research Laboratories, Berkhamsted Hill, Berkhamsted, Herts.

ABSTRACT

The toxicity of the synthetic pyrethroids and natural pyrethrins to animals is reviewed.

The toxicity varies with the vehicle used, the isomer content and the route of administration of the compounds.   As a class, synthetic pyrethroids appear to be particularly safe.

The cat is the most sensitive of the species commonly used in toxicological testing while sheep and cattle are relatively insensitive.

BACKGROUND

Before considering the toxicity of the synthetic pyrethroids it is relevant to review briefly toxicity of the "natural" pyrethrins.

Pyrethrins

The quoted toxicity of natural pyrethrins has varied considerably, which is understandable because of the variety of mixtures of pyrethrins, levels of resinous contaminants and solvents used.

In general the acute LD50 result for the rat has been between 500 and 1500 mg/kg with results of 200 mg/kg and greater than 2600 mg/kg being reported.

Grade of Pyrethrum	Diluent	Py.Content % w/v	Sex	Species	LD50	Conf. Limits	Ref.
PD	Neat	20.3	–	Rat	794.3	604–1045	1
PALE	Neat	20.9	–	Rat	584.3	481–710	1
OR	Neat	27.2	–	Rat	634.0	495–812	1
OR	OPD	20.0	–	Rat	584.3	452–755	1
NP	Neat	77.8	–	Rat	900.0	733–1106	1
Pyrethrin I	DMSO	–	M	Rat	260–420	–	2
Pyrethrin II	DMSO	–	M	Rat	>600	–	2
PALE	Neat	–	–	Rat	710	–	3
OR	OPD	–	–	Rat	820	–	3
PD	PO	–	–	Rat	1870	–	3
OR	PO	–	–	Rat	200	–	3
OR	PO	–	–	Rat	>1500	–	3
OR	PO	–	–	Rat	>2600	–	3
NP	GF	–	F.	Rat	>1400	–	2

Acute dermal toxicity has been studied in the rat and rabbit and in most instances less than 50% kill has been achieved even at the highest levels applied which are up to 5400 mg/kg.

DERMAL LD50 mg/kg

Grade of Pyrethrum	Diluent	Py.Content	Species	LD50	Conf. Limits	Ref.
PD	Neat	20.3	Rabbit	>5000	–	1
PALE	Neat	20.9	Rabbit	>5000	–	1
OR	OPD	20.0	Rabbit	>5000	–	1
NP	Neat	77.8	Rabbit	>19800	–	1
NI	OPD	18.0	Rabbit	>4500	–	1
OR	OPD	20	Rabbit	2060	1100–3680	1
OR	OPD	20		>3160		1
PD	Neat	20.3	Rat	>1500	–	1
PALE	Neat	20.9	Rat	>1500	–	1
OR	OPD	20.0	Rat	>1500	–	1
NP	Neat	77.8	Rat	>5400	–	1
NP	OPD	18.0	Rat	>1350	–	1
OR	OPD	–	Rat	>1800	–	3

There are several early chronic toxicity studies reported with pyrethrins, but by modern standards some of these studies are not adequate.

In the two year rat study there were effects at 5000 ppm but the no effect level is variable in that either 200 or 1000 ppm is quoted.

Limited mutagenicity and teratogenicity data suggests no effects in these studies.

PYRETHRUM CHRONIC TOXICITY

Species	Duration	Dose Route	Result	Ref.
Rat	5 weeks	In diet	8000 ppm few prominent Peyers patches.	3
Rat	13 weeks	Oral	360 mg/kg/day, marked reduction in bodyweight. Liver eosinophilia with early cell necrosis, kidney tubular degeneration.	11
Rat	2 year	In diet	No effect level 200 ppm. Liver bile duct proliferation and focal necrosis at high doses.	9
Dog	13 weeks	In diet	Dose level 5000 ppm. Tremors, ataxia, laboured respiration, salivation mainly in the first month. Slight vacuolation of liver.	3

Isomer Effects

The effect of different isomer ratios with NRDC 143 on the female rat
acute oral toxicity is shown below.

Variable Cis/Trans Ratio – Using 40% Corn Oil Formulations

% cis content	% trans content	Dose range mg/kg	MTD mg/kg	MLD mg/kg	LD50 mg/kg	95% Conf. Limits
80	20	100 – 400	<100	200	224.3	200 – 252
60	40	177 – 707	<177	>353 <500	445.3	397 – 500
50	50	250 – 2000	<250	>500 <1000	1000	733 – 1363
40	60	250 – 4000	>250 <500	>500 <1000	1260	1000 – 1587
30	70	750 – 6000	<750	>750 <1500	1684	1257 – 2255
20	80	3000 – 6000	<3000	>3000 <6000	6000	Maximum volume

The following acute oral LD50 results were reported for mice:

Compound	Species	Sex	Vehicle	Result	Ref.
+ Trans (NRDC143)	Mouse	M	Corn oil	3100	13
– Trans (")	Mouse	M	Corn oil	>5000	13
+ Cis (")	Mouse	M	Corn oil	107	13
– Cis (")	Mouse	M	Corn oil	>5000	13
40/60 ± cis/trans	Mouse	M	Corn oil	490 mg/kg	13

On the basis of these results it is clear that the higher the cis content
the greater the toxicity, both in terms of symptoms and mortality. The toxicity
varies with the amount of cis isomer present, although the variation is not
linear.

This variation also exists in the chronic toxicity tests, for example in the
90 day rat feeding studies, 25:75 dl cis trans isomer ratio material produced a
no effect level of 2000 ppm and 40:60 material produced a no effect level of
600 ppm.

There is a certain amount of published toxicity data on the other
pyrethroids and this has been summarised in the following table.

PYRETHRUM TERATOGENICITY/REPRODUCTION

Species	Duration	Dose Route	Result	Ref.
Rat	2 litters	In diet	5000 ppm reduced bodyweight, no other visible effect.	3
Rabbit	During gestation	Oral in corn oil	90 mg/kg/day, considered unlikely that pyrethrins would induce teratogenic effects in mammals.	3

PYRETHRUM MUTAGENICITY

E.Coli	Test		Non mutagenic	3

SYNTHETIC PYRETHROIDS

There are many synthetic pyrethroids that have insecticidal activity, and many of these have been examined by toxicologists. Unfortunately although they are synthetic, they are frequently not pure in that there are several isomers in each technical product. These isomers can have different toxicological properties, generally the cis isomers are more persistent and more toxic to to mammals than the trans isomers. There is also a variation with other factors of toxicity testing, forexample –

Vehicle effects

There may be a marked effect on toxicity according to the vehicle used, the following results were obtained for NRDC 143 permethrin with a dl cis trans ratio of 25:75.

Acute Rat Oral Toxicity (Female Rats)

Formulation	No. of rats/ group	Dose Range mg/kg	MTD mg/kg	MLD mg/kg	LD50 mg/kg	95% Conf.Limits
110%wv Neat	6	2009–20090	<2009	20090	>20090	Maximum volume
40%wv corn oil	6	2009–8000	<2009	3185	4672	3614–6040
40%wv OPD	6	1268–8000	>1268 <2009	8000	>8000	Maximum volume
40%wv DMSO	6	2009–8000	<2009	5048	>8000	Maximum volume
20%wv glycerol formal	6	1268–5048	<1268	3188	>5048	Maximum volume

TOXICITY OF OTHER PYRETHROIDS

Acute oral LD50 mg/kg

Compound	Species	Sex	Vehicle	Result	Ref.
Allethrin	Mouse	–	Kerosene	480	5
Allethrin	Rat	–	Kerosene	920	5
Allethrin	Mouse	M	Corn oil	500	13
Allethrin	Rat	M	Corn oil	2430	13
Allethrin	Rat	F	Corn oil	720	13
Bioallethrin	Rat	F	Glycerol formal	1030	2
Resmethrin	Mouse	F	PEG	>3200	WRL
Resmethrin	Rat	F	PEG	>3000	WRL
Resmethrin	Rat	F	DMSO	1347	2
Resmethrin	Rat	F	PEG 400	1995	2
Resmethrin	Mouse	M	Corn oil	690	13
Resmethrin	Rat	M	Corn oil	>5000	13
Bioresmethrin	Rat	–	–	>8000	10
Fenothrin	Mouse	M	Corn oil	>5000	13
Fenothrin	Rat	M	Neat	>10000	13
Decamethrin	Rat	M	Peanut oil	52	14
Decamethrin	Rat	F	Peanut oil	31	14
Decamethrin	Rat	F	Arachis oil	40	15
Tetramethrin	Mouse	M	Corn oil	1920	13
Tetramethrin	Rat	M	Corn oil	>5000	13

From these results the mouse is generally more susceptible than the rat.

The results quoted so far relate to laboratory animals, data on toxicity to non laboratory animals of veterinary concern is not as freely available if indeed the work has been done with the majority of these compounds. The following results have been obtained with NRDC 143 25/75 cis:trans

Species	Trial	Route	Vehicle	Result
Sheep	Acute tox.	Intravenous	Corn oil	300 mg/kg minor effects only
Sheep	Acute tox.	Abomasal	Corn oil	800 mg/kg no toxicity
Sheep	Acute tox.	Ruminal	Corn oil	800 mg/kg minor effects only
Cattle	Acute tox.	Ruminal	Corn oil	400 mg/kg tremors/ataxia 800 mg/kg lethal
Cattle	Acute tox.	Abomasal	Corn oil	800 mg/kg no toxicity
Cattle	Acute tox.	Oral	−	1-2 week calves < 1g/kg no toxicity
Dog	Acute tox.	Intravenous	Corn oil	400 mg/kg lethal
Dog	Acute tox.	Intravenous	Corn oil	200 mg/kg no effect
Dog	Acute tox.	Oral	Corn oil	1600 mg/kg no effect
Dog	Sub acute	Oral	Neat	14 days 500 mg/kg no effect
Dog	Sub chronic	Oral	Neat	6 months 250 mg/kg no effect
Cat	Acute tox.	Oral	Corn oil	200 mg/kg lethal

From these results it can been seen that the intravenous toxicity is a hundred times less than for pyrethrins, where doses of 3 to 5 mg/kg are lethal. With sheep and cattle a dose given by the ruminal route is more toxic than by the abomasal route.

Cats are especially sensitive to the synthetic pyrethroids, but this same sensitivity is seen with other classes of compound for example the chlorinated hydrocarbons, DDT or Lindane.

No reference has been made to irritation. Some of the synthetic pyrethroids produce marked irritation especially at high concentrations, others including permethrin are virtually non irritant.

Also no reference has been made to the activity/toxicity relationships, for example Decamethrin is more toxic than many of the other synthetic pyrethroids but it is also more active in certain areas of use, and is thus used at lower concentrations, so the relative safety margin is higher than is at first apparent from the toxicity data.

These facts highlight the problem that toxicity must be reviewed practically with a view to the real risks involved. If the concern is for direct contact or ingestion of the compound by man, then the formulation, concentration and possible routes of absorption are of vital concern, and not just the theoretical toxicity of the technical material.

Similarly, if the concern is for residues and their ingestion by man, then the actual residue levels and their persistence in tissues and ingested materials, must be considered directly, together with an evaluation of chronic toxicity.

254

REFERENCES   Ref.

Toxicity of Various Grades of Pyrethrum to Laboratory Animals   1
J.C. Malone and N.C. Brown
Pyrethrum Post, 9, (3) 3-8, 1968

Toxicity of Natural and Synthetic Pyrethrins to Rats   2
R.D. Verschoyle and J.M. Barnes
Pesticide Biochemistry and Physiology, 2, 308-311, 1972

Mammalian Toxicology of Pyrethrum   3
C.S. Griffin
Pyrethrum Post, Vol.12, No.2, Oct. 1973 50-58

Organic Insecticides   4
Robert L. Metcalf
Interscience Publishers Inc.

Handbook of Toxicology   5
Volume III, National Academy of Sciences, National Research Council
W.B. Saunders Company

The Acute Toxicity of Pesticides to Rats   6
Thomas B. Gaines
Toxicology and Applied Pharmacology, 2, 88-99, 1960

Acute Toxicity Data for Pesticides   7
R. Ben-Dyke, D.M. Sanderson and Diana N. Noakes

Acute Toxicity of Pesticides   8
Thomas B. Gaines
Toxicology and Applied Pharmacology, 14, 515-534, 1969

Toxicological Decisions and Recommendations Resulting from the Safety   9
Assessment of Pesticide Residue in Food
G. Vettorazzi
CRC Critical Reviews in Toxicology, Nov. 1975

A Photostable Pyrethroid   10
M.Elliot, A.W. Farnham, N.F. Janes, P.H. Needham, D.A. Pulman, J.H.Stevenson
Nature, Vol. 246, Nov. 16, 1973, 169-170

The Oral Toxicity of Pyrethrum, Alone and Combined with Synergists and   11
Common Drugs, and Pathological Effects Produced
H. Bond, K. Mauger and J.J. Defeo
Pyrethrum Post, Vol. 12, No. 2, October 1973, 58-63

Pyrethrum The Natural Insecticide   12
John E. Casida
Academic Press 1973

Degradation, Metabolism and Toxicity of Synthetic Pyrethroids   13
Junshi Miyamoto
Environmental Health Perpectives, Vol. 14, 15-28, 1976

KEY TO TABLES

GF	Glycerol Formal
PO	Petroleum Oil
OR	Pyrethrum Oleoresin
NP	Nitromethane Concentrate of Pyrethrins
OPD	Odourless Petroleum Distillate
PD	Partially Dewaxed Oleoresin
Pale	Pale Extract
DMSO	Dimethylsulphoxide
MTD	Minimum Toxic Dose
MLD	Minimum Lethal Dose

PYRETHROIDS, THEIR USE IN THE CONTROL OF ANIMAL ECTOPARASITES

H.D. BAILIE AND J.C. WOOD
Wellcome Research Laboratories, Berkhamsted Hill, Berkhamsted,
Hertfordshire, HP4 2QE, England

ABSTRACT

Four recently discovered photostable synthetic pyrethroids,
permethrin ((NRDC 143) 3-phenoxybenzyl (+) cis, trans -2,2 dimethyl-
3-(2,2-dichlorovinyl)cyclopropane-1-carboxylate); cypermethrin
((NRDC 149) (R,S)- α -cyano-3-phenoxybenzyl (IR,IS)-cis, trans-3-(2,
2-dichlorovinyl)-2,2-dimethylcyclopropane-carboxylate); decamethrin
((NRDC 161) S- α -cyano-m-phenoxybenzyl (IR, 3R)-3-(2,2-dibromovinyl)
-2,2-dimethyl-cyclopropane carboxylate); and fenvalerate (α -cyano-
3-phenoxybenzyl- α -isopropyl-p-chlorophenylacetate) have shown
considerable activity against a number of ectoparasites of animals.
They are likely to provide important alternatives to the present
ectoparasiticides used in veterinary medicine.

Ideally, a veterinary ectoparasiticide should have a high
toxicity to the ectoparasite, low mammalian and avian toxicity,
with low meat, milk and egg residues. For more than a century
natural pyrethrins, extracted from pyrethrum flowers, have been
used as insecticides. These compounds have excellent insecticidal
activity with low mammalian toxicity, but, unfortunately, are not
stable when exposed to light. As a result they have had little
veterinary use because of the cost of the frequent applications
which would be necessary.

A number of synthetic analogues of these natural pyrethrins have
been produced and are known as pyrethroids. The early synthetic
pyrethroids, e.g. resmethrin, bioresmethrin, had greater insecticidal
activity than the natural pyrethrins, but also were not stable in
light. Therefore, as far as veterinary ectoparasites are concerned,
organochlorines, organophosphates and carbamates were relied upon
to achieve control. Within the last few years the

discovery of synthetic pyrethroids, which are relatively stable
when exposed to sunlight, has provided alternatives to these
compounds. Of the photostable synthetic pyrethroids, four have
received most attention as potential veterinary ectoparasiticides.
These are permethrin ((NRDC 143) 3-phenoxybenzyl ($\pm$) cis, trans
-2,2 dimethyl-3-(2,2-dichlorovinyl)cyclopropane-1-carboxylate);
cypermethrin ((NRDC 149) (R,S)-α-cyano-3-phenoxybenzyl (IR,IS)-
cis, trans-3-(2,2-dichlorovinyl-2,2-dimethylcyclopropane-carboxylate);
decamethrin ((NRDC 161) S-α-cyano-3-phenoxybenzyl (IR, 3R)-3-(2,
2-dibromovinyl)-2,2-dimethyl-cyclopropane carboxylate); and
fenvalerate (α-cyano-3-phenoxybenzyl-α-isopropyl-p-chlorophenyl-
acetate).

Some of these synthetic pyrethroids, under a variety of trade
names, are already in use for the control of veterinary ectoparasites.
Permethrin products may contain the compound in a 25:75 cis/trans
isomer ratio or a 40:60 cis/trans isomer ratio. Although changes
in the isomeric ratios of permethrin affect mammalian toxicity as
a previous speaker has explained, we have not found significant
differences in insecticidal or acaricidal activity. Only the
veterinary uses will be discussed here but it is important to note
that these photostable pyrethroids are useful for crop protection
and in industry.

The photostable pyrethroids have shown activity against most
veterinary ectoparasites, and while they are all active at low
concentrations, some show outstanding activity at very low
concentrations. Their wide range of activity can be illustrated
by considering their efficacy against the important veterinary
ectoparasites.

Ticks

Single and multi-host ticks are important ectoparasites in many
countries. Nolan et al (1977) reported that permethrin and
fenvalerate sprayed at 0.025% w/v gave over 98% and 96% control
respectively, and cypermethrin and decamethrin at 0.005% w/v gave
over 92% and 99% control respectively of a susceptible strain of
Boophilus microplus on artificially infested calves. Drummond and
Gladney (1978) reported that 0.025 - 0.1% w/v permethrin sprayed
onto cattle gave significant control of Amblyomma americanum for
two weeks after treatment. A comparative test of ear tags
impregnated with insecticide against the gulf coast tick,
Amblyomma maculatum, on cattle found that 8% fenvalerate tags were

at least as effective as 15% tetrachlorvinphos tags with adequate
residual effect for 11 weeks (Ahrens and Cocke, 1978). Cypermethrin
is recommended for the control of ticks on cattle at a field usage
concentration of 0.015% w/v.

Lice, keds and scab on sheep

Against the sheep biting louse, Damalinia ovis, cypermethrin has
given control at concentrations as low as 1 p.p.m. in a dip, and
concentrations of 5 and 10 p.p.m. showed a persistent effect and
prevented reinfestation for 7 and 19 weeks respectively (Hall, 1978).
Preliminary trials conducted by colleagues at the Wellcome Research
Laboratories, England, and overseas indicate that permethrin is
active against sheep lice and keds (Melophagus ovinus) and that
decamethrin is active against these parasites and also against the
sheep scab mite, Psoroptes ovis.

Flies

The control of flies on livestock has been of interest for many
years, both as an aid to management and in disease control.
Permethrin has an irritating and toxic effect on flies on cattle.
Depending on the fly challenge and weather conditions permethrin
has been shown to control biting flies, e.g. Stomoxys calcitrans
for around two weeks, and non-biting flies, e.g. Musca autumnalis
for one week. Against the horn fly (Haematobia irritans), which
remains feeding and resting on cattle for long periods, three to
four weeks' protection can be expected (Blackman & Hodson, 1977).
Cypermethrin is claimed to give control of biting flies on cattle
for four weeks, and control of non-biting flies for two weeks.
Similar periods of protection with cypermethrin against flies on
horses is claimed. Both compounds are applied to cattle at the
rate of 500 ml 0.1% w/v per animal.

Permethrin is now widely used for the control of flies in
buildings by spraying surfaces with the insecticide. Protection
against flies in buildings can be achieved for four to twelve
weeks with application rates of 25 - 125 mg/m^2. Recent trials with
decamethrin indicate that this compound is also effective in fly

control when applied to buildings. Permethrin when mixed in larval
media at 5 and 10 p.p.m., controlled first and second instar fly
larvae of Musca domestica. However, when fed in an encapsulated
formulation to hens it gave poor results (Townsend & Turner, 1977).

The synthetic pyrethroids do not appear to be good fly larvicides. Economic control of myiasis in sheep by <u>Lucilia</u> spp. is unlikely.

Application of the synthetic pyrethroids to cattle for the control of tsetse flies has given disappointing results. On the other hand, their application to the habitat has given very encouraging results. When tsetse flies (<u>Glossina austeni</u>) were exposed for one minute to plywood treated with permethrin at 500 mg/m^2 100% kill of flies exposed to the surface was still obtained twenty weeks after treatment. Permethrin applied at 50 mg/m^2 to tree bark in a similar test gave 63% mortality 48 hours afterwards, while decamethrin at 10 mg/m^2 continued to give 100% mortality sixteen weeks after application. By comparison, endosulphan and dieldrin at 50 mg/m^2 showed no activity one week after application (Barlow <u>et al</u>, 1977).

Although some systemic activity has been suggested with decamethrin (Schmidt & Matter, 1978) this has not been demonstrated with the other photostable pyrethroids.

Mites

In poultry houses, though the main use of the photostable pyrethroids is likely to be the control of flies, permethrin applied to the buildings is recommended in the U.K. for the control of poultry red mites (<u>Dermanyssus gallinae</u>) at an application rate of 0.1%.

Permethrin sprayed on to poultry at concentrations of 0.125 - 0.5% w/v cleared them of northern fowl mites, <u>Ornithonyssus sylviarum</u>, during the post-test examination period of 77 days. Cypermethrin used at 0.05 - 0.0125% w/v afforded excellent mite control also for a period of not less than 57 days post-treatment. In comparison, carbaryl applied at 0.5% gave similar results (Hall <u>et al</u>, 1978).

Fleas

In dogs and cats, preliminary trials with permethrin and decamethrin have indicated that both compounds have high activity against fleas. With the apparent increase of this parasite in many countries, these compounds could become important in small animal veterinary medicine, particularly when incorporated in plastic collars in which the compound remains effective for several months.

The above examples of activity are not intended to be a comprehensive survey, but are used to illustrate the wide range of insecticidal and acaricidal activity of these compounds.

This range of activity provides an important alternative to the present organochlorines, organophosphates and carbamates, for the future control of veterinary ectoparasites.

Acknowledgements

The authors would like to express their thanks to colleagues at the Wellcome Research Laboratories who provided information on current trials.

References

Ahrens, E.H. and Cocke, J. (1978)
Journal of Economic Entomology, 71, (5) 764-765

Barlow, F., Hadaway, A.B., Flower, L.S., Grose, J.E.H. and Turner, C.R. (1977)
Pesticide Science, 8, 291-300

Blackman, G.G. and Hodson, M.J. (1977)
Pesticide Science, 8, 270-273

Drummond, R.O. and Gladney, W.J. (1978)
The Southwestern Entomologist, 3, (2) 184-189

Hall, C.A. (1978)
Australian Veterinary Journal, 54, 471-472

Hall, R.D., Townsend, L.H. Jr., and Turner, E.C. (1978)
Journal of Economic Entomology, 71, (2) 315-318

Nolan, J., Roulston, W.J. and Wharton, R.H. (1977)
Pesticide Science, 8, 484-486

Schmidt, C.D., and Matter, J.J. (1978)
The Southwestern Entomologist, 3, (2) 133-136

Townsend, L.H. Jr., and Turner, E.C. (1977)
Journal of the New York Entomological Society, 85, (4) 203-204

GENERAL ASPECTS OF FUNGI AND MYCOTIC INFECTIONS

K.H. BÖHM

Institut für Mikrobiologie und Tierseuchen der Tierärztlichen Hochschule Hannover

ABSTRACT

Following brief remarks on the systematics and natural occurrence of fungi, their rôle as causal organisms of infectious diseases is described.

Fungi also cause various other types of damage. Brief comments are made on the usefulness of fungi.

Fungi and mycotic infections

This is a very large field. I shall try to give a survey in a very compressed form.

The systematics of fungi

Traditionally the plant kingdom has been classified into four divisions : Spermatophyta (seed-plants); Pteridophyta (ferns and fern allies); Bryophyta (mosses and liverworts); and Thallophyta (algae and fungi).

Since the end of the last decade taxonomists no longer consider the fungi to be plants. A special Kingdom, Fungi, has been created with some 100,000 species. The division II of this new Kingdom is the Eumycota, the so-called true fungi. Its subdivisions include the yeasts, the dermatophytes, the moulds and the so-called diphasic fungi. These four expressions represent a practical classification, which is very useful for medical and veterinary purposes, but which does not agree with the systematic classification, which is based on botanical criteria. For the botanist the presence or absence of sexual reproduction of an organism is one of the deciding points.

The morphology and physiology of fungi cannot be treated in this lecture.

Natural occurrence of fungi

Fungi have a world-wide distribution. They occur in fluid media, and in moist but also in relatively dry environments. Fungi can be found in soil, in water, on the surface and in the interior of plants, on products of plant origin, on human food and foodstuffs, on animals – from insects up to mammals, including human beings – not only on the skin and on superficial mucous membranes, but also in their internal organs. Spores of fungi are present in the air, in our homes and to heal. Therapy should always be carried out, firstly to shorten the course of the disease and secondly to prevent spore dispersal.

C) <u>Moulds and other fungi</u>

Moulds like members of the genera *Aspergillus*, *Penicillium* and *Mucor* may cause: pneumomycosis in men and poultry, abortion in ruminants and mares, intestinal and subcutaneous infections, etc.

Other fungi, some of them related to moulds, are responsible for diverse diseases of fishes, crustaceans, insects and plants.

D) <u>Diphasic Fungi</u>

Some fungi grow at + 37°C (e.g. yeasts) and at room temperature (e.g. moulds with an air mycelium). The causative agents of histoplasmosis, blastomycosis, sporothrichosis, coccidioidomycosis and chromomycosis belong to the diphasic fungi.

<u>Diagnosis</u>

Diagnosis cannot normally be established without special mycological methods. These include: special stainings for histological examination; Woods-lamp; potassium hydroxide preparations for microscopic examination; culture followed by identification of the isolated fungi; fluorescence microscopy; other serological techniques (agglutination, KBR, etc.); allergic tests.

Only in some rare cases can the diagnosis be made on the basis of clinical examination alone, for example in trichophytosis of cattle.

<u>Specific therapy against fungal infections.</u>

Many preparations are available for local treatment of mycoses. They contain different components such as compounds of phenol, salicilic acid, benzoic acid, mercury, aliphatic carbonic acids, etc. Most of them cannot compete with the modern antimycotica such as Nystatin, Pimaricin and Tolnaftat. These are real antimycotica, i.e. they are not only effective in vitro, but also in vivo. They penetrate the skin and underlying cells and remain for some time in the tissue.

Modern antimycotica with systemic efficacy are Amphotericin B, 5-Fluorcytosin, Griseofulvin and the Imidazolyl-antimycotica Clotrimazol and Miconazol. The latter three are also efficient after local application.

<u>Fungal toxins</u>

Fungi as suppliers of toxins were very popular with the ancient Romans who, from time to time, solved their family and home affairs by means of *Amanita phalloides*, the green death cap.

More than 100 mycotoxins are produced from about 200 microscopic fungi, belonging to more than 20 genera e.g. *Aspergillus*, *Fusarium* and *Penicillium*. In 1951 in France several persons died after *Secale cornutum* poisoning.

Beside their toxic activity, it should be mentioned that fungi as allergens in stables - especially when mouldy hay and straw is used.

Fungi do not contain chlorophyll. Therefore they use as sources of organic compounds those which have been synthetized from green plants. Nitrogen, sulfur, phosphorus, magnesium and other metals can be taken up in an inorganic form. Fungi may be present at temperatures of up to + 60°C and also in extremely cold areas. In acid soil the number of fungi exceeds the number of bacteria. Soils with neutral alkaline pH normally favour the actinomycetes and other bacteria rather than fungi.

Between fungi, bacteria, animals and plants there are many interrelationships. Competition for nutrients between bacteria and fungi is a well-known phenomenon. Sometimes fungi produce inhibiting factors against bacteria and vice versa. On the other hand one of the partners may produce growth factors (vitamins) or may break down various compounds by means of their enzymes.

Fungi and algae form lichens. Beside this symbiotic combination we know the so-called mycorrhizoid fungi. This is a symbiosis between the roots of seed plants (orchids) and fungi. Most forest-trees also have these mycorrhizoid fungi.

But now we should focus on the infectious diseases of animals and human beings caused by fungi:

Infectious Diseases
A) Yeasts
    The most important disease agent for humans is *Candida (C.) albicans*. Other Candida species such as *C. krusei, C. parapsilosis, C. tropicalis, C. stelloidea*, etc. may also cause diseases. They all need additional factors to become pathogenic: Such factors may be general diseases such as diabetes, cancer, leukemia, or high doses of antibiotics and immune suppressive agents. Local factors such as the permanent influence of water on the stratum corneum of the hands are also important.
    The above-mentioned yeasts may cause local or systemic diseases: Septicaemia; Thrush; Genital infections; Eczema; Infections of the nail-bed; Colitis; Endocarditis, etc.
    Cryptococcus neoformans is the aetiologic agent of cryptococcosis, a very dangerous disease.
    In domestic animals yeasts are responsible for
Mastitis in cattle; Trush in poultry and piglets; Abortion in mares, cows and small ruminants; Instestinal mycosis; Eczema; Cryptoccocosis, etc.

The pathogenicity of yeasts is based upon the following factors:
Irritating effect of hyphae in tissues; Destruction of formerly intact surfaces
(skin, mucous membranes) and by this means creating of openings for bacteria;
Capsular substances (*Cryptococcus neoformans*) which inhibit phagocytosis; Pyrogenic compounds.

B) Dermatophytes

About 30 species, most of them belonging to the genera *Microsporum (M.)*,
Trichophyton (I.) and *Epodermophyton* may attack humans, animals or both. These
dermatophytes are classified into three groups according to their natural occu-
rence: anthropophilic, zoophilic and geophilic fungi.

Infection takes place by contact with diseased individuals or with individuals
with a latent infection. In human beings the latter way is less important than in
veterinary medicine. The common use of combs and caps provides an excellent way
for fungal distribution. In animals it is just the same; think of the saddles and
of the grooming equipment for horses. Insects also transmit infection. Places
where animals rub their skin may be infected for months and years with spores and
serve as a source of infection.

Dermatophytes attack the skin, in some rare cases the subcutaneous tissue, and
further the hairs and the nails. The damaging effect of the dermatophytes is based
upon their keratinolytic and other proteolytic enzymes.

In humans nearly every part of the body can be affected with a dermatomycosis.
Infections of the nail beds and deep subcutaneous mycoses, caused by *T. verrucosum*,
are especially protracted. Human infections are often acquired from animals.

Trichophytosis of cattle, mainly caused by *T. verrucosum*, is the number one
dermatomycosis in animals with regard to economic losses as well as to the danger
for humans. Mr. Gründer will present details later. In cats *M. canis* is responsible for the majority of cases.

T. mentagrophytes is representative of species which may attack men, different
domestic and laboratory animals and wild rodents too.

I have chosen the dermatomycoses of horses as an example of an animal mycotic
infection. In pasture especially during the war of 1870/71 and in World Wars I
and II, hundreds and thousands of horses showed severe infections. In many cases,
the animals could not be used for weeks and months. Since feeding and stabling
conditions for horses are now very much better, we see milder forms of the disease.
The preferred localisations are those of saddle and girth. After an incubation
period of 1-2 weeks small papules develop, which may be overlooked easily. Some
days later they become more distinct with erected hairs over them. Later some
yellowish secretion appears, which forms scale and scurf. Itching may be absent.
If no secondary (bacterial) infections complicate the normal progress, the lesions
heal spontaneously after 1-2 months. In some rare cases the eczema shows no tendenc

may cause diseases and complicate diseases.

Other damage by fungi

Fungi can grow on corn and corn products, fruits, potatos, milk and meat. Together with insects and rats, fungi are the most important causes of economic losses of foodstuffs and foods. They can also destroy wood, tissues made from plant fibres, and leather by means of their cellulases and proteolytic enzymes respectively.

Usefulness of fungi. Applied mycology

In ancient times the Chinese, Euripides and Hippocrates mentioned fungi as remedies. In the medicine books of the Middle Ages we find references to certain fungi with pharmacological effects. Fungi and fungal preparations as crude extracts have been used as aphrodisiacs, as hallucinogens (South American), as abortifacients, for stimulating uterus contraction and against heamorrhages. But at the present day too, numerous remedies are prepared from fungi. The alkaloids of the ergot of rye should be mentioned as one example and the antibiotics as another. Some fungi produce cancerostatic substances.

Many species of fungi are edible (mushrooms). Yeasts play a major role in the production of bread and other bakery products. There would be no beer or wine without yeasts! Many kinds of cheese are made with moulds. Vitamins (e.g. riboflavin), enzymes (e.g. pectinase) and other metabolites (e.g. gluconic acid) are made from fungi. Last but not least, fungi are important objects for genetic research, and yeasts are used for testing chemical compounds for mutagenicity.

NEW POSSIBILITIES IN THE TREATMENT OF DERMATOMYCOSES AND OF ASPERGILLUS FUMIGATUS

L. DESPLENTER, D.V.M.

Veterinary Clinical Research, Janssen Pharmaceutica N.V., 2340 Beerse, Belgium

ABSTRACT

Imazalil, an imidazole derivative, is described as a new antimycotic drug for veterinary application. It is highly active against different dermatophytes and against Aspergillus fumigatus.

In clinical trials in cattle and in horses, a cure rate of 88 to 96% is obtained after four applications with the diluted drug emulsion by spraying or wetting the animals.

Another application of imazalil is its vaporization for the prevention of A. fumigatus infection in problem herds. In the different rooms of a chicken hatchery, the Aspergillus contamination is eliminated by vaporization of imazalil. In a broiler farm, the fungal spore load i.e. Aspergillus, Penicillium, and Sco-pulariopsis, is reduced to extremely low levels after vaporization of imazalil.

INTRODUCTION

In the topical treatment of dermatomycoses in farm animals, difficulties may rise, specially if there are extensive lesions or if several animals are involved. To save time and labour, a formulation of an active drug may be developed to treat the animals by means of a knapsack sprayer or a high pressure sprayer.

Another problem in veterinary medecine is the presence of high numbers of Aspergillus fumigatus spores in poultry hatcheries or in poultry farms. This can lead to outbreaks of clinical aspergillosis in the young chickens in ovo or in the recently hatched ones. Even the most severe hygienic conditions are not always able to keep these infections within acceptable limits.

The aim of this study is to prove that with the same drug and the same for-mulation, it is possible to treat both infections: dermatomycosis is cured by

therapeutic treatment and outbreaks of aspergillosis are prevented by the treatment of contaminated rooms.

IMAZALIL: ANTIFUNGAL PROPERTIES

Imazalil-base (R 23979) belongs to the class of β-substituted 1-phenetyl
imidazoles as do miconazole and econazole (Ref. 6). Its chemical name is:
1 - [2-(2, 4-dichlorophenyl)-2-(2-propenyloxy) ethyl] -1H-imidazole.

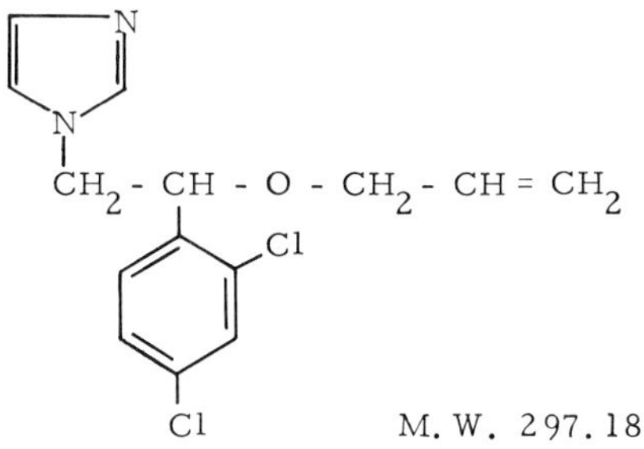

M.W. 297.18

Fig. 1: Structural formula of imazalil

Imazalil-base is a slightly yellowish to brownish solidified oil and is poorly
soluble in water, but very soluble in most common organic solvents.

Its antifungal and antibacterial properties are extensively described by
Thienpont and others (Ref. 8). In vitro, imazalil is very active against different
dermatophytes, A. fumigatus and Ascosphaera apis. Trichophyton mentagrophytes and A. apis are completely inhibited at 0.1 µg/ml. Microsporum canis,
T. rubrum and A. fumigatus are completely inhibited at 1 µg/ml. Yeasts and
other fungi are less sensitive. In vivo, guinea pigs with severe experimental
infections of T. mentagrophytes and M. canis, are treated topically with different
concentrations of imazalil in an ointment base. In the prophylactic experiments
(treatment from day -1), imazalil at 2% cures all animals. Dipping of the
guinea pigs during 5 consecutive days in a 2% emulsion results in a pronounced
improvement of the lesions.

Another striking activity of imazalil is its antifungal activity in the vapour
phase, although its vapour pressure is extremely low (Ref. 10). This fungista-
tic and fungicidal property seems to be limited to a distance of 10 mm. Nevertheless, this vapour phase activity may have an important role when imazalil
is applicated to the hairy skin of animals or is vaporized in rooms such as
chicken hatcheries or poultry farms.

MECHANISM OF ACTION

The mechanism of action of imazalil is based on the inhibition of the biosynthesis of ergosterol in the fungal cell membrane (Ref. 9). This results in an accumulation of lanosterol-like sterols (methyl group on C-14 locus) and leads to functional changes in the permeability of the membrane. This action is specific, since about 600 times more drug is needed to inhibit cholesterol synthesis in cultured mammalian cells than is needed to inhibit ergosterol biosynthesis in Candida cells.

TOLERANCE

The acute, subacute and chronic toxicity studies in several animal species reveal no toxicity at therapeutic dose levels (Ref. 8). The drug produces no teratogenic or mutagenic abnormalities. Drug application to the skin of animals or humans is well tolerated. Even supraconjunctival application of the 0.2% formulation in the eyes of cattle and horses is safe (Ref. 11). Imazalil treatment of the eggs has no influence on the hatching results (Ref. 7).

VETERINARY APPLICATIONS OF IMAZALIL

Because of its high activity against dermatophytes and A. fumigatus, imazalil is selected among other analogues for veterinary development. With the pharmaceutical formulation, clinical trials are carried out for the treatment of dermatomycoses in cattle and horses and for the elimination of A. fumigatus infection from a hatchery and a broiler farm.

The composition of the formulation is:

imazalil	10	g
span 20	48.6	g
tween 20	48.6	g

I. Treatment of dermatophytes in cattle and horses

  A. Cattle (Table 1)

Animal material: 379 cattle, spread over 47 farms, with typical lesions of ringworm infection. The clinical diagnosis is confirmed by direct examination and culture on Sabouraud medium. T. verrucosum is the main aetiologic agent.

Treatment schedule:

Trial A (Ref. 1): once a week during 4 consecutive weeks. At each treatment the animal is sprayed entirely.

Trial B (Ref. 1): twice a week during two consecutive weeks. At the first treatment, the animal is sprayed entirely, but at the following treatments only the lesions and surrounding skin areas are treated.

Trial C (Ref. 3): identical to trial B. This trial is carried out by six practising veterinarians.

Drug application: The 10% formulation is diluted to 0.2% in lukewarm tap water and is sprayed on the animals by means of a knapsack sprayer or a high pressure sprayer. In most instances, at the first treatment, the crusts on the lesions are manually removed by means of a brush or sponge, drenched in the imazalil dilution.

Results: Five weeks after the last treatment, the cure rates in trial A, B and C are respectively 92, 88 and 96%. The evolution of the healing is comparable in the three groups: stabilization within 1 week, improvement of the lesions within 2-3 weeks and new hair growth within 3-6 weeks.

Table 1: Field trials with imazalil in cattle

	Trial A	Trial B	Trial C
Number of animals	165	69	145
Number of farms	15	13	19
Cure rate (5 weeks)	92%	88%	96%
Stabilization	within 1 week		1 week
Improvement	within 2-3 weeks		2-3 weeks
New hair growth	within 3-4 weeks		3-4 weeks

B. Horses (Ref. 2)

Animal material: 9 horses of different breed and with typical ringworm lesions, identified as T. equinum.

Drug application: imazalil 0.2% is applied on the lesions and surrounding skin area with a sponge.

Treatment schedule: twice a week during two consecutive weeks.

Results: in 8 horses, the evolution of the healing is comparable to, and even faster than the healing in cattle. In one horse, new lesions occur because only the lesions without the surrounding skin areas have been treated.

II. Treatment of A. fumigatus infections

The activity of imazalil against A. fumigatus in vitro and its vapour phase

activity make it a useful drug for the treatment of Aspergillus infections in
animal rooms. This activity has been proved in two problem herds: a
chicken hatchery and a broiler farm.

A. Aspergillosis in a chicken hatchery (Ref. 4)

History: Aspergillosis in this hatchery is suspected because of the presence of contaminated eggs and because the chickens, leaving the
hatchery develop clinical aspergillosis within some days after arrival
on the farm.

Hatchery: The hatchery has a total surface of about 275 m^2 and is divided
into three separate rooms: brooding, hatching and packing room. The
hygienic conditions are good and between the hatchings the rooms are
disinfected with formalin and potassium permanganate.

Sampling: In each of the rooms, 30 Petri dishes with Sabouraud medium
are exposed to the air for 15 minutes. After incubation for 2 days at
27°C, the colonies are identified and counted. Each sampling on the indicated
days is done during the hatching and packing of at least 10,000 chickens.

Treatment: Imazalil is vaporized in the rooms by means of a Swingfog
(Motan GmbH, Germany), which produces a mist of droplets of 20 micron
size. This mist gradually settles down on all surfaces. The dosage is
200 mg of active ingredient, diluted in lukewarm tap water, per square
meter of floor surface. The treatment schedule is shown by the arrows
in Figure 2. The first treatment consists of four vaporizations with an
interval of one day. The second treatment, two months later, consists
of two vaporizations with one day interval.

Results: The evolution of the number of A. fumigatus spores is presented
in Figure 2: in the lowest part the number of counted colonies and in the
upper part the number of Petri dishes with massive growth are presented.
- day -7: All 30 Petri dishes show massive growth in the brooding room.
  In the hatching room, 11 Petri dishes have massive growth, while
  622 colonies are counted on the other dishes. In the packing room,
  396 colonies are present, while 18 dishes show massive growth.
- day -6, -4, -2 and 0: Vaporization in the hatchery at 200 mg/m^2.
- day +4: All 90 Petri dishes are completely negative.
- day +12 and +21: The brooding room is negative and only 2 colonies
  are counted in the hatching and packing room.
- day +55: In the brooding, hatching and packing room respectively 24,
  90 and 70 colonies are present. In the packing room, again 16 dishes

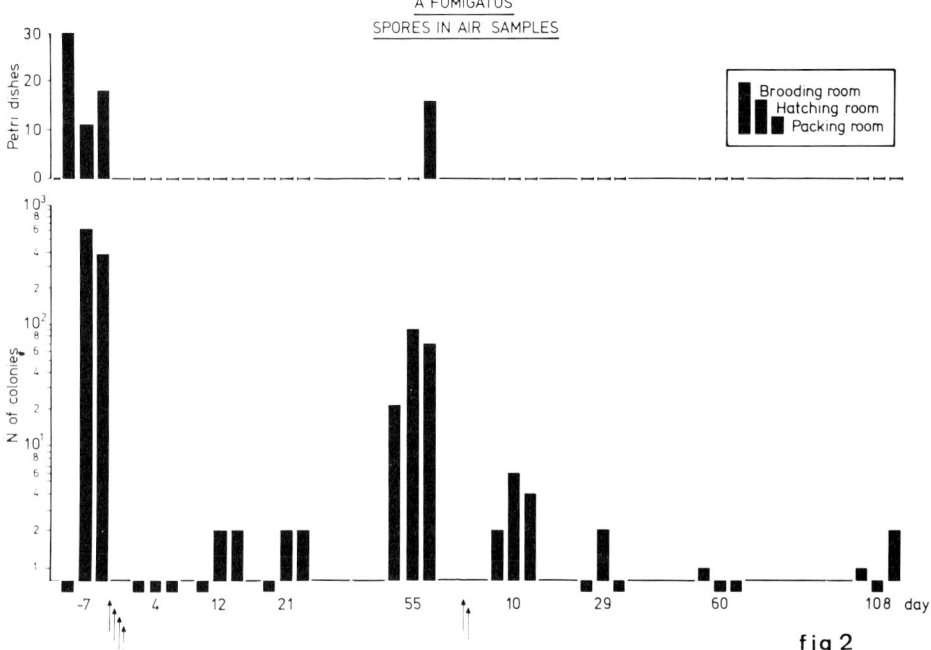

fig 2

have a massive growth of A. fumigatus.

- day +60 and +62: Vaporization of the hatchery at 200 mg/m^2. Day +62 is considered day 0 for the second observation period.

- day +10: In the brooding, hatching and packing room respectively only 2, 4 and 3 colonies are present.

- day +29: Two colonies are present in the hatching room.

- day +60: One colony in the brooding room.

- day +108: One colony in the brooding room and two colonies in the packing room.

Discussion: In this hatchery with severe problems of aspergillosis, four vaporizations with imazalil, eliminate the infection for nearly two months. After two months, the number of Aspergillus spores is highest in the packing room, because in a hatchery this is the most untidy room with a high temperature and relative humidity. Two further vaporizations with imazalil reduce the infection to a very low level for about 3 1/2 months. Only a few colonies are counted and massive growth of A. fumigatus on the Petri dishes is no more observed.

B. Aspergillosis in a broiler farm (Ref. 5)

History: The previous flock of "spring-chicken"-type broilers has been removed because of a severe outbreak of clinical aspergillosis.

Farm: This is a small farm with a total area surface of about 155 m^2, divided into two separate rooms. During the first three weeks the chickens are kept on the floor, whereafter they are moved to a battery room until 7-8 weeks of age.

Sampling: The method of sampling is the same as described for the hatchery. In the floor room, 20 Petri dishes and in the battery room 50 Petri dishes are exposed to the air on day -7, 12 and 46.

Treatment: Imazalil is vaporized with a Swingfog at 200 mg/m^2 on day -2 and 0.

Results (Table 2)

Table 2: Fungal flora in a broiler farm

Fungus	Median number of spores					
	Floor (20 Petri dishes)			Battery (50 Petri dishes)		
	d -7	d +12	d +46	d -7	d +12	d +46
A. fumigatus	3.5 (20)*	0 (0)	0 (3)	0 (22)	0 (0)	0 (1)
Penicillium	3 (18)	0 (0)	0 (3)	2 (41)	0 (0)	0 (5)
Scopulariopsis	17 (20)	0 (0)	0 (5)	11 (47)	0 (0)	0 (5)

( )* : number of positive Petri dishes

- day -7: The previous flock was removed 14 days earlier and the rooms are cleaned and disinfected with an antiseptic. In spite of this cleaning and disinfection, three different fungi are isolated on nearly all Petri dishes: A. fumigatus, Penicillium sp. and Scopulariopsis sp.. The degree of infection is somewhat lower in the battery room than in the floor room: the median number of colonies being 0, 2 and 11 against 3.5, 3 and 17.

- day +12: A new group of 2,000 broilers has been in the floor room on a bedding of wood-shavings for four days. All Petri dishes are completely negative for the three fungi.

- day +46: At that time the broilers are housed on the batteries and the floor room is empty. The number of positive Petri dishes in the floor room is only 3 for Aspergillus, 3 for Penicillium against 5 for Scopulariopsis. In the battery room this is respectively 1, 5 and 5. The number of colonies in these dishes is very low, so that the median value is 0 for all identified fungi.

Discussion: In this farm, aspergillosis would have been a big risk for a new group of young broilers, if the rooms had not been previously treated with imazalil. After the elimination of the Aspergillus infection, the broilers are fattened without any health problem. Even the fungi, which are brought in with the wood-shavings, are completely eliminated by the vaporization with imazalil.

CONCLUSION

Imazalil is an effective drug for the treatment of dermatomycoses in cattle and horses and for the treatment of aspergillosis in animal rooms. In the case of dermatophytes, imazalil is therapeutically active against the fungal infection of the animals. By the treatment of Aspergillus contamination in animal rooms, disease outbreaks of aspergillosis in the animals are prevented with imazalil.

Whether this effect of imazalil is only the result of a direct contact between the fungus and the substance or whether the vapour phase activity of imazalil is also an important factor, remains an open question.

REFERENCES

1. De Keyser, H. Clinical trial on the activity of repeated treatments with imazalil (R 23979) against Trichophyton verrucosum in cattle. Report Janssen Pharmaceutica, April 1979 (V 3171).
2. De Keyser, H. Clinical trial on the activity of repeated treatments with imazalil (R 23979) against Trichophyton equinum in horses. Report Janssen Pharmaceutica, September 1979 (V 3252).
3. De Smet, M., De Vlieger, A., De Wolf, C., Logghe, M., Van Loon, E. and De Smedt, J. Clinical evaluation of imazalil (R 23979) against Trichophyton verrucosum in cattle. Results field trials, Belgium, September 1979 (V 3210).
4. Desplenter, L. and Van Cutsem, J. Activity of imazalil against Aspergillus fumigatus infection in a chicken hatchery. Report Janssen Pharmaceutica, September 1979 (in preparation).
5. Desplenter, L. and Van Cutsem, J. Treatment with imazalil of an Aspergillus fumigatus infection in a broiler farm. Report Janssen Pharmaceutica, September 1979 (in preparation).

6. Godefroi, E.F., Heeres, J., Van Cutsem, J. and Janssen, P.A.J., 1969. The preparation and antimycotic properties of derivatives of 1-phenetyl-imidazole. J. Med. Chem., 12: 784-791.

7. Miltenburg, J. Effect of imazalil spray on eggs with chicken embryos of two and three days old. Report Janssen Pharmaceutica, September 1979 (in preparation).

8. Thienpont, D., Van Cutsem, J. and Marsboom, R., 1979. The biologic properties of imazalil in experimental mycology (in press).

9. Van den Bossche, H., Willemsens, G., Cools, W., Lauwers, W.F.J. and Le Jeune, L., 1978. Biochemical effects of miconazole on fungi. II. Inhibition of ergosterol biosynthesis in Candida albicans. Chem. Biol. Interactions, 21: 59-78. Elsevier/North Holland Scientific Publishers Ltd.

10. Van Gestel, J., Van Cutsem, J. and Thienpont, D., 1979. The vapour phase activity of imazalil (in press).

11. Wouters, L. Irritation study in horses and cattle after supraconjunctival application of imazalil. Report Janssen Pharmaceutica, June 1979 (V 3176).

ACKNOWLEDGEMENT

The author is grateful to Dr. D. Thienpont for his advice in preparing the manuscript, to Dr. H. De Keyser who conducted the clinical trials in dermatomycoses and to J. Van Cutsem for the mycological cultures.

DERMATOMYCOSES OF CATTLE AND THEIR CHEMOTHERAPY

H.-D. GRÜNDER
Medizinische und Gerichtliche Veterinärklinik II (Innere Krankheiten
der Wiederkäuer) der Justus-Liebig-Universität Gießen, Frankfurter
Str. 110, 6300 Gießen, Federal Republic of Germany

Fungal skin infections are caused by Dermatophytes. These particular
forms of Hyphomyces are themselves able to break down keratin enzym-
atically. The exact classification of the Dermatophytes has caused
problems for several decades. The classification according to whether
the fungi are anthropophilic, zoophilic or geophilic is not entirely
satisfactory. Only since the discovery of the complete forms of Trichophyton spp. has it been possible to simplify the situation (GÖTZ,
1978). In cattle the only Dermatophyte infection of importance is
that due to Trichophyton verrucosum, the cause of enzootic ringworm
in cattle. In occasional cases infections are due to other Dermatophytes such as Trichophyton mentagrophytes or Trichophyton rubrum
(WEISS and BÖHM, 1978). These infections are usually caused by cross-
infection from man or domestic animals. The losses due to the damage
caused by Trichophyton infections in breeding and fattening cattle
can only be estimated. Considerable hide damage is caused and this
is only seen after tanning, so that the value of the hide is markedly
diminished. As Trichophyton infection in cattle is a transmissable
zoonosis to man, it is also a public health problem. As Trichophyton
verrucosum often causes a severe infection in man, especially to those
in contact with affected cattle, it would seem advisable that it becomes an officially notifiable disease as regards reporting of outbreaks and erradication schemes.

The causes of the increasing spead of Trichophyton infections in
cattle in West Germany are due to following conditions:

1. Increased stock density.

2. Cattle are being more commonly kept in free-range barns and yards
   than previously.

3. Neglect in treating and eradicating the disease.

The epizootology of ringworm in cattle officially classifies it as
a chronic enzootic infection. Any systematic attack must be aimed at
destroying the source of infection. Experimental and natural infections due to Trichophyton verrucosum are very similar, as regards
clinical symptoms and duration of the disease (GRÜNDER, 1965; LEPPER,
1972 and 1974). After an incubation period of 1 - 4 weeks (on average
3 weeks), round scabby lesions (2 - 3 cm diameter) appear; in the
centre of which, the hair either falls out or breaks off. In the
course of the next couple of months, the ringworm with its typical
round asbestos like scabs (4 - 5 cm diameter) spreads to a greater or
lesser extent over the whole body. KLOBUSIZKY and BUCHWALD (1974) in
their extensive studies of the disease found,that in young cattle the
following areas were mainly affected: Head (26 %), neck (32 %) and
tail (13 %), where as the rest of the body was only 29 % affected.
During the following convalescent period, which also lasts about two
months,the ringworm lesions gradually lose their scabs. Grey flaky
lesions are then left, in which the hair gradually regrows from the
centre outwards. The total duration of the disease, when not complicated by parasitism, mechanical factors or inappropriate treatments
lasts 3 - 6 months.

Trichophyton verrucosum grows in the hair roots and will grow down
as far as to the Stratum spinosum in the cutis. The good symbiotic
relationship between the Dermatomycosis and its cattle host means,
that inflammatory or severe itching reactions do not generally occur;
unlike cases in man. Following recovery from ringworm a strong cellular and humoral immunity usually develops, so that reinfection seldom
takes place, as the further growth of the fungus is prevented by the
occurrence of an allergic inflammatory reaction (LEPPER and ANGER,
1976). As well as the resistence against Dermatomycosis increases
with age in cattle, so that the course of the disease, due to a type
of BLOCH's phenomenon, is considerably shortened and spread consequently diminished.

The epizootology of ringworm in cattle is mainly influenced by the
following factors:

1. Animal management and feeding (stable climate, free-range yards,
   vitamin-A-levels).

2. Number and age of the ringworm susceptible cattle (frequency of changing the numer of cattle and their environment).

3. Increased number of fungal spores in the environment (superinfection).

4. State of immunity.

Veterinary measures used in eradicating outbreaks of ringworm in cattle should have the following aims:

1. The destruction of the existing Dermatophytes.

2. Improvement of skin's resistence to infection.

3. Extermination of Dermatophyte spores in the cattle's environment.

Antimycotic chemotherapy is at present, the main form of treatment for Trichophyton infections in cattle, whereby commercial considerations must be taken as limiting factors, as regards forms and methods of therapy (GRÜNDER, 1972; GRÜNDER and MÜLLER, 1979). In future immunoprophylaxis and immunotherapy methods also may be used (WERNICKE, 1978). The numer of antimycotic drugs is considerable, however most of them do not fulfill the following conditions, required for eradicating ringworm infections in cattle:

1. Good antimycotic activity under controllable conditions.

2. Easy application, which remains on the hair and also penetrates the hair follicles.

3. Non - poisonous, non - residue forming.

4. Economic.

The measures taken to treat Trichophyton infections in cattle depend in the first place on the type of management and the numer of animals affected (Table 1; GRÜNDER, 1972). At the present the favoured methods of treatment are complete body spraying and oral medication.

In the last few years, trials using large numers of antimycotic drugs and different methods of medication have been carried out in the field, using naturally infected cattle. Controlled field-trials using

Table 1: Eradication of ringworm in cattle

Number of infected cattle	Methods for eradication of ringworm in cattle		
	Antimycotic treatment	Raising dermal resistance	Desinfection of the surroundings
Less than 5 animals	Lokal treatment with antimycotic ointments, emulsions or solutions		Not always necessary
Herds with 5 - 20 animals	Antimycotic spraying all animals in the herd or Griseofulvin as feed additive	Not always necessary	After cattle drived to pasture
Herds with 25 - 100 animals	Antimycotic treatment with motor-sprayer or Griseofulvin as feed additive	Correction of vitamin A level in ration	At the same time
Herds or feedlots with steady change of animals	Antimycotic spraying all animals in the herd in monthly intervals	High level of vitamin A in ration	In monthly intervals

Table 2:

Results of therapeutic investigations in naturally ringworm infected cattle after locally application of antimycotic ointments, sprays or solutions

Medicament	Formulation	Number of applications	Number of treated cattle	Ringworm healed %	Control Interval in days
Benzimidazole	5 % ointment	2	91	92	42
	Spray	2 - 3	48	44	42
Aminochinaldine	10 % ointment	2 - 3	44	14	42
Thiabendazole	4 % ointment	2	70	46	49
	5 % solution	1	132	80	42
Amphotenside	Spray	2	33	94	42
Monobenzthione	0,5 - 1 % solution	1 - 2	83	96	30 - 50
Etisazole	1 % solution	2 - 3	151	62	42
Total			652		
Untreated controls				15	30 - 50

Table 3:
Results of therapeutic investigations in naturally ringworm infected cattle after spray-application
of antimycotics

Medicament	Formulation	Number of applications	Number of treated cattle	Ringworm healed %	Control Interval in days
Monobenzthione	0,5 - 1 % solution	2 - 3	244	76	30 - 50
	0,5 - 1 % solution	2	31	77	56
Cyclohexanthio-carbonanilid	0,5 - 1 % solution	3	111	75	42
	1;5 - 2 % solution	3	117	80	42
Etisazole	1 % solution	3	23	70	35
Thymol/Chlorthymol	5 % solution	3	87	66	42
	10 % solution	3	21	77	42
Natamycine	0,1 % solution	2	147	87	56
Total			781	15	30 - 56

Table 4:
Results of therapeutic investigations in naturally ringworm infected cattle after oral Griseofulvin treatment

Medicament	Formulation and dosage	Treatment days	Number of treated cattle	Ringworm healed %	Control interval days
Griseofulvin	Tablets 15 - 35 mg/kg b.w.	18 - 30	5	100	30
	2 % Supplement 10 mg/kg b.w.	30	9	100	30
	2 % Supplement 10 mg/kg b.w.	7	66	92	42
	10 mg/kg b.w.	7	33	91	56
Total			113		
Untreated controls				15	30 - 56

Table 5:
Results of mycologic investigations in naturally with ringworm infected cattle

Medicament	Formulation	Application	Culture of Trichophyton verrucosum			
			before treatment		30 - 56 days after treatment	
			Number of animals	%	Number of animals	%
Etisazole	1 % solution	2 - 3 x brushing	37	70	17	32
Thiadiazine	0,5 - 1 % solution	1 - 3 x brushing	57	90	16	25
Monobenzthione	0,5 - 1 % solution	1 - 2 x brushing	53	74	6	8
Cyclohexanthio-carbonanilid	1 % solution	3 x Spray	43	86	7	14
Griseofulvine	2 % supplement	10 mg/kg b.w. orally for 30 days	8	89	7	78
Natamycine	0,1 % solution	2 x Spray	82	68	8	10
Total			198	83	19	63
Untreated controls			25			63

specially thought-out test-sheets, and non-treated animals as controls were carried out. The clinical course of the disease and its
spontaneous recovery were taken into consideration. Table 2 - 4
show the results obtained during the last few years from different
research-workers. Results of clinical treatments were mainly judged
according to their effect on the course of the disease. In some of
the experiments, the results were checked for fungal growth following
treatment (Table 5).

Results of treatment show some particular differences, in many cases
the rates of recovery could be reproduced. Special attention must be
paid to the age of the experimental cattle and to the time allowed
for the study of the course of the Trichophyton infection. As a result
of the experimental trials over a period of years, the present treatment of ringworm infections in cattle with different antimycotic drugs
can be considered as adequate and economic.

Literature

GÖTZ, H. (1978): Neuere Befunde über Hautkrankheiten durch Dermatophyten. Münch.Med.Wschr. 120, 1379 - 1382

GRÜNDER, H.-D. (1965): Beitrag zur Bekämpfung der Trichophytie beim
Rind. Berl.Münch.Tierärztl.Wschr. 78, 261 - 263

GRÜNDER, H.-D. (1972): Neuzeitliche Behandlung der Trichophytie des
Rindes. Zbl.Vet.Med. 18, Beiheft 17, 106 - 113

GRÜNDER, H.-D. and U. MÜLLER (1979): Behandlungsversuche mit dem anti-
mykotischen Antibiotikum Natamycin bei der enzootischen
Rindertrichophytie. Dtsch.Tierärztl.Wschr. 86 - im Druck -

KLOBUSIZKY, M. and J. BUCHWALD (1974): Prädilektionsstellen des Vor-
kommens der Trichophytieherde bei jungen Rindern und
Ursachenanalyse ihrer Entstehung. Arch.exper.Vet.Med.
28, 409 - 416

LEPPER, A.W.D. (1972): Experimental bovine Trichophyton verrucosum
infection. Res.Vet.Sci. 13, 105 - 115

LEPPER, A.W.D. (1974): Experimental bovine Trichophyton verrucosum
infection. Res.Vet.Sci. 16, 287 - 289

LEPPER, A.W.D. and H.S. ANGER (1976): Experimental bovine Tricho-
        phyton verrucosum infection. Comparison of the rate
        of epidermal cell proliferation and keratinisation in
        non-infected and reinoculated cattle. Res.Vet.Sci. 20,
        117 - 121

WEISS, R. and K.H. BÖHM (1978): Die wichtigsten Dermatophyten und
        Dermatomykosen bei Haustieren. Tierärztl. Praxis 6,
        421 - 433

WERNICKE, R. (1978): Erfahrungsbericht über den Einsatz der sowjeti-
        schen Rindertrichophytievakzine LTF-130 in einem Jung-
        rinderaufzuchtbetrieb der VVB Tierzucht. M.-hefte Vet.
        Med. 33, 28 - 31

PROPERTIES, INDICATIONS AND SIDE-EFFECTS OF MODERN ANTIMYCOTICS

M. PLEMPEL
Institute of Chemotherapy, BAYER AG, 5600 Wuppertal-1 (G.F.R.)

ABSTRACT

Therapeutic management of patients with systemic mycoses continues to be a serious problem due to the lack of oral or parenteral administrable antimycotics that are both, effective and nontoxic.

A comparative assessment of the properties of the systemically active antimycotics

Amphotericin B   5-Fluorcytosin   Miconazole i.v.   Clotrimazol oral

yielded the following classification to be recommended for the treatment of those mycoses of the internal organs which are chiefly encountered in Europe:

Fig. 1a: ANTIMYCOTIC THERAPY IN SYSTEMIC MYCOSES I / CANDIDOSIS

Site and Type of Infection	Therapy of Choice first	second
Septic	5-Fluorcytosin	Amphotericin B Miconazole i.v. Clotrimazole oral
Septic with Endophthalmitis	Amphotericin B + 5-Fluorcytosin	-
Endocarditis	Amphotericin B + 5-Fluorcytosin + Surgery	-
Meningitis	Amphotericin B + 5-Fluorcytosin	Amphotericin B (i.v. and intrathecally) 5-Fluorcytosin Miconazole (i.v. and intrathecally)
Urinary tract	5-Fluorcytosin	Miconazole i.v. Clotrimazole oral
Respiratory tract	5-Fluorcytosin	Amphotericin B Miconazole i.v. Clotrimazole oral
Mucocutaneous	Amphotericin B + 5-Fluorcytosin	Clotrimazole oral
Intestinal	Nystatin oral Clotrimazole oral	5-Fluorcytosin Pimaricin

Fig. 1b: ANTIMYCOTIC THERAPY IN SYSTEMIC MYCOSES II /
         CRYPTOCOCCOSIS, ASPERGILLOSIS AND ENDEMIC PRIMARY MYCOSES

Site and Type of Infection	Therapy of Choice first	second
Cryptococcosis respiratory tract meningoencephal or disseminated	5-Fluorcytosin Amphotericin B + 5-Fluorcytosin	Amphotericin B 5-Fluorcytosin
Aspergillosis respiratory tract	Amphotericin B + 5-Fluorcytosin	Clotrimazole 5-Fluorcytosin
Aspergilloma	Surgery	
Mucor-mycosis	Amphotericin B	-
Histoplasmosis Coccidioidomycosis Paracoccidioidomycosis Blastomycosis	Amphotericin B Miconazole i.v.	-

Some important data concerning Amphotericin B, 5-Fluorcytosin and the imidazoles Miconazole and Clotrimazole are summarized in the following figures:

Fig. 2: AMPHOTERICIN B:
        SPECTRUM OF ANTIMYCOTIC ACTIVITY AND MIC-VALUES

Fungi	MIC-Values in mcg/ml
Dermatophytes	>3
Yeasts (e.g. Cand. alb.)	0.1 - 0.5
Moulds (e.g. Aspergillus fum.)	0.3 - 2
Biphasic fungi (e.g. Histoplasma Coccidioides Paracoccidioides)	0.05 - 1

Fig. 3: AMPHOTERICIN B:
THERAPEUTIC EFFICACY IN SYSTEMIC FUNGAL INFECTIONS
Dosis: 1 mg/kg b.w. in 24 h

Infection	Cure Rate in %
Candidosis	60
Cryptococcosis	60
Aspergillosis	50
Mucor-Mycosis	< 50
Infections by biphasic fungi	60 - 80

Fig. 4: AMPHOTERICIN B:
SIDE-EFFECTS AFTER MAXIMAL DOSAGE OF 1 mg/kg b.w. i.v.

Side-Effects	% of Cases
Fever, cramps, headache, malaise	> 50 - 80

Renal damages
  reversible
  irreversible
  (tubulus-calsinosis
	> 50
	ca. 20

Thrombophlebitis	20

Fig. 5: 5-FLUORCYTOSIN:
ANTIMYCOTIC SPECTRUM OF ACTIVITY AND MIC-VALUES

Fungi	MIC-Values in mcg/ml (Yeast-Nitrogen-Broth)
Candida-species and Torulopsis	0.1 - 2 - 10 - > 25
Cryptococcus neoformans	0.5 - 4 - 15
Aspergillus-species	1 - > 10
Chromomycetes	1 - 10

Fig. 6: THERAPEUTIC EFFICACY OF 5-FLUORCYTOSIN (150 mg/kg/day orally)

Mycosis	Cure-Rate in % of Cases

Candidosis
  respiratory tract
  urinary tract
  mucocutaneous
	80 - 90
	80 - 90
	30

Cryptococcosis
  respiratory tract
  meningoencephal
	> 90
	50 - 60

Aspergillosis	50

Fig. 7: 5-FLUORCYTOSIN:
SIDE-EFFECTS AFTER OPTIMAL DOSAGE REGIMEN
(150 mg/kg/day in 4 Doses)

Side-Effects	% of Cases
Intestinal-tract (Vomitus, pain, diarrhoea)	6
Blood (Leucopenia, thrombopenia, agranulocytosis)	5
Liver (Elevation of transaminases and phosphatase, bilirubinaemia)	5

Fig. 8: CLOTRIMAZOLE AND MICONAZOLE:
THERAPEUTIC EFFICACY IN SYSTEMIC MYCOSES

Mycosis	Therapeutic Efficacy in % of Cases	
	Miconazol i.v.	Clotrimazole oral
Candidosis	60 - 70	60 - 70
Cryptococcosis	?	none
Aspergillosis	?	50
Mucor-Mycosis	?	none
Infections caused by biphasic fungi (Histoplasmosis Cocc., Paracocc.)	50 - 70	?

Fig. 9: CLOTRIMAZOLE (oral):
SIDE-EFFECTS AFTER ORAL APPLICATION IN HUMANS
(3 x 20 mg/kg b.w.)

Side-Effects	% of Cases
Gastro-intestinal tract (Vomitus, pain, loss of appetite)	30
Liver (Elevation of transaminases)	20
Pollakisuria	15

For topical use in mycoses of the skin and topical accessible
mucous membranes the imidazole-antimycotics Clotrimazole and
Miconazole are the drugs of choice in humans, pets and valuable
horses. The imidazoles are characterized by a broad spectrum of
antimycotic activity and a high degree of therapeutic safety.

The only agent which proved to be effective against extended or
deep seated dermatophytoses which are topically inaccessible is
orally administered Griseofulvin.

An unsolved therapeutic problem remains the ringworm-infection
in cattles and sheep, mainly for economical reasons.

The following figure 10 shows the indications of modern antimycotics for topical use in mycotic skin- and mucous membrane-infections:

Fig. 10: ANTIMYCOTIC THERAPY IN SKIN- AND MUCOUS MEMBRANE-
         INFECTIONS

| Mycosis | Therapy of Choice | |
	first	second
Skin-infections		
Dermatophytosis	Imidazoles Griseofulvin orally	Tolnaftate Ectimar (vet.med.only)
Candidosis	Imidazoles	Polyenes Ectimar (vet.med.only)
Chromomycosis	Imidazoles 5-Fluorcytosin locally	Ectimar (vet.med.only)
Pityriasis	Imidazoles	-
Aspergillosis (?)	Imidazoles Ectimar (vet.med.only)	Polyenes
Mucous membrane infections		
Candida and Torulopsis-species		
vaginal	Imidazoles	Polyenes
buccal	Polyenes	Boric acid
Eye and Ear		
Various fungi	Imidazoles	Polyenes

INTRODUCTION TO HUMAN CLINICAL TOXICOLOGY

B. SANGSTER, A.N.P. VAN HEIJST and S.A. PIKAAR
National Poison Control Centre, National Institute of Public Health, P.O. box 1,
Bilthoven.
Department Reanimation and Clinical Toxicology, University Hospital Utrecht,
Catharijnesingel 101, Utrecht. the Netherlands.

ABSTRACT
   Clinical toxicology is a fast developing branch of medical science. In this
article the reasons why are discussed as well as the relationship between clinical
toxicology and other medical, pharmacological and toxicological disciplines. A
picture is sketched of the circumstances under which intoxications in man occur
and what substances are involved. Finally is indicated what preparative work has
to be performed before actual treatment of patients can be started.

INTRODUCTION
   Clinical toxicology is a branch of medical science, that is enjoying an every
year growing attention. One of the causes for this attention is the fact that
medical practitioners see an increasing number of intoxicated patients. This is
also caused by the increasing consciousness of the public about the potentional
hazards of the many substances with which they come into contact. Thus questions
about a possible toxicological origin of certain symptoms and complaints are more
frequently posed.
   This development has led to an increase of clinical and experimental
toxicological research. Also the public authorities are concerned about the
necessity of a good toxicological know-how and they provide facilities and funds
for this purpose. The ultimate goal of this is furthering public health.
   One of the causes of the increasing importance of toxicology is no doubt the
fast development of chemical science that enabled the explosive growth of chemical
industry. Its products changed our society drastically. Examples don't have to be
recalled since they are all too well known. Also the availability of an enormous
number of new, potent medicines is among others a direct consequence of the
development of chemical science.

There are many positive aspects in this changed society, however, the existence of these new products also brought new questions and new problems.

THE RELATIONSHIP BETWEEN CLINICAL TOXICOLOGY AND MEDICAL SCIENCE IN GENERAL

How is clinical toxicology related to other medical disciplines? The answer to this question becomes clear immediately after realising that no such medical specialist as a "clinical toxicologist" exists. For instance there are dermatologists, neurologists, internists, pulmonologists as well as occupational health officers who are interested in toxicology.

Depending on the intoxication any organ or organsystem can be involved and disturbed in its function. One cannot posess specialised knowledge of all medical fields. Internal medicine, however, as a general speciality, is a very good basis for clinical toxicology. Nevertheless one will need consultants who are specialized on the organsystem that is involved by the intoxication. Clinical toxicology is multidisciplinary beyond other specialisms.

THE RELATIONSHIP BETWEEN CLINICAL TOXICOLOGY AND PHARMACOLOGY AND TOXICOLOGY IN GENERAL

What is the relationship between clinical toxicology at one side and pharmacology and general toxicology at the other? The pharmacologist is investigating the effects and workingmechanisms of substances that can be used in the treatment of diseases. These investigations include the consequences of overdosage in which the clinical toxicologist is interested. These effects and their pathophysiological background form the basis for the treatment of the intoxicated patient.

In 1965 the **requirements** for registering new medicines are strengthened. Consequently also more toxicological data were to be provided by the manufacturer. A great problem for the clinical toxicologist is, that of many older drugs these data are often insufficient. As the mechanisms that cause the therapeutical effect in a patient are not necessarily the same as those that cause the symptoms in an intoxicated patient, the clinical toxicologist has to perform experimental research to elucidate the pathophysiology of the intoxication, in order to provide an adequate therapy to the patient who is put under his care.

The task of toxicology as a science is to investigate the influence of all existing substances excluding drugs on man, animal and environment. Realising how many substances there are, this is quite something. Furthermore one has to investigate many aspects of a substance. On the one side there is acute toxicity, at the other hand there is chronic toxicity and of course everything in between. One must also discern ingestion, inhalation and skin contact. There are questions on carcinogenicity and teratogenicity. What is the toxicity of combustion products and so on, and so on.

Clinical toxicology deals with patients to who protective and preventive measures did fail, resulting in actual intoxication. The results of the research mentioned form the basis for the diagnostic and treatment. Generally performing toxicological research does not automatically imply the experimentally testing of methods of treatment. As a result the clinical toxicologist and the general toxicologist not only exchange information, but also experiment together on adequate treatments.

MOST FREQUENTLY OCCURRING TOXICOLOGICAL PROBLEMS

As far as the Netherlands are concerned it is relatively easy to outline the most frequently occurring problems in clinical toxicology as there exists only one information centre, the National Poison Control Centre of the National Institute of Public Health. The figures that will be presented are derived from the number and kind of information provided by this centre (ref. 1). The actual number of real or supposed intoxications is certainly much higher as the centre is not being called for every intoxication. One must consider these figures as an indication of what is going on toxicologically. The picture drawn is rather reliable because only physicians, veterinarians and pharmacists are allowed to call the centre and the general public is excluded.

Data about what kind of patients and their backgrounds are based upon experience at the Department of Reanimation and clinical Toxicology of the University Hospital, Utrecht, and of colleagues throughout the country.

ACUTE INTOXICATIONS IN CHILDREN

Intoxications in children under 10 years of age are almost always accidental. While exploring the house, the garden and the shed the young child encounters a great variety of products that to his opinion requires further investigation. In children this is usually being done by taking the subject into the mouth. The attractiviness is increased when his recent discovery looks like sweets, as happens with medicines. One should realise that children are not discouraged by unappetizing smells or taste. Most accidental intoxications occur at the age of two. Boys are more frequently involved than girls.

In 1978 the centre provided about 7.000 informations concerning children. In more than half of these cases medicines were involved. The greatest number of these informations were about fluoride containing anticariës tablets, 14.7% and analgetics, 11.5%. In 9% psychopharmacons were involved, the majority fortunately the relatively non toxical benzodiazepines. A relatively great number of informations were about vitamin preparations, 8.6%. The oral contraceptives of the mother are quite popular with children, 6.4%.

Another group of substances ingested by children are household products, about
2.500. The greatest category of this group (14.2%) are products on the basis of
petroleum and other aliphatic hydrocarbons such as furniture oil and gasoline.
Several types of washing-preparations are causing intoxications. Dishwashing-
preparations (10.7%), strongly caustic detergents for the dishwashing machine and
all purpose cleaners (6.5%) are quite important. Furthermore children take
pesticides, plants and cosmetics (ref. 2).

ACUTE INTOXICATIONS IN ADULTS

Acute intoxications in adults are almost always intentional. It concerns a
category of patients not known in veterinary medicine, namely people with psychical,
psychosocial or psychiatriacal problems, who intentionally take an overdose of
drugs prescribed to them. Usually this occurs impulsively. The patient almost
never wants to take his life. We therefore prefere to speak of intentional intoxication instead of suicide. Often drinking of alcoholic beverages precedes the
intoxication and mostly more than one substance are ingested.

Unlike with children mostly women intoxicate themselves intentionally. The
number of young patients is strikingly large. The fact that in the Netherlands
just like in the rest of Europe the number of patients in the age 14-18 years is
strongly increasing needs special attention.

The poison control centre provided in 1978 about 3.500 informations concerning
adults. About half of them (46%) were about psychofarmacons. The majority were
benzodiazepines (29%) and tricyclic-antidepressants (9.9%). The number of hypnotic
and sedative drugs was 15.1%, analgetics 15%. Pesticides formed 12.9% of adult
intoxications (ref. 2).

Accidental intoxications in adults are rare in comparison to intentional
intoxications. Mistakes during the preparation or the administration of drugs may
cause accidental intoxications. A second important cause is accidental ingestion
of toxic substances packed in material originally intended for packing food,
(we all know the example of thinner or soldering liquid in a lemonade bottle).
A third situation where accidental intoxications do occur are accidents or fires
in, for instance, factories or ships. This is why the dutch centre is more and
more interested in data about combustion products and their toxicity. These
intoxications do not only create toxicological problems but also organisational
problems. One of the priorities is to measure as soon as possible, what substances
in what concentration are involved. The poison control centre considers it her
task to inform the public authorities that can perform these measurements or that
can order them to be done. This partly being done from self interested motives
because the results of these measurements form the basis of the therapeutical
advice that has to be given. Another priority is the organisation of assistance.

Here also the early information of the responsible authorities is very important. The chance that medical assistance will be provided to all people that have been exposed to the toxic substances (for example onlookers on a fire as well) increases in this way. This is especially important when substances are involved that create serious morbidity after a symptom-free interval, like nitrous fumes (ref. 3).

A last group of intoxicated patients that has to be mentioned are those who are a victim of attempted homicide. In the Netherlands the most commonly used substances are thallium, warfarin, parathion and other cholinesterase inhibitors. Once in a while very rare substances are involved. In these cases high demands are made to the knowledge and inventiveness of the clinical toxicologist (ref. 4).

ACUTE INTOXICATIONS IN ANIMALS

Last year the centre was consulted 308 times by veterinary surgeons. Almost all requests involved small domestic animals. In 45% it concerned intoxications by pesticides. In several cases the intoxication was not accidental, but the result of a deliberate attempt to kill the animal involved. Frequently involved substances were crimidine (19), strychnine (18), thallium (8) and cumarines (14). Drugs were in 66% of the cases involved. Mostly these drugs were intended for the owner and not for the animal. There were no specific drugs that were ingested more often than others. Householdproducts were 17% of the requests for information.

Observing and treating both human and animal patients together can be useful. A good example of this kind of coöperation was a dog that ingested the haloperidol belonging to his owner. This resulted in a severe extrapyramidal syndrome. By putting together veterinary medical knowledge and human clinical toxicological knowledge the diagnosis was made and the animal adequately treated (ref. 5).

THE CLINICAL DEPARTMENT

What does one need to be able to practise clinical toxicology? Quite a lot of patients with acute intoxications do have life threatening disturbances in the function of respiration, circulation and central nervous system. These patients have to be treated at an intensive care department of a hospital.

To be able to transform this intensive care department into a clinical toxicology unit one has to have good and extensive toxicological knowhow and experience at his disposal. This will be discussed lateron. A second important condition is that one has close relations with a toxicological analytical laboratory that may for example be a division of the hospital pharmacy. This laboratory has to be able to provide a 24 hours service and the analytical methods employed does not only have to be reliable but, which is very important, they have to be very fast!

The history taken from the patient or his relatives and the findings at the physical examination are the basis for the diagnosis. Qualitative toxicological analysis is necessary to confirm the diagnosis or to exclude ingestion or exposure to other substances, for example acetaminophen. Close coöperation between clinician and pharmacist, who litteraly has to look over the shoulder of the clinician, is absolutely necessary for an efficient proceeding of this analysis. In several patients more specialised therapies are indicated. These are usually methods to enhance the elimination of the toxical agent such as hemodialysis and hemoperfusion or the administration of specific antagonists such as chelating agents. Besides the severity of the clinical situation the result of quantitative toxicological analysis is the mainstay for the indication for these therapies.

Having close relations with the analytical laboratory of the hospital pharmacy alone is not enough. On needs seperate contacts with other analytical laboratories for less common intoxications that cannot adequately be treated without toxicological analysis, for example herbicides and pesticides. As far as the clinical department in Utrecht is concerned the laboratories involved are the department of residue analysis and the department chemical-foodanalysis of the National Institute of Public Health and the Laboratory for Human Toxicology of the State University of Utrecht.

TOXICOLOGICAL "KNOW-HOW"

Last but certainly not least what is most essential in clinical toxicology will be discussed. Knowledge of symptoms, diagnostics and treatment of intoxications. The National Poison Control Centre performs as far as the Netherlands are concerned the function that it provides this knowledge to all physicians, veterinary surgeons and pharmacists free of charge.

The Centre consists of an information department where 24 hours a day information can be obtained by telephone (030-742200 and 742875). The Centre can only function in an optimal way when answers to questions can be given promptly. It is a matter of course that quite a lot of preparatory work has to be done to make this possible.

This preparatory work is being done by the Documentation department, that feeds the information department with data. These data are in the first place obtained from literature and are brought together on files. This year computerising of all data has started. A lot more has to be done because a caller almost never asks for information about symptoms and therapy of an intoxication by a specific substance. Usually he only knows the name of the product involved. Therefore the documentation department has to feed the information department with data on products, their composition and toxicity, in order to be able to give a proper answer to the questions the way they are posed. This can only be done when industries are willing to place data concerning the often secret composition of their products at the disposition of the Centre. In the Netherlands much

296

coöperation is being encountered in this respect. The fact that these data are only used for providing information about toxicity and therapy and that therefore secrecy is maintained is of great importance. Also the fact that the centre is a governmental institution is important in this respect.

Providing information is one thing. Another thing is that one has to evaluate whether the information provided fits in what happens with the patients or has to be revised. This is also a task of the documentation department. A questionnaire is being sent to anybody who called for information. The questions concern the clinical picture that occurred and the result of the therapy advised. As 80% of these questionnaires is received back the data thus obtained are of great help in improving the quality of the information provided.

Once in a while it becomes evident that a specific intoxication is always very severe or that the therapy available is insufficient. When this occurs the centre can initiate animal experimental research in order to investigate the pathophysiology or the therapy of the intoxication involved. Also it can be necessary to perform clinical research to get a better insight in what is going on in the patients themselves. Because of the close contacts that exist between the poison control centre and the department of reanimation and clinical toxicology it is possible, thanks to the willingness of many colleagues to transfer their patients to this department, to observe and treat in a relatively short period of time large numbers of patients with a specific intoxication. After finishing the investigation it was not necessary any more to concentrate all cases at one place in the Netherlands because the improved therapy was worked up into the files of the centre.

CONCLUSION

An overall picture is given of all the preparative work that has to be done and the contacts that have to be made before clinical toxicology as a distinct medical disciplin can begin to function. All these things are necessary and have a high priority. However the essence of the work and therefore the interest of the clinical toxicologist is the intoxicated patient itself aswell physically as psychically.

REFERENCES
1. HEIJST, A.N.P. VAN, J.M.C. DOUZE and S.A. PIKAAR.
   Nationaal Vergiftigingen Informatie Centrum.
   Ned. T. Geneesk. 120, 206-209 (1976)
2. HEIJST, A.N.P. VAN. Berichten uit het RIV 1978, p. 35-36.
   Staatsuitgeverij 's-Gravenhage 1979.

3. SANGSTER, B., A.N.P. VAN HEIJST, S.A. PIKAAR. Poison Control Centers and Calamities. Vet. Hum. Toxicol. 20, 419-420 (1978).

4. SANGSTER, B., T.J.F. SAVELKOUL, M.G. NIEUWENHUIS, J. VAN DER SLUYS VEER. Two cases of carbachol intoxication. Neth. J. Med. 22, 27-28 (1979).

5. LEEUW, B. DE, B. SANGSTER. Severe extrapyramidal syndrome in a dog caused by a Haloperidol (Serenase[R]) intoxication. Vet. Quart. 1, 134-137 (1979).

LE CENTRE NATIONAL D'INFORMATIONS TOXICOLOGIQUES VETERINAIRES DE L'ECOLE
NATIONALE VETERINAIRE DE LYON.

(THE NATIONAL INFORMATION CENTRE ON ANIMAL TOXICOLOGY OF THE LYON NATIONAL
VETERINARY SCHOOL).

G. LORGUE, D. COURTOT, G. KECK, P. JAUSSAUD.
Laboratory for Toxicology, Ecole Nationale Vétérinaire de Lyon, Marcy l'Etoile,
69260 Charbonnières les Bains (France)

ABSTRACT

The "Centre National d'Informations Toxicologiques Vétérinaires" was officially
created in 1976.

The aims of the centre are :

- to give answers by telephone on urgent toxicological problems, or in written
form for more complete information on toxicology.

- to establish files on the main forms of poisoning and to set up a permanent
information system. This information begins from today in the form of the review
"Notes de Toxicologie Vétérinaires".

- to contribute to the training and teaching of future veterinary practitioners.

To achieve these aims the centre has a bibliographical file, a PDP 11 DIGITAL
Computer. At the moment there is a distinct shortage of staff. The extention of the
centre will be undertaken by a team of 3 or 4 students.

The centre is officially open to everybody. A telephone stand-by is maintained
every day from 7.30 am to 6.30 pm hours except Sundays and public holidays. During
closing hours a telephone answering machine records the calls.

The centre is allied with the toxicological analysis laboratory which carries
out 9,000 analyses a year and acts as a "relay" to advise the veterinary practitioner when poisoning is suspected.

The summary of activity shows 1,485 requests for information during the period
from July Ist 1978 to June 30th 1979, 50 % coming from veterinary surgeons, 16 %
from private individuals, 19 % from the Directions Départementales des Services
Vétérinaires (Regional Boards of Veterinary Services).

These figures show that even if there are still many imperfections and gaps to
fill, the work of the Centre meets a true need on the part of the veterinary profession.

The Centre National d'Informations Toxicologiques Vétérinaires was officially conceived at the Ecole Nationale Vétérinaire de Lyon on August 14th 1976.The compilation of the bibliographical files and of the basic library took almost two years' work. It is necessary to emphasize that the Centre could have only been set up and have existed thanks to both the moral and financial support of the Direction des Services Vétérinaires (Veterinary Services Board). We should like to express thanks to all those who in one way or another have helped us at any time.

First of all we shall briefly attempt to outline the aims, the facilities and also the running of the Centre. Then secondly we will sum up its activities during the period from July 1st 1978 to June 30th 1979.

I - THE AIMS, THE FACILITIES AND THE RUNNING OF THE CENTRE.

A - The Aims.

The aims can be easily brought together under three headings.

1) In the short run.

The Centre is above all a telephone centre where the veterinary practitioner may obtain a quick and efficient answer to his very urgent toxicological problems. It also serves as a postal base to which the veterinary practitioner may make enquiries concerning toxicology, especially when he is not in a great hurry and wishes to acquire certain essential knowledge.

In order to achieve these aims the Centre must possess a store of sufficiently important bibliographical data which must be both easily accessible and quickly usable.

2) In the medium term.

The Centre :

- will choose from this store of bibliographical data the basic references on the main forms of poisoning, concerning both domestic and other animals. These will then be analysed and files drawn up. These files may be sent out to the veterinary practitioner upon request in the form of a photocopy.

- is setting up a permanent information system on toxicology, which allows the practitioner to get hold of new facts and to acquaint himself with current problems in animal toxicology. This information is available from today onwards by means of the Centre's published review, "Notes de Toxicologie Vétérinaire".

3) In the long run.

- We expect to be able to organise various seminars and advanced courses in animal toxicology.

- By its own observations in the field, by the results of various analyses and by the references they provide, the Centre will be able to provide a much greater contact between the student and his future practice. Thus acting as a base for research and particularly for doctoral theses on veterinary matters this Centre will contribute towards the teaching and training of the future members of our profession.

B - The Facilities.

At the present moment these include :

1) Bibliographical files.

The basic file, which is made up of index cards in the sphynxo system, currently comprises :

. 20,000 permanently filed references,

. 6,000 references in the pre-filing stage,

  15,000 articles repints, microfilms or photocopies duly analysed and
    filed,

.   150 toxicological files on the most common forms of poisoning.

The Centre has very recently purchased a P D P 11 Digital computer which will be extended by a hard disc unit in 1980. The first program, which will be operational from October 1st 1979, will allow the handling of all telephone and written enquiries. The actual bibliographical data will begin to be put into the computer during next year.

2) The library.

At the moment the Centre has a small library at its disposal containing about 170 works on Toxicology. This may indeed appear insufficient, but taking into account our budgetary constraints, the high cost of books has prevented us from doing any more in this respect.

3) Staff.

Three veterinary teachers and one researcher share the task of answering telephone calls and written enquiries, of creating data files and of reading and analysing the articles. They are helped by a part-time secretary. However, there is a distinct lack of human resources here, since the running of the Centre represents only a small part of the activities of these people.

When finances have permitted, this Centre has benefited from contributions by students of our school. These students have produced some excellent work. If we are to look towards a foreseeable extension of this means of giving information, it would be useful, if not essential, to be able to train and continuously maintain a team of 2 to 4 students.

C - The running of the Centre.

- The Centre is open to everybody. Until now, however, only the veterinary profession has been officially informed of its existence by one circular. No publicity or announcements have been made to private individuals.

- A telephone stand-by is maintained every day from 7.30 am to 6.30 pm,excluding Saturday afternoons, Sundays and public holidays. An answering machine records all calls during closing hours or on any day when the stand-by does not operate. We do intend to operate a complete stand-by using a group of students who will first undergo a period of induction. Starting this up will depend upon the Centre's financial situation in the months and years to come.

- In 1976 the Centre adopted the structure of a non-profit making organisation as governed by the act of 1901. It was indeed very urgent to find a solution to an ever-disquieting financial situation. The subsidy from the Direction des Services Vétérinaires had gone down by a half whereas operating costs,especially telephone calls, were on the increase. Acting as such a non-profit making institution, an appeal was launched to the practising veterinary surgeons, who were the main users. In return for paying a subscription the Centre guarantees :

. The publishing of a review, "Notes de Toxicologie Vétérinaire",

. The free mailing of toxicological files.

- The Centre is allied with the toxicological analysis laboratory. In this respect it acts as a "relay" when poisoning is suspected to advise the practitioner on how to conduct an enquiry, on taking samples, or it serves to transmit the results of urgent analyses. From July 1st 1978 to June 30th 1979, 1088 cases of isolated or collective animal poisoning were examined by the laboratory. This represents approximately 9,000 toxicological analyses performed on biological samples.

- Lastly, the C.N.I.T.V. should essentially be a means of contact for all those who are concerned with animal toxicology, whether they be practitioners, researchers, teachers or students...

The Centre has formed some excellent contacts with animal toxicologists abroad — in the U.S.A., Holland, Belgium and in Canada. It is also in liaison with French Human anti-poison Centres. Our medical colleagues, especially those of the Lyon anti-poison centre, have given us invaluable help through their advice and friendship. May they thanked very sincerely.

II - SUMMARY OF ACTIVITIES DURING THE PERIOD FROM JULY 1ST 1978 TO JUNE 30TH 1979

During this period, the Centre received 1,485 enquiries, divided up into :

- 1,374 telephone calls,
- 111 written enquiries.

From this summary, the following general observations can be made :

1) Type of Enquirers (Table I)

They are mainly veterinary practitioners, either rural or veterinary surgeons for small animals (50 percent of enquiries) who address requests to the Centre. Next there are the Directions Départementales des Services Vétérinaires (Regional Boards of Veterinary Services - 18.8 percent). These percentages are approximately

TABLE I - Telephone calls and written enquiries for the period
July 1st 1978 to June 30th 1979

Type of enquirer	Telephone calls		Written enquiries		Total enquiries	
	Number	%	Number	%	Number	%
Veterinary practitioners	698	50,8	52	46,8	750	50,5
Regional Boards of Veterinary Services	262	19,1	17	15,3	279	18,8
Veterinary Schools	18	1,3	8	7,2	26	1,7
Vets-Pharmaceutical Industries	22	1,6	1	0,9	23	1,5
Vets-livestock food Industries	10	0,7	2	1,8	12	0,8
Anti-poison centres, Doctors, Chemists	108	7,9	5	4,5	113	7,6
Farming organisations	14	1,0	1	0,9	15	1,0
Individuals	220	16,0	14	12,6	234	15,7
Miscellaneous (insurance companies	22	1,6	11	9,9	33	2,2
TOTAL	1 374		111		1 485	

TABLE II - Types of animal involved

Species	Telephone enquiries	Written enquiries	Total
Cattle	406	53	459
Sheep	66	4	70
Pigs	32	1	33
Horses	72	6	78
Goats	14	1	15
Dogs	276	17	293
Cats	58	3	61
Farmyard Animals	32	5	37
Rabbits	12	-	12
Winged Game	6	1	7
Ground-Game	6	1	7
Fish	56	2	58
Miscellaneous Animals	50	4	54
Humans	38	-	38

TABLE III - Types of toxic agents involved
Types of inquiry

	Number	Percentage
- Pesticides	377	25,4
- herbicides	94	6,3
- insecticides	65	4,4
- fungicides	6	0,4
- anticoagulant ratpoisons	72	4,8
- convulsion-inducing poisons (strychnine, metaldehyde, crimidine)	82	5,5
- those which cannot be precisely determined	58	3,9
- Plants	104	7,0
- Medecines	278	18,7
- Lead	41	2,8
- Copper	21	1,4
- Mercury	10	0,7
- Fluorine	4	0,3
- Household products	20	1,3
- Fertiliser	6	0,4
- Miscellaneous	171	11,5
- Cases of pollution	78	5,2
- General enquiries	201	13,5
- Non-established causes	174	11,7

the same as those observed in previous years.

A considerable increase can be observed in calls coming from private individuals (15.7 percent against 8 percent in 1977). These are usually from farmers who have traced us through practitioners or through farming organisations.

Calls from anti-poison Centres (7.6 percent) are also on the increase. These inquiries are mainly concerned with the accidental swallowing by children of medecines for animal consumption, and to a lesser extent with cases of animal poisoning.

2) Types of animal involved (Table II)

The two most involved types of animal are bovines and dogs. It must be stressed at this point that very urgent enquiries, i.e. where the practitioner, after having made the diagnosis, wants to give the animal the appropriate treatment immediately, are relatively few in number and mainly concern dogs.

Generally, our colleagues, above all those in rural practice, are notified too late and they finish up with dead animals. However, they still consider it necessary to obtain information in order either to make or to confirm their diagnosis, to prevent any further accidents which may arise.

It is also worth noting that the high occurrence of poisoning of cattle and dogs could stem from the fact that these species of animal are naturally inclined to eat absolutely anything. We have thus had cattle eating over 20 kg of sticks of explosives (TNT), polystyrene tiles ..., puppies swallowing petrol, washing powder, and of course the whole range of pharmaceuticals to be found in the family chemists, especially neuroleptics.

Under the heading of Miscellaneous animals there are guinea-pigs, snakes, tortoises... (indeed it is strange to see the types of animal some people can keep in an appartment), as well as those animals living in zoos.

Under the heading of humans we have filed calls concerning the danger of foods contaminated by pharmaceutical, pesticides or industrial residues. These are generally few in number but nevertheless create problems which are difficult to solve.

3) Types of Enquiry - Types of toxic agent involved (Table III)
- It can be observed that in 11.7 percent of suspected cases no toxic substance whatsoever could be found.
- 13.5 percent of calls involve general requests for information, such as the kind of appropriate samples from the living or dead animal in order to carry out toxicological or histological analyses for diagnosis.
- Cases of pollution - enquiries relate to how the veterinary practitioner should act in practise and in legal terms, and these involve the kind of samples to take and how to store them.
- suspected cases of pesticide poisoning are very frequent, representing 25.4

percent of enquiries. Herbicides are most frequently involved, with aryloxyacids
particularly from the group of phenoxyacetates (2.4 D, 2.4.5.T). This is essentially due to their very widespread use, and although suspected cases are frequent with this type of by-product, confirmed cases of poisoning are much less
frequent. The same can be said for other herbicides, such as atrazine and sima-
zine. However, nitrophenolic pesticides by-products (DNOC), dipyridilium (Paraquat) and Sodium Chlorate are fatal in all cases. Suspected cases of poisoning
by insecticides, although less frequent than the others, are still quite considerable. These are mainly due to lindane and parathion, and are probably linked
to the very frequent use of these compounds.

Cases of poisoning by fungicides are very rare. This is due to the fact that
most of them are not very toxic. Anticoagulant rat poisons are often responsible
for poisoning among dogs and to a lesser extent among cats or other animals. It
is illogical to observe that the main culprit, namely coumafene, is sold by many
firms as totally harmless to domestic pets.

Calls concerning suspicion of convulsion-inducing poisons (strychnine, metaldehyde, crimidine) are in fact less frequent than the large number of actual cases of these products in domestic carnivores. Veterinary practitioners are mostly
confronted with this problem almost daily and they know all about it. Strychnine,
which is used in France to destroy pests, especially the fox, is in reality almost on open sale, and to say the least, either accidental or malicious poisoning
is commonplace. It would be much better if legislators could someday become aware
of the high toxicity of this substance and would very severely limit its use.

Poisoning by plants, which was very common in 1976 during the drought, is on
the decrease. It must be stressed, however, that we are convinced that the enquiries made to the centre represent only a small part of the true situation.
- Frequent examples of poisonous plants are the Dog's Mercury and Colza, to a
lesser extent the oenanthe, acorns, hemlock, yew and black night-shade. The latter
mainly relates to ensilages which are contaminated with large quantities of this
plant.
- We have been struck by the large number of cases of poisoning by medicated products (18.7 percent). The main cause with cows and sheep is tetramisole. By itself
or in conjunction with bithionol sulfoxyde, this antiparasitic kills several
thousand animals a year in France.

Treatment against cattle grubs using organic phosphorus compounds is equally
responsible for serious poisoning in cows, especially those of the Charollais
breed. Furoxone continues to take its toll of accidents among fattening calves.
To this one may add the medecines swallowed willingly by puppies which are normally consumed by their owners. Therapeutical mistakes are just as frequent in all
species of animal.

- Lead and copper are the two metals which, in cows and sheep respectively, involve the majority of fatal accidents, often involving more than one animal. In the large majority of cases this involves accidental poisoning by the swallowing of minium or of copper sulphate.

TO CONCLUDE,

The "Centre National d'Informations Toxicologiques Vétérinaires" was established as a useful tool for the veterinary practitioner in cases of animal poisoning. We do not know if we have succeeded, because the task is a mammoth one. There are still many imperfections and gaps to fill, commonly due to a lack of means. However, the good wishes and the many expressions of thanks from our colleagues show us that it meets a real need in the profession.

RECENT TRENDS IN ANIMAL POISONING

D.J. HUMPHREYS

Physiology and Chemistry Department, The Royal Veterinary College, Royal College Street, London, NW1 OTU (U.K.)

ABSTRACT

   The materials causing poisoning, in both individual species and in domestic animals as a whole, in the U.K. during the last thirty years have been studied. Although lead has remained the dominant overall cause of intoxication, other agents appear to have become relatively more important in recent years. The main hazards to cattle, pigs and poultry have probably remained essentially unchanged. However, in line with the decreasing general importance of arsenic as a toxic agent, copper and Brassica species have become the most significant problem in sheep. Although numerical data is unavailable for these species, the causes of intoxication in cats and dogs have been considered.

INTRODUCTION

   Individual case reports, details of consecutive cases published by University laboratories and, in the United Kingdom, annual reports of the Chief Veterinary Officer and, more recently, the Veterinary Investigation Diagnosis Analysis (VIDA) data of the Ministry of Agriculture, Fisheries and Food contain information on materials causing poisoning in animals. Unfortunately, the apparent relative importance of various materials gathered from these publications may not be representative of the overall situation in the field. Despite this, due to the relevance of the information to those teaching toxicology and to practising veterinary surgeons, an attempt has been made to define the materials causing intoxication in animals and any trends that have developed during the last thirty years in the U.K. The main source of information employed has been the annual reports of the Chief Veterinary Officer and, for the period 1975 to 1978, the VIDA data.

Fig. 1 summarises the data for cattle, sheep, pigs and birds collectively for the period 1949-1978. This shows that the number of lead poisoning incidents confirmed by the Veterinary Investigation Centres in the U.K. increased considerably from

1949-1963, and decreased gradually thereafter. During the latter period, the total number of poisoning incidents tended to follow the pattern noted for lead. However, the former have not continued to decline in recent years. This is due to the

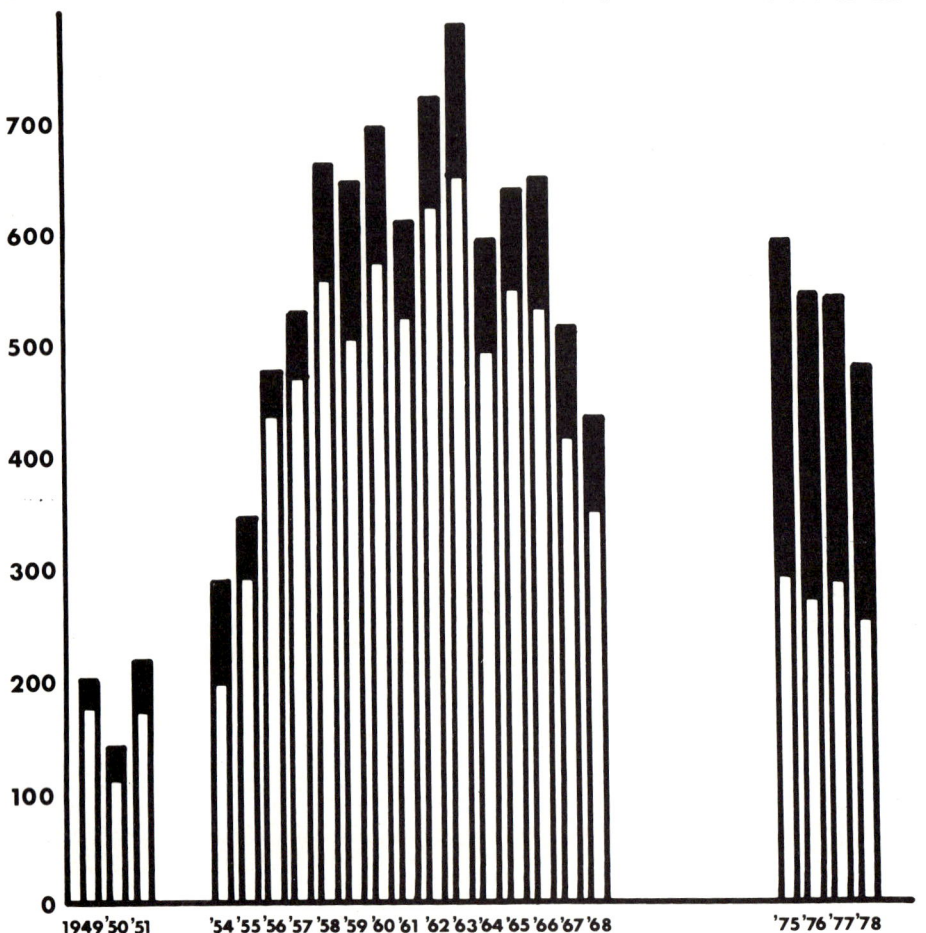

Fig. 1. Total number of confirmed poisoning incidents involving ☐ lead, and ■ all other materials, in all animals between 1949 and 1978.

relatively greater contribution made to the total losses due to intoxication by materials other than lead.

Due to differences in the nature of the materials involved and in the detail available, when defining the substances causing intoxication and apparent differences between animal species the situation from 1949-1958, 1959-1968 and 1975-1978 must be considered separately. During 1949-1958 the apparent order of decreasing relative importance for the main toxic agents affecting animals collectively was lead, arsenic, zinc phosphide and phosphorus. The Chief Veterinary Officers reports for this period do not include data for individual species.

However, the 325 consecutive cases investigated by Orr (1952) suggest that lead was
the most important single cause of poisoning in cattle and that arsenic was also an
important hazard, while sodium chloride, <u>Taxus</u> <u>baccata</u>, phosphorus, copper and
nicotine also affected this species. The rodenticides phosphorus and zinc phosphide
and, although less important, sodium chloride were the main problem with poultry.
Sodium chloride and, to a lesser extent, lead affected pigs; while arsenic
represented by far the most serious difficulty with sheep. Data for individual
species are also unavailable for the period 1959-1968. However, lead apparently
remained the dominant overall toxic agent while arsenic, although still a
significant hazard, was usually less important than copper. Zinc phosphide, which
was no longer used as a rodenticide, was not included in data for this period.
Phosphorus, although still causing some losses, was of only relatively minor
importance. The situation between 1975-1978 is represented in Figs. 2, 3 and 4.
Fig. 2 includes the data for the number of confirmed incidents involving chemicals
in all animals from the 1976 VIDA. The numbers of plant poisoning incidents in
this figure have been compounded from the 1976 VIDA and the Animal Diseases Report
of the Ministry of Agriculture for 1978. The latter, which is the only available
source of such information, deals with the incidence of plant poisoning during the
two years April 1st, 1975 – March 31st, 1977. These values have been halved to give
average annual figures, rounded up to a whole number, and added to the appropriate
data from the 1976 VIDA to give the composite picture in Fig. 2. Fig. 2 indicates
that although lead remains the dominant individual problem sodium chloride, copper,
organochlorine and organophosphorus compounds, arsanilic acid and arsenic, basic
slag and mercury are also important. A number of other chemicals which are not so
important individually, and are dealt with later, also represent a significant
collective present day hazard. Fig. 2 shows that although <u>Pteridium</u> <u>aquilinum</u>,
<u>Brassica</u> species, <u>Senecio</u> <u>jacobea</u>, <u>Quercus</u> species, <u>Taxus</u> <u>baccata</u> and <u>Umbelliferae</u>,
such as <u>Oenanthe</u> <u>crocata</u>, were the most important individual plants, other species
also produce intoxication in animals.

The materials affecting individual species during 1978, which can be taken as
typical of recent years, are shown in Figs. 3 and 4. It can be seen that lead
remains the main hazard to cattle while <u>Pteridium</u> <u>aquilinum</u>, <u>Senecio</u> <u>jacobea</u> and
arsenic are also noteworthy. A variety of other plants and chemicals, which are
individually relatively less important make a significant collective contribution
to cattle losses. The possible identity of these plants is apparent from Fig. 2.
These chemicals that are grouped together and are not otherwise specified in the
VIDA (chemicals NOS) can include ammonium salts, basic slag, copper, fluoride,
mercury, molybdenum, organochlorine, organophosphorus and phenolic compounds,
phenothiazine and urea. The most important hazards to poultry were chemicals NOS,
lead and organochlorine and organophosphorus compounds.The former category would
include sodium chloride which is the most important single cause of poisoning in

310

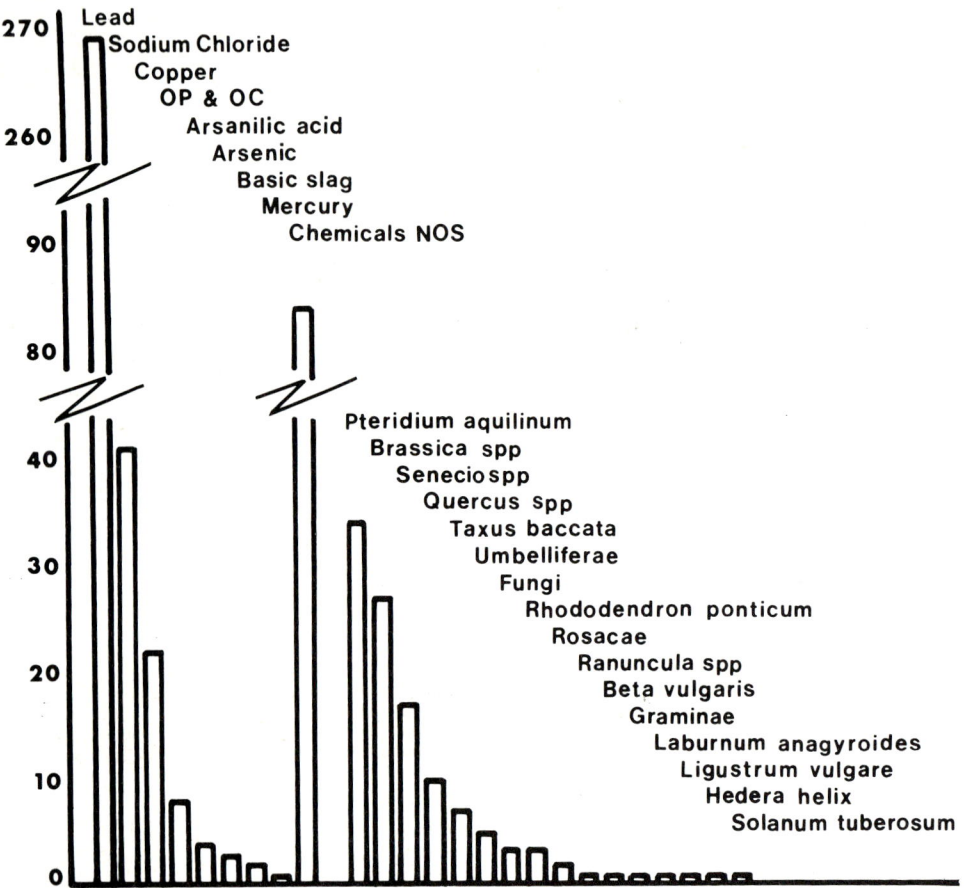

Fig. 2. The number of poisoning incidents due to various materials in all
animals during 1976. NOS - not otherwise specified.

poultry and which accounted for 55% of the recorded poisoning incidents in this
species compared with 19% for lead from 1975-1977. Ammonia, arsenic, mercury,
arsanilic acid, chloralose, ethylene glycol, metaldehyde, polychlorinated biphenyls
and sulfa drugs also affect birds. Although sodium chloride is the most important
problem, arsanilic acid also prevents a noteworthy hazard to pigs. Chemicals NOS
affecting this species include copper, hydrogen sulphide, hypochlorite, iron, lead,
mercury, nitrite, organochlorine and organophosphorus compounds, coal tar products,
furazolidone, procaine and warfarin. Oenanthe crocata, Pteridium aquilinum,
Solanum tuberosum (sprouting and green potato), and mouldy cereals also cause losses
in pigs. Although copper represents the most important single cause of poisoning in
sheep, Brassica species and, to a lesser extent, basic slag, Pteridium aquilinum,
lead, organochlorine and organophosphorus compounds are also noteworthy. Unspecifi
agents affecting this species include the chemicals arsenic, cobalt, lead, seleniu

carbon tetrachloride, formaldehyde and xylene, and the plants <u>Dryopteris</u> <u>filix-mas</u> and <u>Quercus</u> species.

The other species worthy of consideration, but for which numerical data are unavailable, are cats and dog. Materials that have caused intoxication in cats

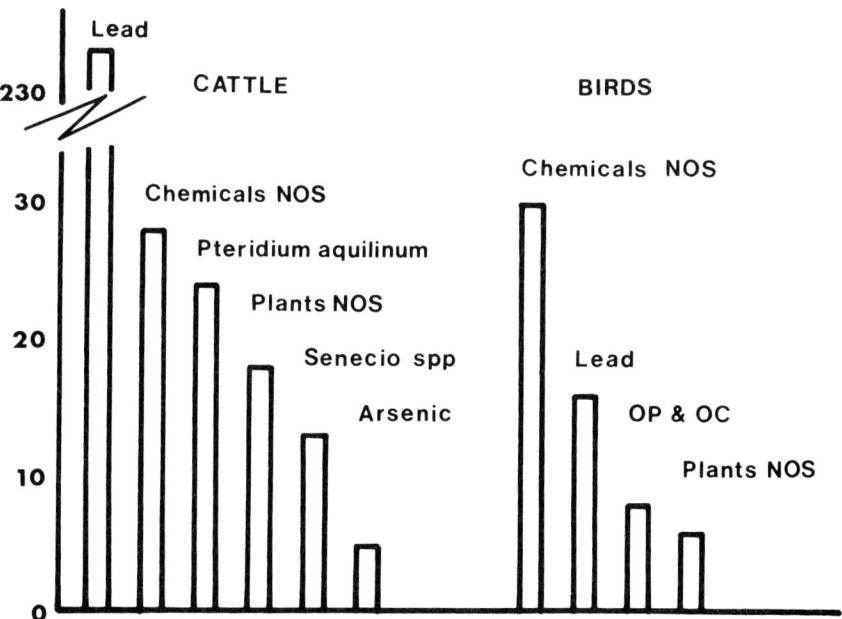

Fig. 3. Number of confirmed poisoning incidents due to various materials in cattle and birds during 1978. NOS - not otherwise specified.

include rodenticides, aspirin and paracetamol employed in owner medication, benzoic acid meat preservative, barbiturates and chloral hydrate euthanasic agents in meat, benzyl benzoate, carbon monoxide, ethylene glycol, metaldehyde in proprietary slug baits, nitrite in preserved meat, pentachlorophenol wood-preservative in sawdust litter, organochlorine and organophosphorus compounds, paraquat, strychnine, and vitamin A in liver. House plants such as <u>Solanum</u> <u>pseudocapsicum</u>, can also prove hazardous to this species. The materials affecting dogs include lead, mercury, sodium chloride, rodenticides, acrolein liberated from overheated fat-containing cooking pans, barbiturates, chloral hydrate and fluoroacetamide in meat, ethylene glycol, a variety of human medicaments, metaldehyde, nicotine, organochlorine and organophosphorus compounds, paraquat, strychnine, theobromine in chocolate, and plants such as <u>Laburnum</u> <u>anagyroides</u> and <u>Rhododendron</u> species.

Despite the difficulty of obtaining data representative of the situation in the field some tentative conclusions may be drawn from available information. Although

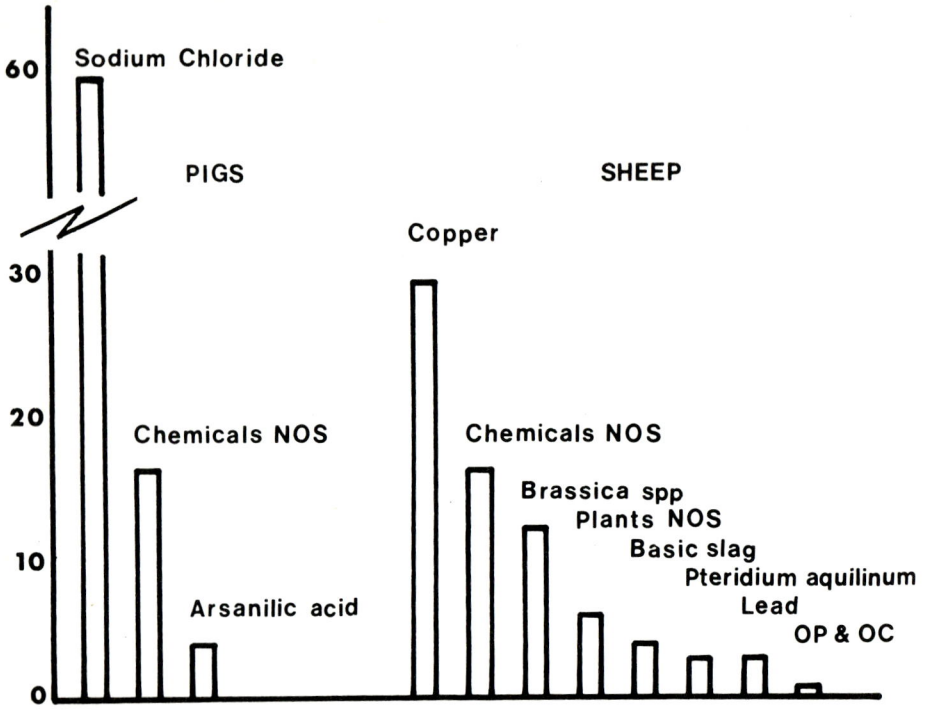

Fig. 4. Number of confirmed poisoning incidents due to various materials in
pigs and sheep during 1978. NOS - not otherwise specified.

the number of confirmed incidents of poisoning involving this material increased
considerably during 1949-1963 and declined thereafter lead has remained the dominant
individual toxic factor throughout the period considered. The total number of confirmed poisoning incidents also declined after 1963 but, due to the increasing
relative importance of materials other than lead in recent years, this trend has
not been maintained. The most important toxic materials recorded during 1949-1958;
1959-1968 and 1975-1978 were lead, arsenic, phosphorous, zinc phosphide and sodium
chloride; lead, copper, arsenic and sodium chloride; and lead, sodium chloride,
copper, Pteridium aquilinum, Brassica species, Senecio jacobea, Quercus species
and organochlorine and organophosphorus compounds. Poisonous plants, which were
probably equally important then, were not included in the data for the two earlier
periods. The rodenticides phosphorus and zinc phosphide were only significant
hazards during 1949-1958; and arsenic has become rather less important over the
years. Copper, which became noteworthy from 1959 onwards, remains an important
toxic agent. The toxicological significance of the pesticides warfarin, organochlorine and organophosphorus compounds and of mycotoxins has become apparent in
recent years. Considering individual species, lead has remained the most important
toxic agent to cattle throughout. The other important individual hazards to this

species have been arsenic, <u>Pteridium aquilinum</u>, <u>Senecio jacobea</u> and <u>Quercus</u> species. Although other materials have become relatively more important in recent years, the main toxic hazards to cattle have probably remained essentially unchanged. During 1975-1978 inclusive, lead, <u>Pteridium aquilinum</u> and <u>Senecio jacobea</u> accounted for 74%, 9% and 5% of the cattle poisoning incidents confirmed by the Veterinary Investigation Centres in the U.K. In poultry, phosphorus, zinc phosphide, sodium chloride and lead were probably the most important individual toxic agents during 1949-1958. During 1975-1977 inclusive, sodium chloride, lead and organochlorine and organophosphorus compounds were responsible for 55%, 19% and 7% of recorded poultry poisoning incidents. It appears that while sodium chloride and lead have remained important throughout, the nature of the pesticides affecting birds has changed. In the case of pigs, during 1949-1958 sodium chloride and lead were probably the greatest problem, and between 1975-1977 sodium chloride and arsanilic acid were implicated in 69% and 7% of confirmed poisoning losses in this species respectively. Although sodium fluoride, zinc phosphide, and phosphorus poisoning have been replaced by arsanilic acid, organophosphorus compound and warfarin intoxication in more recent years, sodium chloride has remained the main toxic hazard to pigs. Arsenic appears to have been by far the most important toxic agent to sheep during 1949-1958 whereas during 1975-1977 inclusive, copper and <u>Brassica</u> species which were the most important problems accounted for 35% and 14% of confirmed sheep poisoning losses respectively.

ACKNOWLEDGEMENTS

The author wishes to thank Mr. J.B.J. Stodulski for preparing the figures, Mr. D. Woulds for photographic assistance, Mrs. M. Howes for typing the manuscript, Mr. G. Davies and Mrs. J. Whaley for providing some of the data, and Professor D.G. Harvey for reading the manuscript.

REFERENCES
Orr, A.B. (1952) Veterinary Record 64: 339.
VIDA. Ministry of Agriculture, Fisheries & Food. The Epidemiology Unit, Central Veterinary Laboratory, Weybridge, Surrey, England.

POISONING OF DOMESTIC ANIMALS AS AN INDICATION OF ENVIRONMENTAL POLLUTION

M. DEBACKERE

Institute for Veterinary Pharmacology and Toxicology

Faculty of Veterinary Medecine, R.U.G.

Casinoplein 24, B-9000 GENT (Belgium)

ABSTRACT

Environmental pollution control becomes more and more a general hygienic problem
For some industrial pollutants their perciptible properties will be sufficient to
alarm human beings residing in the vicinity of the industrial plant. For others
with a cumulative character the presence of domestic animals as indicators can
be of great value. In this paper a survey will be given of some environmental
pollutions which occured in our country and which could be detected thanks to
poisonings in animals. Among them heavy metals and other metalloids or non metal
pollutants. The particular sensitivity of some livestock species is discussed also

INTRODUCTION

Already in the fifth century A.D. the Roman Emperor Justinian the Great included
in the Corpus Juris Civilis 'Aerem corrumpere non licet', it's forbidden to pollute
the air. (ref. 10)

The anthropogenic air pollution provoked through civilisation has occupied
mankind already during two millennia. Air pollution control, however has become
a general hygienic problem only during the twentieth century.

In the beginning of the revolutionary changes in industry attention was drawn
only to the possible direct dangers of air pollutants for human beings. Gradually however, dangers and damages were increasing in such a manner that they
led to a deterioration in the quality of the human environment. Considerable
progress has been made in the protection of the environment and the fight
against air pollution, only starting after the end of the second world war, on
the one side because of the improvement of the analytical methods used for
detection and control, on the other side thanks to the efforts of a wide variety
of different individuals and groups which have forced National Governments to
pay careful attention to the environment by the promulgation of legislations.
(ref. 13)

Therefore, notions such as emission and immission are used since that time. Both processes lead to economic and social harmful consequences such as damages to vegetation and adverse effects on human and animal health.

AIR POLLUTION AND ITS CONSEQUENCE FOR MEN AND ANIMALS

Mainly three sources can be held responsible for the pollution of the atmosphere through emissions of air pollutants.

Besides the combustion of fossil fuels for house heating and the exhaust emissions from motor vehicles, industrial emissions contribute to a great extent to the pollution with a wide variation of toxic substances in very different compositions and concentrations. (ref. 19)

Air pollution by industrial sources however also means an intermediate step in the pollution of water and soil because the greatest number of pollutants emitted are deposited. These superficial deposits on plant foodstuffs, consumed by humans are commonly removed or reduced in concentrations by washing or discarding the surface layers. The deposits on feed plants consumed by domestic animals on the contrary are not removed by washing and are therefore ingested along with the plant tissues. Therefore one can say in the case of air pollution that intoxications will be provoked predominantly by inhalation for human beings and by ingestion for domestic animals. Investigations for the damages in animals and animal production due to industrial air pollution however remained for a long time neglected by the environmental toxicology. Only step by step it was accepted by toxicologists and veterinary clinicians that neither the deposit of dust nor the inhalation of gases, but the intake of specific toxic or accumulative pollutants with fodder plants was the most suitable source of industrial poisoning in domestic animals. With the industrial revolution after the second world war however experiences have learned that the presense of domestic animals in the neighbourhood of industrial plants can be a very helpful aid for the detection of emissions and immissions of toxic substances.

DOMESTIC ANIMALS AS INDICATORS

For the detection of most current gaseous pollutants the smell or the irritation of the respiratory tract will be sufficient to alarm population. In the case however of the immission of substances without perciptible properties but with a very strong cumulative character the presence of domestic animals on pastures in the vicinity of the immission sources can be of an unexpected value. By eating day by day the contaminated vegetation as such a progressive accumulation will occur till the no effect level will be surpassed and clinical symptoms will appear, even at a stage that human beings will not have any idea about the presence of an environmental pollution.

In this paper we will give a survey of some important environmental pollutions which occurred during the last years in the Flemisch Countryside of Belgium with severe dangers for humans and which were diagnosed at our laboratory thanks to the clinical symptoms and toxicological analytical data in poisoned domestic animals.

EMISSIONS OF HEAVY METALS

Copper

In 1971 and 1974 our laboratory was consulted in connection with the death of different sheep. All animals were grazing on pastures in the vicinity of a copper smelting works. As well the clinical signs as the postmortem changes were characteristic for a chronic copper poisoning. (ref. 4) Liver copper concentrations were determined in five animals and varied between 900 and 2300 ppm on a dry weight basis. The sheep liver stores copper more readily than that of other animal species and a copper concentration of 30-150 ppm dry weight is normally present. (ref. 3) When it reaches 400 ppm dry weight, the animal is predisposed to copper poisoning. Analyses of soil samples showed values between 18 and 130 ppm against 3-10 ppm for immissionfree areas. Grass samples contained as much as 100 ppm copper on a dry weight basis.

Sheep are more susceptible than any other animal species to excess copper especially when molybdenum is deficient in their diet and the copper-to-molybdenum ratio is greather than 10:1. (ref. 5) Forage copper levels of 20 ppm on a dry matter basis are critical for sheep and levels of 30-40 ppm are toxic without discussion. This means that already small increases above the normal grass copper levels of 8-15 ppm, will be toxic for sheep and therefore sheep can be accepted as a very good indicator for environmental pollutions by copper emissions.

Lead

During the last years we detected two serious cases of environmental lead immissions thanks to several outbreaks of poisoning in domestic animals. Air pollution was provoked in one case by motor vehicle emissions and in the other by fumes and dusts emitted from a non-ferrous metal smelter, both the most important sources of current air pollution by lead as mentioned by Murozumi. (ref. 15)

In the first case six calves showed over a period of three weeks severe signs of central nervous stimulation and acute death occured. All animals were obliged to graze on a pasture in the north-eastern corner of a speedway crossing at maximum 200 meter of the speedway border. Besides the clinical symptoms and post mortem findings which let suspect a lead poisoning, chemical analysis gave following results : liver and kidneys 5-15 and 13-32 ppm respectively on a wet weight basis, grass and soil samples till 80 and 140 ppm respectively on dry weight basis. According to Ter Haar (ref. 18) 30% of the tetra-ethyl-lead used in Petrol are deposited as inorganic lead on the vegetation on either side of the roadway. The lead content decreases rapidly, however, with distance from the roadway. Motto (ref. 14) found levels as high as 225 ppm dry weight grass immediately adjacent to roadways decreasing to 50 ppm at 68 m from the road.

The second case however was one of the heaviest industrial lead pollutions ever known in Belgium.

During the spring of 1973 ten milch-cows on the same farm suddenly over a period of one week showed very severe signs of intermittent central nervous convulsions. Local investigations revealed that all animals since two to three weeks were fed with hay forage coming from pastures arounding one of the greatest non ferrous metals smelters of Belgium. During the following six months a total of 19 cows died on different farms all situated within maximum two kilometers from the lead industry. Liver and kidney levels reached 165 and 520 ppm respectively on wet weight basis. Also seven horses died with the typical sign of paralysis of the recurrent laryngeal nerve and aspiration pneumonia. Liver and kidney levels rised to 96, respectively 52 ppm wet weight.

There are some contradictory conclusions with regard to the susceptibility between domestic animals for lead poisoning. Some authors (ref. 6, 16) pretent that horses can tolerate a double dose in comparison to cattle. Aronson (ref. 1) found that the exposure for 2 months of a dosage of 5-6 mg/kg proved lethal in some cattle, while only 1,7 mg/kg fed for several months was fatal to horses. However a consideration of the grazing habits of horses precludes any firm conclusions. (ref. 2) Horses will pull forage together with the roots and eat the roots with the attached soil which usually contains far greater amounts of lead than the forage itself. Moreover, poisoning in cattle is mostly acute, in horses more chronic. In the opinion of some authors (ref. 11) cumulative toxicity of lead takes place as well in cattle as in horses. In cattle, lead accumulation evolves progressively without symptoms till liver levels attein their limit at which moment clinical signs of central nervous system stimulation are exhibited with an acute character. In horses on the other hand clinical signs appear already very early and evolve parallel with the accumulation but they show more peripheral nerve involvement and gastrointestinal disturbances.

Normal lead concentrations in forages from immissionfree areas in our country amount to an everage of 10 ppm dry weight basis. We know that pasture grass containing between 50 and 80 μg lead/gr dry weight is toxic to cows and to horses

and the total diet for humans even residing near smelters, only consists for a
small fraction of food grown in the vicinity, and this is washed before its
consumption. We therefore can agree that horses and cattle are very good indicators
for an environmental lead pollution already before resident population would be
affected.

EMISSIONS OF OTHER POLLUTANTS

Besides heavy metals a lot of other substances can pollute the environment in
the form of gases, fumes or dusts. For three of them we have known a series of
environmental pollutions which were detected thanks to the presence of animals.

Arsenic

In April 1971 about 10 to 15 million of bees died on their first flight after
their winter sleep. This occurred in an area eastwards to south-eastwards of
the same smelter as already cited for lead. Blossoms of willow-trees, the only
flower at that moment, contained 15 to 54 ppm arsenic on dry weight basis. A
concentration of 0,23 µg Arsenic was found per bee. Industrial poisoning due to
arsenic-bearing emissions is one of the most commonly occuring industrial poisonings in bees because bees are very susceptible to arsenic. (ref. 9) An amount
of 0,7 - 0,6 µg arsenic per bee is found in poisoned bees, while for normal
bees these amounts vary between 0 and 0.05 µg per bee.

Cyanides

Two cases of severe cyanide poisoning caused by industrial pollution were
identified at our laboratory. In both cases several cows, pigs and even water
birds died immediately after drinking water of a watercourse in the neighbourhood
of a metal cleaning factory. For the first one pollution was caused by fumes
escaping from the factory through windows just above the course, the second was
provoked by polluted waste waters. Concentrations varied between 14 and 54 mg
cyanides per liter, while quality criteria for farmstead uses recommend that
levels above 0,2 mg/l are grounds for rejection of a supply. (ref. 17)   The
minimum lethal dose given per os is of the order of 1-2 mg/kg body weight.
(ref. 12)

Fluorides

For fluoride emissions also some livestock species, in particular cattle and
more specifically milch-cows, are very good indicators, at the one side because
they are vegetarians and at the other side because they show a very active
calcium metabolism. In our country also we were recently confronted with some
severe environmental fluoride pollutions.

A first case was characterized by a very extensive spread and was caused by an enamel factory. Different cows, sheep and horses had to be slaughtered and at least 500 animals, mostly milch-cows were affected by fluorosis. In humans, however there were no definite proofs for fluorosis till now. Further details of this case will be published in a separate paper but fluoride determinations revealed concentrations till 125 ppm for urine, 400 ppm for grass-forage and 15 000 ppm for bone samples. Based on the dental lesions the beginning of the fluoride overload seemed to have occurred already 4 years earlier.

Another case was limited to one farm situated around a brickworks. (ref.7,8) The total herd consisted of 18 lactating cows 17 of which were affected. All the pastures of the farm were situated around the plant.

Most reviews indicate that natural pasture fluoride contents are between 5 and 10 ppm (dry weight). A concentration of 30 ppm in forage is accepted as the upper non-damaging limit for dairy cows. (ref. 10) For all the pastures examined this level was reached or exceeded during different months. Clay and stone dust originating from coal mines, both used in the brick fabrication process, contained 307 respectively 652 ppm fluoride.

In living animals diagnosis of fluorosis can be made by dental examination and fluoride determinations of the urine. According to Clarke (ref. 4) values of 15 ppm and above are considered as indicating ingestion of abnormal quantities of fluoride, while values above 10 ppm are suspect. Others (ref. 10) accept concentrations under 10 ppm as normal for non-polluted areas. All animals showed concentrations above 15 ppm so that there was no doubt that the total herd was affected by fluorosis.

Based on the dental lesions it could be concluded that the fluorosis was endemic to the farm since the first incisors were already affected only for the animals born and reared on the farm. From the data of eruption and crown formation it could be calculated that fluoride pollution started already 5 years before.

In this limited time we have tried to give a survey of a series of environmental pollutions from our experience as veterinary toxicologist. Some of them represented a very serious danger for human beings, but they could be detected already before damages were provoked to humans, thank to the occurrence of poisonings in domestic animals. These cases prove that animals can be very sensitive indicators and that for the study of environmental pollutions the co-operation between environmental toxicologists and veterinary toxicologists can be of great value for the protection of human health.

REFERENCES

1. A.L. ARONSON. Amer. J. Vet. Res., 33 (1972), 627.

2. A.L. ARONSON. "Outbreaks of Plumbism in Animals, associated with industrial Lead Operations" in "Toxicity of Heavy Metals in the Environment", F.W. Oehme, 1978, Marcel Dekker Ed. New York.

3. B.W. BUCK. "Copper/Molybdenum Toxicity in Animals" in "Toxicity of Heavy Metals in the Environment", F.W. Oehme, 1978, Marcel Dekker Ed. New York.

4. E.G.C. CLARKE and M.L. CLARKE. Veterinary Toxicology, 1975, Baillière Tindall Ed. London.

5. I.J. CUNNINGHAM. N.Z. J. Sci. Tech., 27 (1946), 372.

6. P.W. DANCKWORTT. Dtsch. Tierärztl. Wschr., 47 (1939), 277.

7. M. DEBACKERE and F.T. DELBEKE. Intern. J. Envir. Studies, 11 (1978), 245.

8. M. DEBACKERE and F.T. DELBEKE, Intern. J. Envir. Studies, 13 (1979), 225.

9. J.A. DOLOTOVSKAYA. Bull. Apic. Inform., 5 (1962), 9.

10. H.D. GRÜNDER. "Fluorimmissionwirkungen auf Rinder", Habilitationsschrift (Hannover 1970).

11. P.B. HAMMOND and A.L. ARONSON. Ann. N.Y. Acad. Sci., 111, (1964), 595.

12. H.J. HAPKE. "Toxikologie für Veterinärmediziner", 1975, F. Enke Verlag, Stuttgart.

13. L. HODGES. "Environmental Pollution", 2nd Ed., 1977, Holt, Rinehart and Winston Ed. New York.

14. H.L. MOTTO, R.H. DAINES, D.M. CHILKO and C.K. MOTTO. Environ Sci.Technol., 4, (1970), 231.

15. M. MUROZUMI, CHOW, J. TSAIHWA and C. PATTERSON. Geochem. Cosmochim. Acta, 33, (1969), 1247.

16. O. ROEMMELE. Tierärztl. Umschau, 5, (1950), 109.

17. I. SUNSHINE. Handbook of Analytical Toxicology, 1969, The Chemical Rubber Co, Ohio, p. 754.

18. G. TER HAAR. "Lead in the Environment" in "Lead", T.B. Griffin and J.H. Knelson, 1975, Georg Thieme Verlag Stuttgart.

19. J. TESINK. Tijdschr. Diergeneesk., 92, (1967), 1751.

EFFECTS OF LEVAMISOLE ON RESPONSES OF FLUKE-INFECTED AND FLUKE-FREE RATS AND CATTLE TO *SALMONELLA DUBLIN*

M.M. AITKEN, P.W. JONES and D.L. HUGHES

A.R.C. Institute for Research on Animal Diseases, Compton, Nr. Newbury, Berks., U.K.

SYNOPSIS

The predisposition of fluke-infected rats and cattle to lethal or persistent infection with *S. dublin* may be due to impairment of immune responses, including bacterial phagocytosis by neutrophils. Levamisole given before challenge with *S. dublin* reduced the mortality rate in rats but not in cattle. Immunostimulant effects of levamisole were not detected in cattle.

ON LONG TERM TOXICITY OF ZINC-ETHYLENDITHIOCARBAMATE (ZINEB) IN CHICKENS TREATED SINCE THEIR FIRST DAY OF LIFE

M. GENNARO SOFFIETTI

Istituto di Patoligia generale ed Anatomia patologica Veterinaria, Torino (Italia)

ABSTRACT

Chicks were fed ad libitum from the age of 1 day with poultry feed containing Zineb at 2.1%. The animals were observed after 2, 3, 10, 12, 18 and 24 months. After 2 months a thyroidal struma was already manifest and it grew progressively worse in time.

One thyroid was found to weigh 43.38 g after 10 months of treatment. Histologically a picture of colloidal struma was found, characterized by a striking cellular desquamation in the alveoli and hyperplasia of the epithelium of the follicles which after 18 and 24 months' treatment assumed papillomatous-like aspects associated with large interstitial hemorrhages and sclerosis of the intrafollicular wall.

The microfollicular formations were still quite numerous. Zineb residues in thyroids were determinated. It is concluded that this research is interesting both in its toxicological and comparative pathological aspects.

INVESTIGATION OF THE RESIDUAL AMOUNT OF THE ß-BLOCKING AGENT CARAZOLOL
IN TISSUES OF PIGS

W. BARTSCH, K. KOCH, K. VOLLERS, G. SPONER and K. DIETMANN
Forschungslaboratorien der Boehringer Mannheim GmbH (G.F.R.)

Abstract
   Carazolol, an extremely potent ß-blocking agent (ref. 1;2), is used
for the prevention of sudden death and in emergencies in pigs (ref.3).
In relation to the usual food intake in humans, the ADI-values are not
reached at all (37 %, 2 hours after administration). From the point of
view of food regulations it seems, therefore, to be acceptable to waive
the specific withdrawal period between administration and slaughtering.

Introduction
   The ß-blocking agent carazolol is useful in pigs for the prevention
of sudden cardiac death and disorders due to stress situations. For
all drugs administered in emergencies, the residual amount of drug in
the tissues must be investigated in order evaluate the risk to humans
who eat meat from such treated animals.

Method
   The effective dose (1 mg per 100 kg i.m. body weight) was injected
as ^{14}C-carazolol into castrated boars. The pigs were stressed by
transport in a lorry for 90 min and were killed at 2 (n = 6), 8 (n =
2) or 16 hours (n = 2) after carazolol administration. The ^{14}C-ac-
tivity counted in the different tissues was assumed to be representi-
tive of the residual amount of carazolol.

Results and discussion
   The amount of the drug was determined in muscle, liver, kidney and
fat, which are all of interest for human intake. Taking into account
the usual daily intake (see below), the theoretical total intake of
carazolol is shown in fig. 1 (4.44 mcg for 2 hours). The acceptable
daily intake (ADI-value) was calculated according the following equa
tion:

$$\text{ADI-Value} \quad = \quad \frac{20 \text{ mcg/kg p.o. (N E D R) x 60 kg (H B W)}}{100 \text{ (safety factor)}} \quad 12 \text{ mcg}$$

N E D R = No effect dose rabbit; H B W = human body weight.
The values for carazolol-equivalent in mg/1000 g tissue are as follows:

Tissue(usual daily intake in g by humans)	Hours after injection		
	2	8	16
Muscle (300)	1.77	0.4	0.08
Liver (100)	28.40	4.82	11.18
Kidney (50)	17.52	3.67	3.69
Fat (50)	3.71	13.62	0.014

In terms of the usual food intake, the amount which might be ingested 2 hours after injection would be 37 % of the ADI-value, and after 8 or 16 hours only 12 %.

Reference: 1 = W. BARTSCH, K. DIETMANN, H. LEINERT, G. SPONER; Arzneim. Forsch./Drug. Res. 27, 1022 - 1026 (1977). 2 = R.B. INNIS, F.M.A. CORREA and S. H. SNYDER; Life Sciences 22, 2255 - 2264 (1979).3 = E. u. K. FIEBIGER, K.J. NITZ, K. VOLLERS, W. BARTSCH; Tierärztl. Umschau 33 Jg. 10, 531 - 536 (1978).

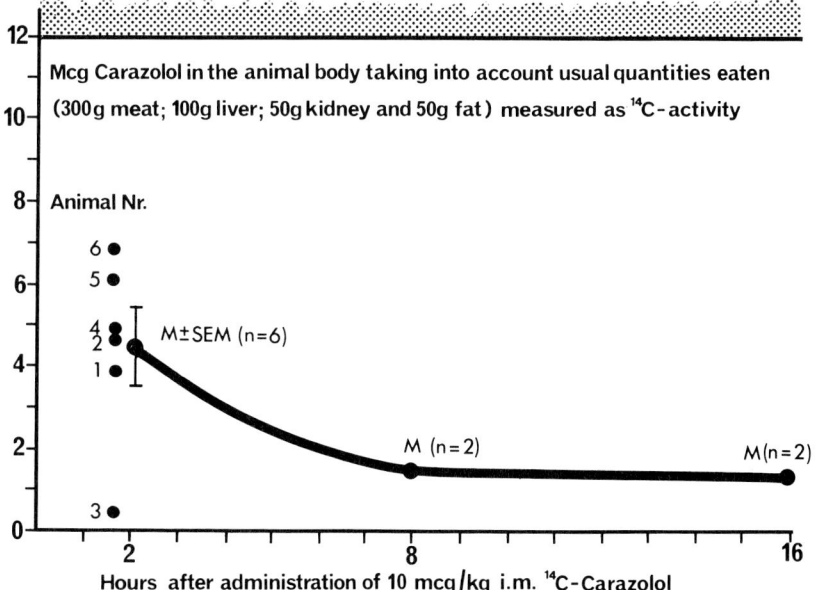

Mcg Carazolol in the animal body taking into account usual quantities eaten (300g meat; 100g liver; 50g kidney and 50g fat) measured as ^{14}C-activity

Animal Nr.

M±SEM (n=6)

M (n=2)   M(n=2)

Hours after administration of 10 mcg/kg i.m. ^{14}C-Carazolol

SULFUR-CONTAINING AMINO ACIDS AS PRECURSORS OF BRONCHIAL-SEEKING METHYL SULFONE METABOLITES OF 2,4',5-TRICHLOROBIPHENYL IN MICE

Å. BERGMAN[1], I. BRANDT[2], Y. LARSSON[2] and C.A. WACHTMEISTER[1]

1) Section of Organic Chemistry, Environmental Toxicology Unit, Wallenberg Laboratory, University of Stockholm, S-106 91 Stockholm, Sweden.
2) Department of Pharmacology, Biomedical Centre, Faculty of Veterinary Medicine, The Swedish University of Agricultural Sciences, Box 573, S-751 23 Uppsala, Sweden.

ABSTRACT

In order to investigate the origin of the sulfur atom in methyl sulfone metabolites of polychlorinated biphenyls, groups of mice were dosed with 2,4',5-trichlorobiphenyl and ^{35}S-methionine or ^{35}S-cysteine. Control groups received the labelled amino acids only. The biphenyl used is known to be metabolized to two methylsulfonyltrichlorobiphenyls, which accumulate in the murine lung. Thus, extracts of lungs were analyzed by partition between hexane and sulfuric acid, thin layer radiochromatography (TLRC), gas chromatography (GC) and mass fragmentography (MF). The lungs of mice injected with both trichlorobiphenyl and ^{35}S-labelled methionine or cysteine contained radioactive compound(s) soluble in conc. sulfuric acid. TLRC of a re-extract from diluted sulfuric acid gave a radioactive spot at $R_f = 0.21$ corresponding to the R_f-value of 4-methylsulfonyl-2,4',5-trichlorobiphenyl. The corresponding extracts of mice treated with the labelled amino acids only did not contain any significant amounts of radioactivity. GC and MF verified the occurrence of one major and one minor methylsulfonyltrichlorobiphenyl in the TLRC-spots with $R_f = 0.21$.

INTRODUCTION

The transformation routes of foreign compounds in vivo to sulfur-containing metabolites such as thiols, methyl sulfides, methyl sulfoxides and methyl sulfones have attended great interest during the latest years. We recently showed that polychlorobiphenyls (PCB) with specific chlorination patterns (chlorine atoms at least in positions 2,4',5 and hydrogen atoms in positions 3,3',6 and 6') are metabolized to methyl sulfones, which are accumulated in the bronchial mucosa of mice (except for 2,2',4,4',5,5'-hexachlorobiphenyl, which is most probably accumulated in the lung as such)[1]. Methyl sulfone metabolites of PCB have also been identified in adipose tissue of seals from the Baltic Sea[2], in faeces from mice treated with some single PCB's[3-5] and in milk and adipose tissue of a PCB-exposed Japanese woman[6].

In human lung tissue, these metabolites have not yet been identified, but in connection with PCB intoxication in man, clinical symptoms and pathological changes in the respiratory tract have been described[7]. These lesions may be correlated to the accumulation of methylsulfone metabolites observed in the bronchial mucosa.

The present investigation was performed in order to study if the sulfur atom in methionine and cysteine could be transferred to PCB during its transformation to methyl sulfones. 2,4'5-Trichlorobiphenyl, known to give methyl sulfides and sulfones[1], was given to mice followed by injection of ^{35}S-labelled methionine or cysteine. Control groups were treated with the labelled amino acids only.

RESULTS AND DISCUSSION

Hexane extracts of lungs from mice of each group were rocked with conc. sulfuric acid and the radioactivity was measured in the hexane phase. None of the two experimental and two control groups showed any activity in this fraction. The acidic phases were diluted with water and re-extracted with hexane followed by radioactivity determination. A high concentration of radioactivity was found in these extracts of the lungs of mice given 2,4',5-trichlorobiphenyl and ^{35}S-methionine or ^{35}S-cysteine, while no activity was present in the corresponding fractions of the control groups. Methyl sulfones of PCB are known to be solubilized in conc. sulfuric acid and the above results thus indicate the formation of ^{35}S-labelled methylsulfonyltrichlorobiphenyl(s). The extracts containing activity were transferred to TLC-plates and eluted with hexane:ethyl acetate (4:1). Radioactive material was localized with radiochromatogram scanning and autoradiography. Radioactive spots at R_f = 0.21 in the TLC-plates of both experimental groups were observed and correlated to that found for 4-methylsulfonyl-2,4',5-trichlorobiphenyl (R_f = 0.21). The labelled spots were scraped off, extracted and analyzed by GC. Two peaks within a narrow range were observed, the major one (with the longer retention time) showing the same retention time as 4-methylsulfonyl-2,4',5-trichlorobiphenyl. Mass fragmentography confirmed the occurrence of this compound in both extracts analyzed. The minor compound was shown to be an isomeric sulfone (MF). In conclusion, the present study shows that the sulfur atoms of both methionine and cysteine can be precursors of the methyl sulfone groups of methyl sulfones derived from PCB.

REFERENCES AND ACKNOWLEDGEMENTS

1. Å. Bergman, I. Brandt and B. Jansson, Toxicol. Appl. Pharmacol., 48, 213 (1979). - 2. S. Jensen and B. Jansson, Ambio, 5, 257 (1976). - 3. T. Mio, K. Sumino and T. Mizutani, Chem. Pharm. Bull., 24, 1958 (1976). - 4. T. Mizutani, K. Yamamoto and K. Tajima, J. Agric. Food Chem., 26, 862 (1978). - 5. T. Mizutani, Bull. Environm. Contam. Toxicol., 20, 219 (1978). - 6. S. Yoshida and A. Nakamura, J. Food Hyg. Soc., 19, 185 (1978). - 7. N. Shigematsu et al., Environm. Research, 16, 92 (1978).

The study was supported by the Research Committee of the National Swedish Environment Protection Board. Dr B. Jansson is acknowledged for running the mass spectra.

THE EFFECTS OF POLYCHLORINATED NAPHTALENES (PCN) ON METAMORPHOSIS OF RANA
AGILIS TADPOLES

S. SIVIERI BUGGIANI

Institute of General Pathology and Pathological Anatomy, Veterinary Medicine
Faculty, Pisa (Italy)

ABSTRACT

   Rana agilis tadpoles exposed to concentrations of 0.1 and 0.05 ppm of
commercial PCN (Halhowax 1014) metamorphosed 3 weeks later than a control group.
Histological changes in the endocrine glands were also noted.

INTRODUCTION

   PCNs are known in veterinary pathology and in occupational medicine as
causative agents of X-disease of cattle and chloracne in humans (1,2).

   They are industrial compounds with physical and chemical properties similar
to organohalogenated pollutants, widely used in a variety of technical products.
They are introduced into the environment unintentionally via industrial discharges. Recently PCNs have been reported to be present in environmental samples
together with other chlorinated pollutants such as the PCBs and PCTs (3,4).

   Up to the present little has been known about the environmental behaviour,
fate and toxicity of the PCNs, and more attention should be given to establishing
the biological signifiance of PCN pollution (5).

   This synopsis summarizes the effects of low levels of a commercial PCN, Halhowax 1014, on frog (Rana agilis) tadpoles.

MATERIAL AND METHODS

   Four groups of 40 tadpoles (5 days old) were placed into 4 glass fish ponds
(50x35x20 cm) with gravel and some stones on the bottom, previously thoroughly
cleaned. Water was added to a suitable volume.

   The tadpoles were hatched in the laboratory from a batch of eggs laid by only
one frog, and collected from an unpolluted pool which also supplied the water
used in the experiment.

   The tadpoles were fed with boiled lettuce and fish food, and maintained at
room temperature (15°-21°) for 12 weeks.

   One group of tadpoles was retained as control. The other 3 groups were exposed respectively to concentrations of 0.2, 0.1, and 0.05 ppm of Halhowax 1014 in water. The highest of these concentrations proved to be fatal for 52% of larvae after 18 h.

This group was removed from the experiment. All the other tadpoles survived throughout the experiment. At the end of the experiment they were euthanized and fixed in 80% alcohol for histological investigation.

RESULTS AND DISCUSSION

The tadpoles maintained in clean water developed normally, being lively and reacting to stimulation. Those which developed in water containing PCN metamorphosed 3 weeks later than the control group. They reacted slowly to any stimulatic and had darker pigmentation. There was no difference between the groups treated with 0.1 and 0.05 ppm. However, tadpoles in a test group treated with KI and PCN started to metamorphose after 48-72 h.

From these findings it appears that PCN acts on the endocrine system which controls metamorphosis. It seems that the effect of PCN is a reversible one and can be counteracted by inorganic iodine.

The hypothesis of interference could be supported by research on different kinds of animal exposed to products closely related to PCNs such as PCB (6.7).

Histological changes in the endocrine glands were also noted.

REFERENCES

1. SMITH, H.A. and JONES, T.C., 1971. Veterinary Pathology, 2nd Ed. Lea & Febiger.

2. PATTY, F.A., 1967. Industrial Hygiene and Toxicology Vol. II. Interscience Publ., New York, London, Sydney.

3. VANNUCCHI, C. et al., 1978. Chemosphere, 6: 483.

4. McINTYRE, A.D. and MILLS, C.F., 1975. Ecological Toxicology Research Vol. VII. Plenum Press, New York, London.

5. IN CHU et al. 1977. Bull. Environ. Contam. Toxicol., 18 (2): 177.

6. JEFFERIES, D.J. and PARSLOW, J.L.F., 1972. Bull. Environ. Contam. Toxicol., 8: 306.

7. MOCCIA, R.D. et al., 1977. Science, 198: 425.

ORAL REHYDRATION TREATMENT OF PIGLET DIARRHOEA

R.J. BYWATER

Beecham Pharmaceuticals Research Division, Walton Oaks, Tadworth, Surrey.

Piglets with diarrhoea following experimental infection with enteropathogenic E.coli were given access to either a Glucose-Glycine Electrolyte Solution (GGES*) or to water. All were allowed to suckle normally. The mortality in the GGES group was significantly lower than in the control group, and the weight gain in severely diarrhoeic piglets was also greater in the treated piglets.

Gnotobiotic piglets challenged with pig rotavirus were given access to either ad lib GGES or milk. The GGES piglets showed uninterrupted growth in comparison with the controls.

It was concluded that oral rehydration with the GGES was effective in piglets with diarrhoea following either E. coli or rotavirus infection.

INTRODUCTION

Oral fluid replacement as a treatment of dehydration in diarrhoea has been successfully used in man (Ref.1) and in calves (Ref.2).

The principle is that active absorption of glucose and glycine in the small intestine is accompanied by water and sodium movement, which reverses the net loss occurring in diarrhoea. The present experiments were designed to show whether oral rehydration was effective in piglets with diarrhoea due to either enteropathogenic E. coli or rotavirus.

METHODS, RESULTS AND CONCLUSIONS

The GGES used* contained in the dry state, glucose (67.53%); sodium chloride (14.34%); glycine (10.3%); citric acid (0.81%); potassium citrate (0.21%) and potassium dihydrogen phosphate (6.8%). A weight of 64 g of the powder in 2 litres of water gave an isotonic solution.

E. coli experiment   Colostrum deprived piglets were challenged with a culture of enteropathogenic E. coli, and piglets were then given access to GGES or water in cube drinkers. A high proportion of challenged piglets showed diarrhoea within 12 hours. The results are shown in Table 1.

*Lectade ® ; Beecham Scour Formula ®; Resorb ®

Table 1. Mortality and weight gain in piglets experimentally challenged
with E. coli (*P<0.05)

	GGES	Control
Number	96	95
Mortality	11.6%	24%
Weight gain in piglets scouring >3 days (g/day ± SEM)	178* ± 5.8	150 ± 6.6

Rotavirus experiment Hysterectomy derived piglets were maintained in isolators,
and were challenged with pig rotavirus. This challenge had been shown to give
acute diarrhoea with weight loss lasting three days, followed by spontaneous
recovery. Piglets were either given continued milk feeding (controls) or were
given GGES ad lib for 3 days. On day one milk was withheld; and on day 2 and 3
milk was given at half strength.

The results (Fig.1) showed that the weight loss seen in the control pigs was
minimised in the pigs given access to GGES, showing that any mucosal damage caused
by rotavirus was insufficient to impair the rehydration produced by GGES.

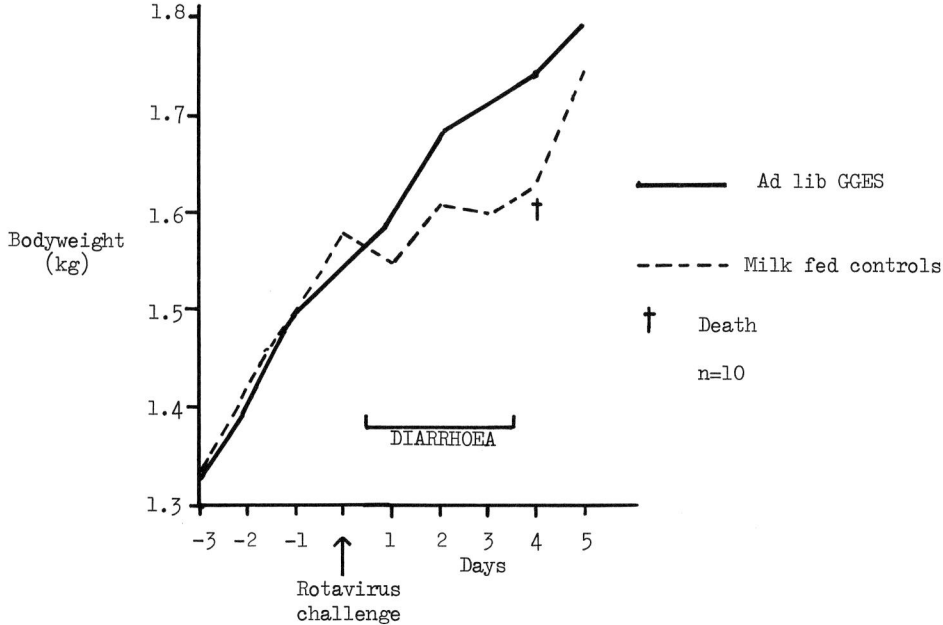

Fig.1 Weight gain in gnotobiotic piglets challenged with rotavirus. Controls were
milk fed, GGES had milk withheld for 1 day, and were given ad lib GGES for
3 days.

It was concluded that GGES was effective in either rotavirus or E. coli diarrhoea
in piglets.

REFERENCES   1. Nalin, D.R. & Cash, R.A. (1970) Trans.Roy.Soc.Trop.Med. 64, 769
2. Bywater, R.J. (1977) Am J Vet Res, 38, 1983

THE EFFECT OF AMMONIUM IONS ON THE MOTILITY OF THE SMALL INTESTINE

S. GARWACKI, K. SOWA and M. DUTKIEWICZ
Institute of Animal Physiology, Agricultural University, Warsaw, Poland.

ABSTRACT

Experiments are presented which show ammonium chloride as a stimulator of
intestinal motility. It is suggested that ammonium facilitates the action of
acetylcholine.

INTRODUCTION

Increased concentrations of ammonia in the blood of animals cause changes in
cell metabolism, and modify the effects of hormones and the action of the central
and peripheral nervous systems. Ammonia is always present in the intestinal contents and in the intestinal wall. Our experiments were aimed at establishing the
effects of ammonia on small intestine motility. They were carried out on three
sheep fitted with canulae into the distal duodenum. Hyperammonemia in sheep was
induced by a rapid intravenous injection or continuous infusions of ammonium
chloride. In order to define the "pure" intestinal effect of ammonia and the
possibility of its modification by drugs, experiments were also made in vitro
using rabbit and guinea pig intestines.

RESULTS

Intravenous injections of ammonium chloride (0.5-1.0 m mol/kg) or continuous
infusing to give blood ammonia concentrations of 0.3-0.5 m mol/dcm^3 caused a
marked increase in the amplitude of intestinal motility in sheep. Atropine in
large doses (0.5-1.0 mg/kg) prevented this effect. In vitro guinea pig and rabbit
intestines also responded to ammonium with an increase in the amplitude of motility. In the case of guinea pig, there was also an increase in tonus of the
smooth muscles. The stimulation of intestinal motility in some cases was preceded
by a transitory lowering of the muscular activity. Hexamethonium (5.0 mg/dcm^3)
and atropine (0.5 mg/dcm^3) blocked the effects of ammonia in vitro. It seems that
the observed stimulation of intestinal motility was mediated through an increased
sensitivity of the post-synaptic membrane to acetylcholine. It is unlikely, however, that ammonia affects only the cholinergic transmission in the intestinal

wall. Results from previous experiments indicate that the action of ammonia on rumen motility and metabolism in the whole animal is observed when smaller concentrations of ammonium chloride than 0.3 m mol/dcm^3 blood are present.

CONCLUSION

The findings suggest that stimulation of intestinal motility by the ammonium ion is mediated by facilitating the acetylcholine action on the intestine.

THE EFFICACY OF DISTOJECT[R] AGAINST ADULT *F.hepatica* IN CATTLE, EXCRETION IN MILK
AND TOLERANCE FOR THE MUSCLE FOLLOWING INTRAMUSCULAR ADMINISTRATION OF A DOSE OF
3 mg/kg.

C.A. LADAGE and H.A. van RIESSEN
ACF Chemiefarma NV, Maarssen (The Netherlands)

ABSTRACT

The injectable formulation Distoject[R] of the new anti-liver-fluke compound
nitroclofene is highly active against (adult) liver flukes in cattle after intramuscular administration of 3 mg/kg. The bio-availability of the compound is good.
Nitroclofene, - mainly eliminated with faeces and urine -, is excreted in milk
in only minor amounts.
The formulation has minor irritant effects on muscle.

INTRODUCTION

During the development of the new injectable anti-liver-fluke compound
nitroclofene for treatment of fascioliasis in ruminants, not only the efficacy
and tolerability, but also to the pharmacokinetic and pharmacodynamic behaviour
of the compound has been given much attention (1).

In this paper some efficacy results in cattle are presented as well as results
of experiments in respect of bio-availability of the compound in cattle, excretion
in milk and the tolerance for the muscles at the site of injection.

RESULTS

The results of the experiments are presented in Table 1 and in the Figures 1
and 2. The results with regard to the tolerance for the muscle are presented in
a paper published elsewhere in these Proceedings of the EAVPT Congress.

SUMMARY

The results presented in Table 1 show that after intramuscular administration
of Distoject[R] the dose of 3 mg nitroclofene/kg was highly active against

adult *F.hepatica* in cattle. Since 10-11 weeks after treatment 91% of the treated animals were free from *Fasciola* ova it may be assumed that also a good efficacy against younger flukes is obtained.

At the dose of 3 mg/kg a good bio-availability was obtained (Figure 1) while only minor amounts of nitroclofene were excreted in the milk, whereupon it was rapidly eliminated (Figure 2).

After intramuscular injection of 12 ml in the neck of cattle the irritancy to the muscle was comparable with that resulting from injection of a commercially available oxytetracycline formulation, whereas the reactions were much milder than after injection of chloramphenicol.

Table 1

Efficacy of nitroclofene in cattle with an adult liver_fluke infection

Exp.No	Dose_range mg/kg	n	External efficacy (weeks p.t.) *				
			2	4	5_6	8	10_11
1	2.5_2.7	24	96	96	83	79	75
1	2.8_3.2	81	99	99	95	93	91
2	2.8_3.1	15	100	100	100	100	nt
3	2.8_3.1	15	100	94	100	94	89
Mean	2.8_3.2	111	99.3	98.5	96.4	94.1	90.7

* : Reduction in EPG is not calculated as a positive effect

REFERENCE

(1) Ladage, C.A., 1979. The development of a new injectable anti-liver-fluke compound. Ph.D. Thesis, Utrecht University.

Figure 1

concentration in plasma (mg/l)

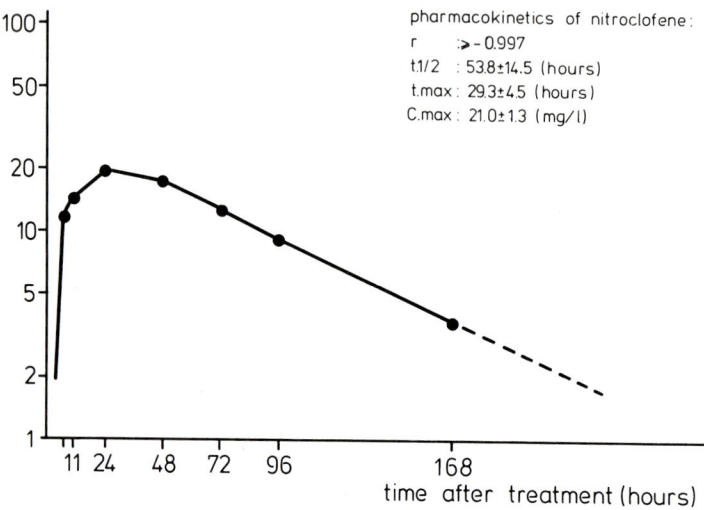

pharmacokinetics of nitroclofene:
r : > - 0.997
t.1/2 : 53.8±14.5 (hours)
t.max : 29.3±4.5 (hours)
C.max : 21.0±1.3 (mg/l)

time after treatment (hours)

Figure 2

concentration in milk (mg/l)

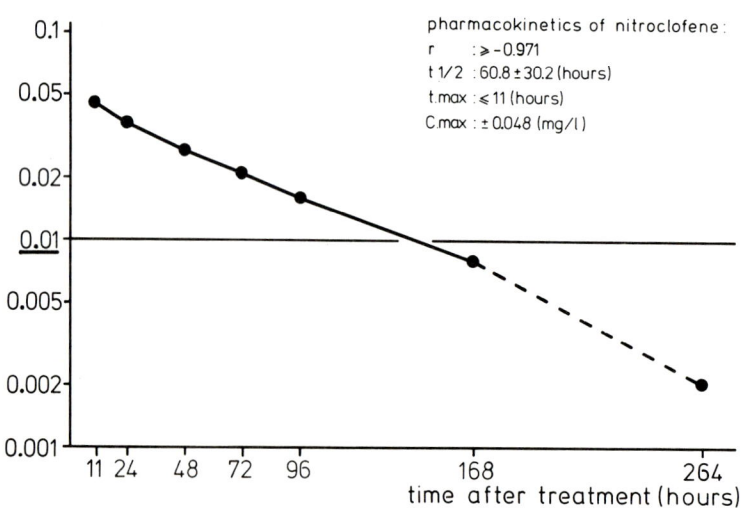

pharmacokinetics of nitroclofene:
r : > - 0.971
t 1/2 : 60.8±30.2 (hours)
t.max : ⩽ 11 (hours)
C.max : ± 0.048 (mg/l)

time after treatment (hours)

TRANQUILLIZER RESIDUES IN SLAUGHTER PIGS

M.OLLING, R.W.STEPHANY and A.G.RAUWS

National Institute of Public Health, Bilthoven, The Netherlands

ABSTRACT

Analytical methods have been developed to determine the content of veterinary tranquillizers azaperone and propiopromazine. Kidney tissue proved to be the most suitable sampling material to detect residues of these tranquillizers. The methods are applied to random sampled kidneys from locally produced or imported pigs, obtained from two slaughter houses in The Netherlands.

INTRODUCTION

Transport stress is an important cause of quality loss or even mortality in slaughter pigs (1). Tranquillizers are used to prevent or diminish this effect. The extent of this practice is not exactly known, its impact on public health still less (2). The effectiveness of tranquillizers is questioned (3) and selective breeding (4) or more careful transport (5) might provide alternatives. Here the results are presented of a pilot study of the presence of tranquillizer residues in slaughter pigs.

MATERIAL AND METHODS

Azaperone (Stresnil[R], Janssen, Beerse (Belgium)) was determined in 5 or 10 g of kidney tissue. An alkaline homogenate was ground with sand and anhydrous sodium sulfate. The dry mixture was extracted with petroleum ether. Clean up by back extraction and chromatography on alumina followed. The extract residue was analyzed by gas liquid chromatography (column: 3% OV 17 on Gas Chrom Q) using an alkali flame ionization detector. Besides azaperone in this also the active biotransformation product azaperol was detected and quantitated (6). In the range 20-100 ng/g the recovery for both substances was $70 \pm 15\%$ (mean $\pm$ s.d.). The lower limit of detection (10 g sample) was 20 ng/g.

Propiopromazine (Combelen[R], Bayer, Leverkusen (G.F.R.)) was determined in 5 g of kidney tissue. The extraction and clean up procedure was as described for azaperone. The extract residue was chromatographed on polyamide thin layer plates (solvent: cyclohexane/methanol/chloroform/ammonia - 90/20/20/0.25 - v/v/v/v). After drying the the spots on the plate were quantitated by fluorescence densitometry. In the range 20-200 ng/g the recovery was $75 \pm 8\%$ (mean $\pm$ s.d.). The lower limit of detection was 2 ng/g.

RESULTS

Azaperone plus azaperol were determined in 27 samples from the slaughter house in Oss and 29 samples from the slaughter house in The Hague (7). Propiopromazine was determined in the same 29 samples from The Hague and 14 samples from Oss. The results are shown in Figure 1. The concentration ratios meat/kidney and liver/kidney, found in model experiments with pigs are given in Table 1.

Table 1

Tranquillizer concentrations in meat and liver relative to those in kidneys (mean ± s.d.)

	Azaperone + Azaperol	Propiopromazine
meat/ kidneys	0.11 ± 0.04	0.46 ± 0.29
liver/ kidneys	0.47 ± 0.17	1.52 ± 0.13 (8 h post inj.) 4.86 ± 3.10 (24 h post inj.)

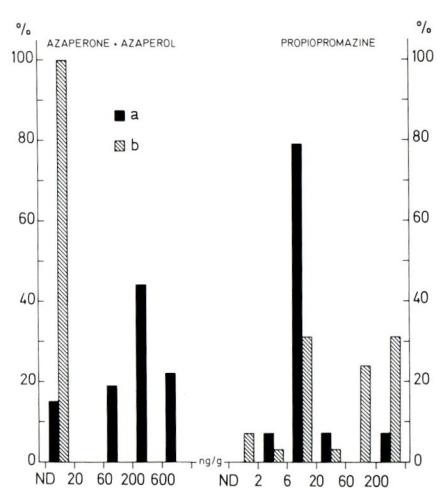

Figure 1

Residues of tranquillizers in kidneys of slaughter pigs
a : Dutch pigs (slaughter house in Oss)
b : German pigs (slaughter house in The Hague)
ND: Not detectable

CONCLUSIONS

1. The analysis of random samples showed that the use of tranquillizers in transport of slaughter pigs is by no means neglegible.

2. Although the present exposure of the human population to tranquillizers in meat and meat products probably is harmless, extension of the practice to more species of slaughter animals may not be so, and therefore will require careful toxicological evaluation.

REFERENCES

1. Lendfers, L.H.H.M.: De gevoeligheid van het Nederlandse slachtvarken voor transportinvloeden. Dissertatie Utrecht, 1974

2. Grossklaus, D.: Schlacht- u.Viehof Z. 1973, 79-84

3. Dantzer, R.: Ann.Rech.Vét. 5, 465-505 (1975)

4. Eikelenboom, G. et al.: Proc.Int.Pig.Vet.Soc.Congress 1978, p. T 8.

5. Reuter, G., Stolle, A.: Schlacht.Vermarkt. 1975, 151-156

6. Rauws A.G. et al.: Toxicol.Appl.Pharmacol. 35, 333-339 (1976)

7. Rauws, A.G., Olling, M.: J.Vet.Pharmacol.Ther. 1, 57-62 (1978)

EFFECT OF INJECTION SITE ON BIOAVAILABILITY OF AMINOPENICILLINS IN CALVES

G.H. PALMER

Beecham Pharmaceuticals - Research Division, Tadworth, Surrey, England

ABSTRACT

The effect on bioavailability of route (intramuscular or subcutaneous) and site (anterior, midline, posterior) of administration of aminopenicillins was assessed in calves. Results indicate that bioavailability is affected by route, site, penicillin used and may be modified by the pharmaceutical preparation used.

SYNOPSIS

Introduction

It is widely assumed that bioavailability resulting from intramuscular administration of a drug is greater than by the subcutaneous route. In man there are indications that for some drugs bioavailability is affected by site or position in the body as much as by route of administration.

There has, however, been no systematic study of this phenomenon in animals. The following experiments were carried out to provide some information relating to the effect of injection site and route for the aminopenicillins in calves.

Methods

1. Calves (40 - 65 kgs) were dosed in various sites by intramuscular and subcutaneous routes with preparations of the aminopenicillins; ampicillin or amoxycillin.

2. Bioavailability was assessed by microbiological assay (B subtilis - agar diffusion precision ± 5 - 10%) on serum.

3. The preparations used were:

   (a) Sodium ampicillin solution in water (SA)[*]

   (b) Ampicillin trihydrate in an oily suspension (PIS)[*]

   (c) Amoxycillin trihydrate in an aqueous suspension (CAS)[*]

   All doses were given at 7 mg penicillin (free acid) per kg bodyweight.

Results

Experiment 1

This was a preliminary study with PIS in a group of 12 calves to compare intramuscular and subcutaneous dosing in various sites. Intramuscular dosing into the gluteus medius was shown to be more likely to be intramuscular than intermuscular and was used as a standard comparator.

338

Table 1   Penbritin Injectable Suspension 7 mg/kg Calves 37 ± 1 kg

Treatment	Peak mcg/ml	% AUC 0 - 24 hrs
IM gluteus medius	3.9	100
IM rump	4.6	105
SC rump	3.3	84
SC over ribs	4.6	109

Experiment 2

This study was carried out to assess position in the body, i.e. anterior, mid-line or posterior, using PIS. In essence neck (IM) was higher than rump (IM) whilst SC (midline) was higher than rump (IM). There was, therefore, an interaction between site and route. Also sodium salt was less influenced by site or route than PIS.

Experiment 3

This experiment was carried out to compare bioavailability for different routes in the same position in the body (i.e. neck versus rump, IM versus SC) using CAS.

Table 2   Clamoxyl Aqueous Injectable Suspension 7 mg/kg Calves 40 ± 1 kg

Treatment (n = 6)	Peak mcg/ml	% AUC 0 - 24 hrs
IM rump	3.0	100
SC rump	2.8	106
IM neck	3.8	129
SC neck	2.8	104

In essence IM dosing gave higher values than corresponding SC doses and neck (IM) was higher than rump (IM).

Conclusions

For the aminopenicillins:

1. Site and route influence bioavailability.

2. Sodium salts (soluble) are less influenced than suspensions.

3. Different penicillins (or formulations?) may be influenced by different sites/routes.

4. Overall, neck IM in the calf shows maximum bioavailability irrespective of drug, physical form or formulation.

*   (a) Penbritin Veterinary Injectable (Beecham)
    (b) Penbritin Injectable Suspension (Beecham)
    (c) Clamoxyl Aqueous Injectable Suspension (Beecham)

WHOLE AUTORADIOGRAPHIC STUDY OF THE DISTRIBUTION OF ^{14}C-CARBARYL IN THE QUAIL

M. SANOU, P. BENARD, V. BURGAT-SACAZE, J.P. BRAUN and A.G. RICO

Laboratoire de Radioéléments, Ecole Vétérinaire, Toulouse (France)

ABSTRACT

Autoradiographs of laying quails treated orally with 1 naphtyl-N-methyl ^{14}C carbamate (carbaryl ND) showed that the labelled product was carried to and persisted in the central nervous system, that relatively important fixation occurred in the kidney and the liver, and that radioactivity accumulated in the oviduct and was progressively transferred to the eggs. Various accidents due to toxicity (change in the behaviour of the animals, diminution of fertility, malformation of the young), already reported by different authors, can be accounted for in the light of these data.

INTRODUCTION

Carbaryl (1-naphtyl-N-methyl-carbamate) or Sevin is an anticholinesterasic insecticide widely used in phytotherapy for the treatment of fruit and other crops and also in veterinary medicine as external antiparasitic. This wide use results in the regular intake of this insecticide by wild birds. The toxic effects of carbamate on birds have recently been studied in the quail (ref. 5).

METHODS

Carbaryl ^{14}C at 100 µCi.kg^{-1} was administered orally to 20 laying quails, kept in individual cages.

The birds were sacrificed 1, 3, 5, 8, 12, 24, 48 and 96h, and 8 and 15 days later. Eggs were collected up to 13 days after the labelled compound had been administered.

All the biological material was treated by macroscopic autoradiography according to ULLBERG's technique (ref. 6) with a cryomicrotome PMV 450.

RESULTS AND DISCUSSION

Quail

The autoradiographs showed that absorption of radioactivity takes place rather quickly after the animals have been dosed. Thus, one hour after the treatment, low activities were detected in the whole organism. Two organs in particular fixed radioactive metabolites, i.e. the hepatic and renal parenchyma. However, radioactivity did not accumulate but disappeared quickly from these organs.

In the central nervous system, the highest activity was reached 5 h after the treatment. This fixation in the central nervous system was very persistent since 15 days after administration, the encephalon was the organ containing the strongest activities. This fact is interesting as several authors have noticed important biochemical changes in this tissue due to accidental or experimental intoxication. In particular, it has been reported that the administration of this insecticide to quails (30 mg.kg^{-1}) entails a significant inhibition of the nervous acetyl--cholinesterasic activity (ref. 1). This could explain the behavioural changes recorded by different authors, at least to a certain extent.

Eggs

Two facts should be noted : an accumulation of radioactivity in the oviduct and a progressive transfer into the eggs. The accumulation of radioactivity in the oviduct is progressive until 12 hours after the treatment. After this time, the organ is still clearly labelled.

The kinetics of incorporation into the eggs is more interesting to study. In all the animals observed, the ovarian membrane is generally hardly marked. However, radioactivity appears more concentrated in the follicles about to be detached. Hence the accumulation of radioactivity in the ovarian follicles can happen only if the latter are mature. The movement of the labelled metabolites at this stage of development of the eggs is confirmed by studying the eggs laid by the animals. In those collected the day after administration of the drug, the yolk was weakly labelled except on the germinative disk. In the eggs laid on the eighth day, the whole yolk fixed radioactivity.

These data are interesting in connection with reproductive disturbances in birds reported by different authors to be caused by this insecticide. ANDRAWES et al. have shown that the radioactivity found in the yolk corresponds to active metabolites. In the same way, several authors (ref. 2) have described a diminution of the hatchability of eggs.

REFERENCES

1. BURSIAN, S.J. and ENDENS, F.W., 1978. The effect of acute carbaryl administration on various neurochemical and blood chemical parameters in the Japanese quail. Toxicol. Appl. Pharmacol., 46: 463-473.

2. DeROSA, T., TAYLOR, D.H., FARRELL, M.P. and SEILKOP, S.D., 1976. Effects on reproductive biology of the Coturnix. Poultry Science, 55: 2133-2141.

3. GHADIRI, M., GREENWOOD, D.A. and BINNS, W., 1967. Feeding of malathion and carbaryl to laying hens and roosters. Toxicol. Appl. Pharmacol., 10:392.

4. HARRISSON, I.R., 1961. Further observations on 1-naphtyl-N-methyl Carbamate as a veterinary insecticide. Vet. Rec., 73: 290.

5. LORGUE, G., DELATOUR, P., COURTOT, D., GASTELLU, J. and DUPAS, J.C., 1974. Recherches sur les effets toxiques sur la caille des résidus de carbaryl, insecticide du groupe des carbamates. Bull. Soc. Sci. Vét. et Méd. Comparée Lyon, 76: 187.

6. ULLBERG, S., 1954. Studies on the distribution and fate of ^{35}S-labelled benzyl penicillin in the body. Acta Radiol., suppl. 118: 1-110.

DISTRIBUTION OF ^{14}C MEBENDAZOLE IN GUINEA-FOWL AS STUDIED BY WHOLE BODY AUTO-
RADIOGRAPHY

P. BENARD, M. SANOU, V. BURGAT-SACAZE, J.P. BRAUN and A.G. RICO

Laboratoire de Radioéléments, Ecole Nationale Vétérinaire, Toulouse (France)

ABSTRACT

[14]C-Mebendazole was administered orally to 12 adult guinea fowls. The animals
were sacrificed at different times and then treated by whole body autoradiography
according to ULLBERG's technique.

The results show that Mebendazole is not absorbed very much. A marked elimination
via the bile is described. Ten days after the administration of the drug, only
the liver and the retina were still labelled.

INTRODUCTION

Mebendazole or methyl-5-benzoyl-benzimidazole-2-carbamate, is a potent, orally
active, broad spectrum anthelmintic, used in humans and many animal species
(dogs, horses, pigs, sheep, birds; ref. 1).

The purpose of this survey was to study by whole body autoradiography the
distribution of this drug labelled with ^{14}C in the guinea fowl after oral administration.

Its toxicity as well as its pharmacokinetics in different species are fairly
well known. Mebendazole is usually well tolerated.

METHOD

[14]C-Mebendazole was administered orally to 12 young adult guinea fowls. The
dose was 12 mg per animal and the activity 100 µCi.kg^{-1}.

The animals were sacrificed 24, 28 and 72 hours and 8, 10 and 15 days after
drug administration. They were plucked, deepfrozen and treated by whole body
autoradiography according to ULLBERG's technique (ref. 2).

RESULTS AND DISCUSSION

The autoradiographs revealed :

From a kinectic point of view :

After 24 hours weak and comparable activity was noted in the blood and muscles.

The liver and the kidney are the organs which fixed the highest radioactivities. Moreover, there was considerable excretion in the bile and high activities were detected in the lumen of the digestive tract.

After 10 days traces of radioactivity were found mainly in the liver and the kidney, and in the digestive tract.

These results support what is already known about this compound in other species, i.e., low intestinal absorption and strong bilary elimination (entero-hepatic cycle).

In the tissues, there was slight fixation by the muscles. Radioactivity was always present in the liver, where it could be detected 10 days after drug administration.

Particular localizations:

An observation recorded here for the first time is the strong affinity of this drug for the retina and most probably for the melanic pigments, since 10 days after administration of the labelled product, the eye as well as the tegument of the head were still clearly labelled.

Bearing in mind these metabolic data, one can assert that 15 days after the treatment, the residues of Mebendazole in the tissues of the guinea fowl can be considered as negligible.

REFERENCES

1. MARSBOOM, R., 1973. Toxicologic studies on Mebendazole. Toxicol. Appl. Pharmacol., 24: 371-377.

2. ULLBERG, S., 1954. Studies on the distribution and fate of ^{35}S labelled benzyl penicillin in the body. Act. Radiol., 118: 1-110.

IMMUNOSUPPRESSION BY THE ORGANOTIN COMPOUNDS DI-N-BUTYLTINDICHLORIDE AND DI-N-OCTYLTINDICHLORIDE

Willem Seinen and André H. Penninks

Working-Group Pathology-Toxicology, Faculty of Veterinary Sciences,

State University Utrecht

ABSTRACT

Di-n-butyltindichloride (DBTC) and di-n-octyltindichloride (DOTC) represent a new group of organometallic compounds with anti-lymphocytic properties. In rats they induce lymphocyte depletion in thymus and thymus-dependent areas of peripheral lymphoid organs, without signs of myelotoxicity or a generalized toxicity. As a consequence of their selective lymphocytotoxic action, they induce immunosuppression. The similarity of effects upon rat and human lymphocytes suggests that DBTC and DOTC acts in the same manner in rat and man and offers the possibility of a therapeutic use of these compounds.

INTRODUCTION

Di-n-butyltin and di-n-octyltin compounds have primarily used in industry, in particular, they act as heat stabilizers of poly (vinyl chloride) (PVC) plastics (ref. 1,2). Since these compounds induce lymphocyte depletion in thymus and thymus-dependent lymphoid areas (ref. 3,4) they represent a new group of antilymphocytic agents. Following administration (oral and intravenous), lymphoid atrophy occurs at concentrations that do not compromise other organ systems. For example, rats fed a diet containing 50 or 150 mg DOTC/kg for 4 weeks showed a reduction in the total number of thymocytes of 33 and 6% respectively. The viability of these cells was also dose-relatedly decreased. Like the number and viability of thymus cells, the number and viability of spleen and peripheral lymph node cells was also decreased by DOTC, but less severely so. However, the number and viability of bone marrow cells was not affected by DOTC and DBTC treatment.

Via the spleen colony assay of Till and McCulloch (ref. 5) effects on bone marrow stem cells were excluded (ref. 6). This indicates a selective effect of DBTC and DOTC on thymus and thymus-dependent lymphocytes, which is not mediated by an increased release of glucocorticosteroids, since thymus atrophy is also observed in adrenalectomized rats (ref. 3).

In this study, it was demonstrated that in rats, the immune response is distinctly disturbed by DBTC and DOTC, especially in those reactions in which T-lymphocytes participate.

RESULTS

The immune function studies carried out and the effects of DBTC and/or DOTC are summarized in Tabel 1.

Tabel 1.   The effect of DBTC or DOTC on various immune functions of rats

Cell-Mediated Immunity	Effect	Reference
In vivo		
- delayed type hypersensitivity to tuberculin	+	7
- allograft rejection	+	7
- graft-versus-host reaction	+	8
- resistance to Listeria monocytogenes infection	+	9
In vitro		
- lymphocyte transformation by Phytohemagglutinin (PHA) and Concanavalin A (Con A)	+	8
Humoral Immunity		
In vivo		
- thymus-dependent antibody synthesis to sheep red blood cells (SRBC)	+	7
- thymus-independent antibody synthesis to E.coli lipopolysacharide (LPS)	-	7
In vitro		
- plaque formation against SRBC	+	7
- transformation of lymphocytes by LPS	-	8
Phagocytosis by macrophages of carbon particles	-	7
Sensitivity to LPS	+	9

A dose-related suppression of cell-mediated immunity occurred in such manifestations as tuberculin hypersensitivity, skin graft rejection, graft-versus-host reactivity and lymphocyte transformation by the T-cell mitogens phytohemagglutinin (PHA) and Concanavalin A (Con A). The resistance against a Listeria monocytogenes, also a T-cell dependent phenomenon, was dose-relatedly decreased. The resistance against a Salmonella dublin strain was decreased by DBTC and DOTC, but this may also be related to an increased susceptibility to Salmonella dublin endotoxin, since these organotin compounds induce a hypersensitivity for E.coli lipopolysacharide (LPS) in rats.

Inhibition of the humoral immunity is shown by a reduction of plaque-forming cell numbers in the spleen as well as by a reduction of the hemagglutinin and hemolysin titers against sheep red blood cells (SRBC) in the serum of DBTC and DOTC exposed rats. In contrast to this inhibition of the antibody response on the thymus-dependent antigen SRBC, the response on the thymus-independent antigen E.coli LPS, nor the mitogenic response of spleen cells on E.coli LPS was suppressed by treatment of rats with DBTC or DOTC. The blood clearance of carbon particles was not impaired by DOTC treatment, nor were the blood monocyte numbers affected by DBTC or DOTC treatment. Therefore it is concluded that these compounds impaire T-lymphocytes and spare B-lymphocytes, which is in agreement with the lymphocyte depletion observed selectively in thymus and thymus-dependent areas of peripheral lymphoid organs of rats exposed to these compounds.

In vitro DBTC and DOTC are extremely cytotoxic both for rat and human lymphocytes. Rat thymocyte survival decreased in a dose-related and time-dependent fashion when cultured in the presence of graded amounts of DBTC or DOTC. A concentration as low as 0.5µg DBTC/ml. medium still greatly decreased the survival of rat thymocytes (ref. 8). Although, the viability of human thymocytes was less reduced than rat lymphocytes, the human cells were definitely damaged by the organotin compounds. They lost their ability to form E-rosettes with SRBC and showed a tendency to aggregate upon exposure to DOTC and DBTC. E.rosette formation was already decreased at concentrations as low as 0.02µg DBTC/ml. A direct cytotoxicity of DBTC and DOTC on lymphocytes is also demonstrated in ^{3}H-thymidine incorporation studies. DNA-synthesis of human as well as rat thymocytes was already inhibited at levels of 0.02μg DBTC and 0.1μg DOTC/ml medium. These results indicate a comparable effect of organotin compounds upon human and rat lymphocytes.

REFERENCES

1. Ross, A. (1965). Ann. N.Y. Acad. Sci. USA. 125 : 107
2. Piver, W.T. (1973). Environ Health Perspect 4 : 61
3. Seinen, W.,Willems, M.I. (1976). Toxicol. Appl. Pharmacol. 35 : 63
4. Seinen, W.,Vos, J.G., Van Spanje, I., Snoek, M.,Brands, R., Hooykaas, H. (1977). Toxicol. Appl. Pharmacol. 42 : 197
5. Till, J.E., McCulloch, E.A. (1961). Radiat. Res. 14 : 123
6. Seinen, W.,Penninks, A.H. (1979). Ann. N.Y. Acad. Sci. USA. 320 : 499
7. Seinen, W., Vos, J.G., van Krieken, R., Penninks, A.H., Brands, R., Hooykaas, H. (1977). Toxicol. Appl. Pharmacol. 42 : 213
8. Seinen, W., Vos, J.G., Brands, R., Hooykaas, H. (1979). Immunopharmacol. 1 : 343
9. Seinen, W. (1979). Immunologic Considerations in Toxicology. Ed. R.P. Sharma. CRC Press. Inc. In Press.

AN INVESTIGATION INTO THE ROLE OF E.COLI-ENDOTOXIN IN THE PATHOGENESIS OF
COLIFORM MASTITIS

J.H.M. VERHEIJDEN[*], A.S.J.P.A.M. van MIERT[**] and C.T.M. van DUIN[**]

[*] Department of Herd Health and Ambulatory Clinic, Yalelaan 20, Utrecht

[**] Institute of Veterinary Pharmacology and Toxicology, Biltstraat 172, Utrecht

ABSTRACT
    In the present study, it could be demonstrated that the symptoms of generalized
disease associated with E.coli-endotoxin induced mastitis are not due to circulating
endotoxin.

INTRODUCTION
    In a previous study (9) it was found that the effect of E.coli OIIIB4
lipopolysaccharides (LPS) on several clinical and clinical-chemical parameters is
markedly dependent on the route of administration (either intravenously or
intramammarily) and on the dose of LPS used. In particular it was found that after
intramammary administration of LPS there is no marked effect on rumen motility.
This is in contrast to the general theory (I) (2) (3) (8) (10) that the symptoms of
generalized disease are caused by absorption of LPS from the udder. Further
research was therefore conducted on the role of LPS in the pathogenesis of
coliform mastitis.

MATERIALS AND METHODS
    The pyrogen used was a purified LPS from Escherichia coli OIIIB4 (Difco
Laboratories, Detroit, Michigan, U.S.A.). Methods for maintaining glassware and
solutions free of bacterial pyrogen contamination, for preparing leucocytic
pyrogen and for recording body temperature and rumen motility have been described
by Van Miert and Atmakusuma (4) and Van Miert et al. (5) (6) (7). Plasma zinc
concentrations were determined by atomic absorption spectophotometry (Perkin-
Elmer, model 305B).

RESULTS
    There was a strong similarity between the effects of intravenous infusion of
leucocytic pyrogen and intramammary administration of LPS on body temperature,
rumen motility and plasma zinc concentration of goats. In contrast, intravenous
administration of LPS, either by means of a single injection or infused, produced
different effects on these parameters.
    Goats that were tolerant to a single injection of LPS were also tolerant to an
intravenous infusion of LPS. However, in cows the intramammary administration of
one fifth of the dose LPS to which the animals were made tolerant produced a
maximum effect on body temperature and plasma zinc concentration (fig. I).

DISCUSSION
    On the basis of the above findings it is postulated that the symptoms of
generalized disease associated with E.coli-endotoxin induced mastitis can not

be ascribed to circulating endotoxin, although it is impossible to preclude that occasionally small quantities of endotoxin from the udder are absorbed in the circulation.

It is plausible, that in patients suffering from clinical mastitis the symptoms of generalized disease are predominantly a result of the formation of leucocytic (endogenous) pyrogen in the udder and its subsequent absorption into the circulation. Further research to validate this hypothesis is recommended.

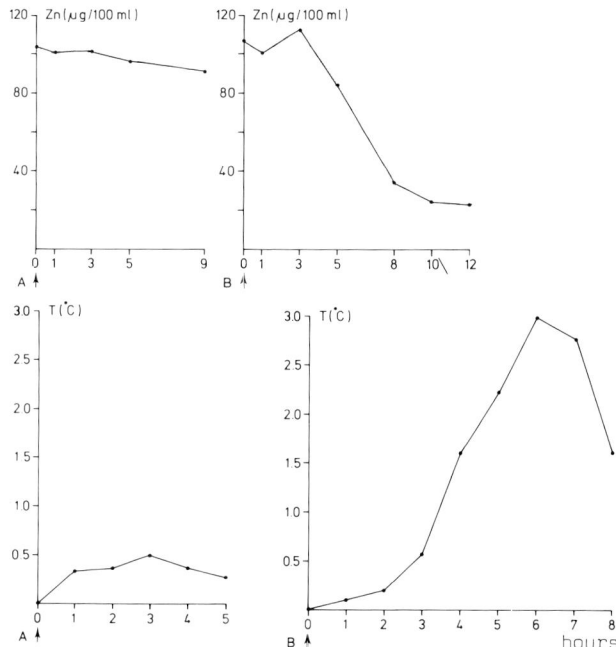

fig.1.The effect on body temperature (T) and plasma zinc concentration (Zn) of three cows made tolerant to endotoxin by daily intravenous injections of 6.4 µg/kg LPS E.coli O111B4: A. the effect of a single intravenous injection of 6.4 µg/kg LPS E.coli O111B4 (↟)
B. the effect of intramammary administration of 0.6 mg LPS E.coli O111B4 (↟↟)

REFERENCES
1. Burvenich, C.: Vlaams Dierg. Tijdschr. 47 (1), 53 (1978)
2. Carroll, E.J., Schalm, O.W., and Lasmanis, J.: Am. J. Vet. Res. 25, 72I (1964)
3. Jain, N.C., and Lasmanis, J.: Res. Vet. Sci. 24, 386 (1978)
4. Miert, A.S.J.P.A.M. van, and Atmakusuma, A.: Zbl. Vet. Med. A 17, 174 (1970)
5. Miert, A.S.J.P.A.M. van, Duin, C.T.M. van, and Veenendaal, G.H.: Zbl. Vet. Med. A 23, 8I9 (1976)
6. Miert, A.S.J.P.A.M. van, Essen, J.A. van, and Tromp, G.A.: Arch. Int. Pharmacodyn. I97, 388 (1972)
7. Miert, A.S.J.P.A.M. van, Wal-Komproe, L.W. van der, and Duin, C.T.M. van: Arch. Int. Pharmacodyn. 225, 39 (1977)
8. Radostits, O.M.: Can. Vet. Journal 2, 40I (1961)
9. Verheijden, J.H.M.: Further investigations into some aspects of acute coliform mastitis in cattle. Thesis Utrecht (1979)
10. Ziv, G., Hartman, I., Bogin, E., Abidar, J., and Saran, A.: Theriogenology 6, 343 (1976)

A CLINICAL TRIAL OF OXATOMIDE IN CANINE ATOPIC DERMATITIS

A.T. YOXALL

Department of Clinical Veterinary Medicine, University of Cambridge (U.K.)

ABSTRACT

Canine atopic dermatitis was utilised as a spontaneous animal disease model in which to assess the clinical efficacy of a novel antiallergic compound, oxatomide. In a double-blind cross-over study oxatomide was significantly better than placebo in controlling the clinical signs of this condition.

INTRODUCTION

Oxatomide (1-(3-(diphenyl methyl)-1-piperazinyl)propyl)-1,3-dihydro-2H-benzimidazol-2-one), is a novel, orally-active antiallergic compound, synthesised by Janssen Pharmaceutica, Beerse, Belgium. The antiallergic capability of this compound had been shown to be mediated by its ability to inhibit mast cell histamine release together with an ability to block H_1 histamine receptors. Good results had been obtained in several models of hypersensitivity, including rat cutaneous passive anaphylaxis, rabbit anaphylactic bronchoconstriction, systemic anaphylaxis in the guinea pig and prevention of histamine release in dogs after injection of cremophor EL. Toxicity studies in mouse, rat, guinea pig and dog had indicated that the compound was safe for clinical use.

The problem was to identify a spontaneously-occurring disease condition in a domestic animal that could be used as an analogue for an allergic condition occurring in man, in which the efficacy of the compound could be assessed prior to large scale clinical trials in man.

The model - Canine Atopic Dermatitis

Canine atopic dermatitis presents many similarities to atopic dermatitis in man, and presents problems to the clinician, in that control of symptoms normally calls for continuous administration of corticosteroids. For this reason it was considered justifiable to utilise this condition for the evaluation of the clinical efficacy of oxatomide.

Design of the trial

Several tests, useful in man for the diagnosis of atopic disease, were evaluated
in the dog. They were found to be unreliable in performance or interpretation in
the dog. (Tests included total IgE level, using anti-human IgE; RAST test (anti-
human IgE); intradermal skin sensitivity testing; mast cell degranulation test;
delayed skin blanch to acetylcholine).

Light microscopic examination of thin sections, prepared as for electron
microscopy, proved to be a useful diagnostic aid.

In view of the non-specific nature of the clinical signs, and lack of a definitive
diagnostic test, a diagnostic screen was devised (Figure 1). On the basis of clinical
and laboratory findings, each case was given a numerical score, according to a
defined scoring system. The attending clinician was provided with active drug or
a placebo of identical appearance, sufficient for 14 days' treatment, at a dose
rate of 2 mg/kg body weight. After 14 days, the animal's score was reassessed, and
a cross-over to either active drug or placebo was made for a further 14 days, at
the end of which time the score was reassessed once more.

RESULTS

23 cases completed the trial. The mean reduction in clinical score following
14 days' placebo treatment, before or after cross-over, was 4 score points. The
mean reduction in score following 14 days' oxatomide treatment was 12 score points.
(The maximum score for any case was 37 points prior to treatment). These results
indicated that oxatomide was significantly superior to placebo (at the 5% level)
in ameliorating the clinical signs of canine atopic dermatitis.

DIAGNOSTIC SCREEN FOR ATOPIC DERMATITIS

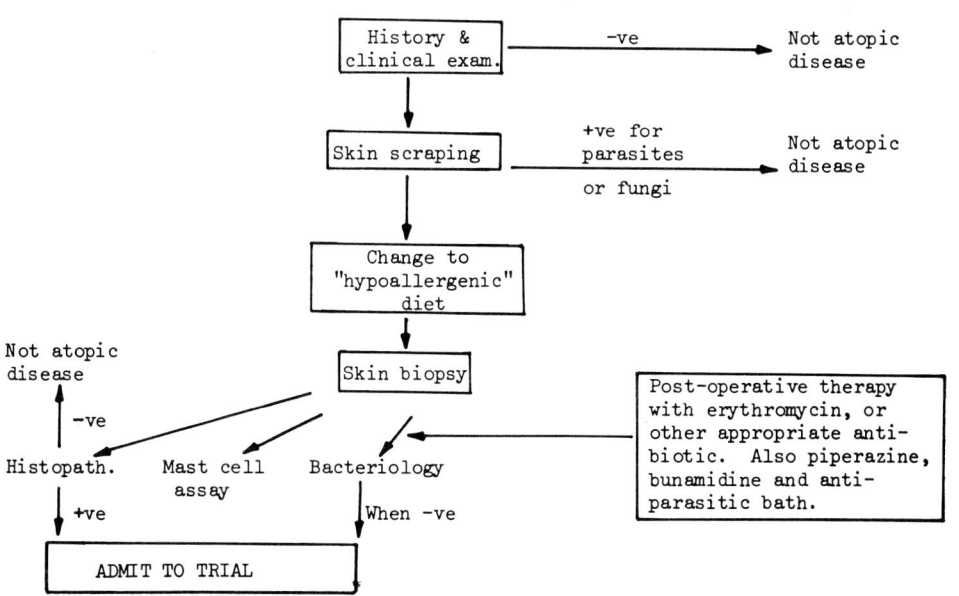

INTRAMUSCULAR BIOAVAILABILITY, SERUM DRUG LEVELS AND LOCAL IRRITATION OF SEVERAL
OXYTETRACYCLINE VETERINARY INJECTABLE PRODUCTS IN COWS

G. ZIV

Ministry of Agriculture, Kimron Veterinary Institute, Bet Dagan, Israel

ABSTRACT

Large variations were found among 13 injectable veterinary products of oxytetracycline with respect to the intramuscular bioavailability profile, peak serum drug
level and degree of irritation at the intramuscular injection site. The intramuscular bioavailability and local irritation of injectable veterinary oxytetracycline products appears to be largely formulation-dependent.

INTRODUCTION

Injectable oxytetracycline (OTC) products for animal use are presented either
in dry form to be reconstituted with water immediately before treatment or in a
ready-for-use form in which various concentrations of the drug are solubilized
in organic solvents. The latter forms are generally preferred by the majority of
users because of convenience, longer shelf-life and economic considerations but
they possess poorer absorption characteristics and may produce variable degree of
pain and damage at the injection site. The present communication deals with the
comparative intramuscular bioavailability, serum OTC levels and local irritation
of several of these products in dairy cows.

MATERIALS AND METHODS

Studies were conducted with 13 commercial OTC products, 9 of which contained
the drug solubilized in polyethylene glycol, in 2 products polyvinyl pyrrolidone
constituted 15% to 18% of the organic solvent and 2 products were presented in
dry form. Each product was first injected intravenously (i.v.) to a group of
Israeli-Friesian cows and 5 to 6 days later each cow was injected i.m. at two or
three sites with the same product and dose used i.v. Serum drug levels were
determined and the area under the concentration-time curve (AUC) of the drug
after i.v. injection was considered to represent the product's absolute bioavailability. The relative i.m. bioavailability was calculated from the AUC
measured after i.m. injection. Local irritation at the injection site was
subjectively assessed by the degree of swelling and oedema resulting 24, 48 and
72 hours after i.m. injection. Four categories were used:
none, mild, severe and very severe local reactions.

RESULTS

Data presented in Table 1 show the following:

a) Among the 13 products examines, large variations were found in the i.m. bioavailability, C max values and degree of local irritation;

b) A good correlation was not found between drug concentration in the product and the relative i.m. bioavailability. For example, Product C, containing 50 mg OTC/ml resulted in a mean i.m. bioavailability of 63% whereas products I and K, containing 150 mg and 200 mg OTC/ml, respectively, were 50% and 72% intramuscularly bioavailable. Product E, showing the lowest bioavailability value (15%) contained 100 mg OTC/ml;

c) Products F and G, containing the drug solubilized in PVP, produced the highest C max values and did not result in local irritation;

d) All the products containing PEG as a major component of the organic solvent produced local irritation;

e) The two water soluble products examined were not absorbed better than the PEG-containing products, causing mild to severe local irritation.

DISCUSSION

Clinical equivalency of competing brands of the same drug is of great importance to the practicing veterinarian. For many drugs it is not possible to make such a comparison directly, but the study of blood levels and the product's bioavailability after administration to groups of animals give a measure of physiological equivalence. The present study showed that OTC preparations which are administered i.m. at the same dose, and even those containing the same quantity of active drug and are thus generically equivalent, cannot be assumed to be associated with the same therapeutic performance measured either as clinical effect or as resultant blood level. In many cases the differences are not marked, but, in others, potential or real clinical differences may result. Where an antibiotic may be critical to the proper treatment of a disease, the clinical efficacy can be greatly modified by the rate and extent of absorption of the active species into the systemic circulation. The present findings bring evidence that the absorption characteristics of the products tested and, consequently the potential therapeutic performance and duration of drug residues at the i.m. injection site can be markedly affected by the materials and methods used in its manufacture. This type of evidence has implications for the developmental pharmacist, government regulatory bodies and above all to the clinician. The plethora of evidence linking therapeutic performance of antibacterial drugs with their pharmaceutical formulation indicates that different preparations of a drug should be assumed to be different therapeutically until proven the same.

TABLE 1 - Intramuscular bioavailability, serum drug levels and local irritation of several oxytetracycline veterinary injectable products in dairy cows

Product code	Solvent	OTC conc. in product (mg/ml)	Dose (mg/kg)	No. of cows used	Relative i.m. availability (% of i.v. AUC) Mean	SD	Mean C_{max} (mcg/ml)	Duration (hours) of serum drug levels at ≥ 2 mcg/ml	≥ 1 mcg/ml	Local irritation
A	PEG(a)	50	8.5	4	53	15	1.75	0	4.5	Severe
B	PEG	50	10	4	69	15	2.25	3	6.5	Mild
C	PEG	50	10	6	36	11	1.25	0	2.5	V. severe
D	PEG	100	10	6	38	6	1.15	0	1.5	V. severe
E	PEG	100	8	6	15	4	0.65	0	0	V. severe
F	PEG	100	10	6	32	11	1.40	0	6.0	V. severe
G	PVP(b)	100	8	4	64	12	2.75	4	10.0	None
H	PVP	100	10	6	78	9	3.15	6	12.0	None
I	PEG	150	8.5	7	50	14	1.65	0	10.0	Severe
J	PEG	150	8	5	28	9	0.80	0	0	V. severe
K	PEG	200	7.5	4	72	7	2.00	3	8	Mild
L	Water for injection		8	8	28	9	1.35	0	4	Severe
M	Water for injection		10	6	32	7	1.85	0	8	Mild

(a) Polyethylene glycol
(b) Polyvinyl pyrrolidone.

SUBJECT INDEX